ORTHOPEDIC CLINICS OF NORTH AMERICA

www.orthopedic.theclinics.com

Global Perspectives in Orthopedic Surgery

April 2020 • Volume 51 • Number 2

ELSEVIER

1600 John F. Kennedy Boulevard • Suite 1800 • Philadelphia, Pennsylvania, 19103-2899.

http://www.orthopedic.theclinics.com

ORTHOPEDIC CLINICS OF NORTH AMERICA Volume 51, Number 2
April 2020 ISSN 0030-5898, ISBN-13: 978-0-323-73391-5

Editor: Lauren Boyle
Developmental Editor: Kristen Helm

Orthopedic Clinics of North America (ISSN 0030-5898) is published quarterly by Elsevier Inc., 360 Park Avenue South, New York, NY 10010-1710. Months of issue are January, April, July, and October. Business and Editorial Offices: 1600 John F. Kennedy Blvd., Suite 1800, Philadelphia, PA 19103-2899. Customer Service Office: 3251 Riverport Lane, Maryland Heights, MO 63043. Periodicals postage paid at New York, NY and additional mailing offices. Subscription prices are $344.00 per year for (US individuals), $786.00 per year for (US institutions), $403.00 per year (Canadian individuals), $960.00 per year (Canadian institutions), $471.00 per year (international individuals), $960.00 per year (international institutions), $100.00 per year (US students), $100.00 per year for (Canadian students), $220.00 per year for (international students). Foreign air speed delivery is included in all *Clinics* subscription prices. All prices are subject to change without notice. **POSTMASTER:** Send change of address to *Orthopedic Clinics of North America*, **Elsevier Health Sciences Division, Subscription Customer Service, 3251 Riverport Lane, Maryland Heights, MO 63043. Customer Service (orders, claims, online, change of address): Elsevier Health Sciences Division, Subscription Customer Service, 3251 Riverport Lane, Maryland Heights, MO 63043. Tel: 1-800-654-2452 (U.S. and Canada); 314-447-8871 (outside U.S. and Canada). Fax: 314-447-8029. E-mail:** journalscustomerservice-usa@elsevier.com **(for print support);** journalsonlinesupport-usa@elsevier.com **(for online support).**

Reprints. For copies of 100 or more, of articles in this publication, please contact the Commercial Reprints Department, Elsevier Inc., 360 Park Avenue South, New York, NY 10010-1710. Tel.: 212-633-3874; Fax: 212-633-3820; E-mail: reprints@elsevier.com.

Orthopedic Clinics of North America is covered in *MEDLINE/PubMed* (*Index Medicus*), *Cinahl, Excerpta Medica, and Cumulative Index to Nursing and Allied Health Literature.*

EDITORIAL BOARD

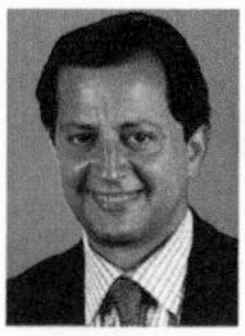

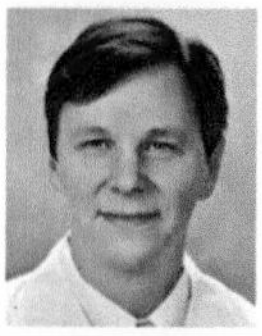

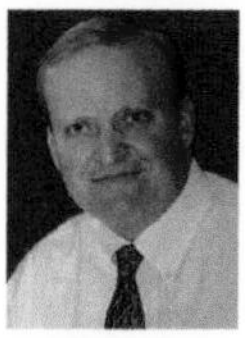

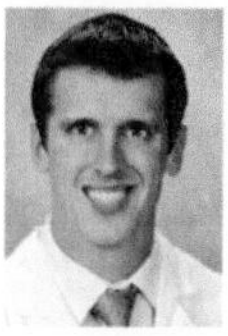

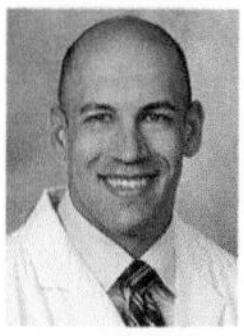

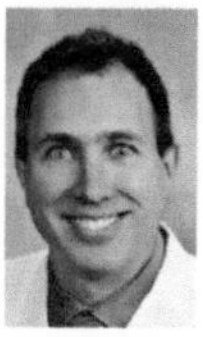

CONTRIBUTORS

AUTHORS

MOHAMMAD S. ABDELAAL, MD
Department of Orthopedic Surgery, Rothman Institute at Thomas Jefferson University, Philadelphia, Pennsylvania, USA

THOMAS R. ACOTT, MD
The Core Institute, Phoenix, Arizona, USA

SYED S. AHMED, MBChB, LLM, MSc, FRCS (Tr & Orth)
Post CCT Fellow, Lower Limb Arthroplasty, University College London Hospital, London, United Kingdom

DANIEL BAUMFELD, MD, PhD
Department of the Locomotor Apparatus, Adjunct Professor, Federal University of Minas Gerais, Belo Horizonte, Brazil

KEITH R. BEREND, MD
JIS Orthopedics, New Albany, Ohio, USA

MATHIAS P. BOSTROM, MD
Professor of Orthopaedic Surgery, Chief of Adult Reconstruction and Joint Replacement Service, Hospital for Special Surgery, New York, New York, USA

CHRISTOPHER BRAY, MD
Department of Orthopedic Surgery, Prisma Health Upstate, Steadman Hawkins Clinic of the Carolinas, Greenville, South Carolina, USA

JORGE CHAHLA, MD, PhD
Assistant Professor, Midwest Orthopaedics at Rush, Rush University Medical Center, Chicago, Illinois, USA

NICHOLAS CHANG, MBBS, MSc, FRCSC
Clinical Fellow, Roth McFarlane Hand and Upper Limb Centre, St. Joseph's Health Care, Western University, London, Ontario, Canada

SHI-MIN CHANG, MD, PhD
Professor and Director Doctor, Department of Orthopedic Surgery, Yangpu Hospital, Tongji University School of Medicine, Shanghai, People's Republic of China

JOSEPH T. CLINE, MD
Medical Resident, The University of Tennessee-Campbell Clinic Department of Orthopaedic Surgery and Biomedical Engineering, Memphis, Tennessee, USA

JOSE CARLOS COHEN, MD
Chief, Foot and Ankle Service, Federal University Hospital of Rio de Janeiro (UFRJ/ HUCFF), Rio de Janeiro, Brazil

DAVID A. CRAWFORD, MD
JIS Orthopedics, New Albany, Ohio, USA

CLAIRE DONNELLEY, BS
Department of Orthopaedic Surgery, University of California, San Francisco, San Francisco, California, USA

SHOU-CHAO DU, MD
Lecturer and Vice-Director Doctor, Department of Orthopedic Surgery, Yangpu Hospital, Tongji University School of Medicine, Shanghai, People's Republic of China

CESAR EDUARDO CASTRO FERREIRA MARTINS, MD
Foot and Ankle Surgeon, Curitiba, Paraná, Brazil

ERIC FORNARI, MD
Co-Director, Pediatric Orthopedic Surgery, Children's Hospital at Montefiore, Associate Professor, Albert Einstein College of Medicine, Bronx, New York, USA

MATTHEW N. FOURNIER, MD
PGY-5 Orthopaedic Resident, University of Tennessee-Campbell Clinic Department of Orthopaedic Surgery and Biomedical Engineering, Memphis, Tennessee, USA

LISA G.M. FRIEDMAN, MD, MA
Midwest Orthopaedics at Rush, Rush University Medical Center, Chicago, Illinois, USA

GRANT E. GARRIGUES, MD
Associate Professor, Midwest Orthopaedics at Rush, Rush University Medical Center, Chicago, Illinois, USA

ELIZABETH B. GAUSDEN, MD, MPH
Orthopaedic Surgery Fellow, Hospital for Special Surgery, New York, New York, USA

JEFFREY A. GREENBERG, MD, MS
Partner, Indiana Hand to Shoulder Center, Indianapolis, Indiana, USA

FARES S. HADDAD, BSc, MD(Res), MCh(Orth), FRCS(Orth), FFSEM
Professor of Orthopaedics and Sports Surgery, University College London Hospital, London, United Kingdom

ZHI-YONG HOU, MD, PhD
Professor and Director Doctor, Department of Orthopedic Surgery, Third Hospital of Hebei Medical University, Shijiazhuang, People's Republic of China

SUN-JUN HU, MD, PhD
Associate Professor and Vice-Director Doctor, Department of Orthopedic Surgery, Yangpu Hospital, Tongji University School of Medicine, Shanghai, People's Republic of China

GRAHAM J.W. KING, MD, MSc, FRCSC
Medical Director, Roth McFarlane Hand and Upper Limb Centre, St. Joseph's Health Care, Professor, Western University, London, Ontario, Canada

LAURENT LAFOSSE, MD
Chairman of the Clinique Générale, Clinique Générale, Alps Surgery Institute, Annecy, France

ANDRÉ VITOR KERBER C. LEMOS, MD
Foot and Ankle Surgeon, UNIFESP – Federal University of São Paulo, São Paulo, São Paulo, Brazil

BASSAM A. MASRI, MD, FRCSC
Orthopedic Surgeon, Professor and Head, Department of Orthopedic Surgery, University of British Columbia, Vancouver, British Columbia, Canada

BENJAMIN M. MAUCK, MD
Instructor, University of Tennessee-Campbell Clinic Department of Orthopaedic Surgery and Biomedical Engineering, Memphis, Tennessee, USA

SILVANA TEIXEIRA DE MIRANDA, PT
Physical Therapist, Federal University Hospital of Rio de Janeiro (UFRJ/HUCFF), Rio de Janeiro, Brazil

SAAM MORSHED, MD, PhD, MPH
Department of Orthopaedic Surgery, University of California, San Francisco, San Francisco, California, USA

CAIO NERY, MD, PhD
Associate Professor, Foot and Ankle Clinic, UNIFESP – Federal University of São Paulo, São Paulo, São Paulo, Brazil

NATHAN N. O'HARA, MHA
Department of Orthopaedics, University of Maryland School of Medicine, Baltimore, Maryland, USA

CHRISTOPHER PEDNEAULT, MDCM, FRCSC
Clinical Fellow, Department of Adult Hip and Knee Reconstruction, University of British Columbia, Vancouver, British Columbia, Canada

CARY S. POLITZER, MD
Resident, Department of Orthopaedic Surgery, University of California, San Diego, La Jolla, California, USA

AJAY PREMKUMAR, MD, MPH
Orthopaedic Surgery Resident, Hospital for Special Surgery, New York, New York, USA

CAMILO RESTREPO, MD
Department of Orthopedic Surgery, Rothman Institute at Thomas Jefferson University, Philadelphia, Pennsylvania, USA

HEATHER J. ROBERTS, MD
Department of Orthopaedic Surgery, University of California, San Francisco, San Francisco, California, USA

MATTHEW R. SCHMITZ, MD
Chair, Department of Orthopaedics, San Antonio Military Medical Center, Houston, Texas, USA

JACOB SCHULZ, MD
Albert Einstein College of Medicine, The Children's Hospital at Montefiore, Bronx, New York, USA

RICHARD M. SCHWEND, MD
Professor of Orthopaedics and Pediatrics, Department of Orthopaedics and Musculoskeletal Sciences, University of Missouri Kansas City, Kansas University Medical Center, Children's Mercy Hospital, Kansas City, Missouri, USA

ADAM SEAL, BS
Medical Student, University of Tennessee-Campbell Clinic Department of Orthopaedic Surgery and Biomedical Engineering, Memphis, Tennessee, USA

PETER F. SHARKEY, MD
Professor of Orthopaedic Surgery, Sidney Kimmel Medical College, Rothman Institute at Thomas Jefferson University, Philadelphia, Pennsylvania, USA

DAVID W. SHEARER, MD, MPH
Department of Orthopaedic Surgery, University of California, San Francisco, San Francisco, California, USA

RICHARD A. SMITH, PhD
Professor, University of Tennessee-Campbell Clinic Department of Orthopaedic Surgery and Biomedical Engineering, Memphis, Tennessee, USA

STEFAN ST GEORGE, MD
Orthopedic Resident, Department of Orthopedic Surgery, University of British Columbia, Vancouver, British Columbia, Canada

EMMANUEL THIENPONT, MD, MBA, PhD
Cliniques Universitaires Saint Luc, Brussels, Belgium

THOMAS W. THROCKMORTON, MD
Professor, University of Tennessee-Campbell Clinic Department of Orthopaedic Surgery and Biomedical Engineering, Memphis, Tennessee, USA

ERICKA VON KAEPPLER, BS
Department of Orthopaedic Surgery, University of California, San Francisco, San Francisco, California, USA

KEVIN C. WALL, MD, MPH
Resident, Department of Orthopaedic Surgery, The University of Alabama at Birmingham, Birmingham, Alabama, USA

NAE WON, BA, MPH
Department of Orthopaedic Surgery, University of California, San Francisco, San Francisco, California, USA

KHALED M. YAGHMOUR, MBBS
Foundation Doctor, University College London Hospital, London, United Kingdom

CONTENTS

Preface: Global Perspectives in Orthopedic Surgery xv
Frederick M. Azar

Knee and Hip Reconstruction
Patrick C. Toy and William M. Mihalko

Challenges to Implementing Total Joint Replacement Programs in Developing Countries 131
Christopher Pedneault, Stefan St George, and Bassam A. Masri

In this review article, the authors present the many challenges that orthopedic surgeons in developing countries face when implementing arthroplasty programs. The issues of cost, sterility, and patient demographics are specifically addressed. Despite the many challenges, developing countries are beginning to offer hip and knee reconstructive surgery to respond to the increasing demand for such elective operations as the prevalence of osteoarthritis continues to increase. The authors shed light on these nascent arthroplasty programs.

The Changing Face of Infection, Diagnosis, and Management in the United Kingdom 141
Syed S. Ahmed, Khaled M. Yaghmour, and Fares S. Haddad

Prosthetic joint infection is still a rare but devastating complication following total hip and knee arthroplasty. The incidence of prosthetic joint infection ranges from 2% to 4% in primary procedures as opposed to nearly 20% in revisions. The challenges that arise here include mainly diagnostic uncertainty, management in immunocompromised patients, recurrent infection, infection around a well-fixed implant, and substantial bone loss, and require careful preoperative assessment and well-defined management plans. This article summarizes recent developments in the diagnosis and management of this increasingly prevalent issue specifically focusing on outcomes following debridement, antibiotics, and implants retention and one-stage revision procedures.

Unicompartmental Knee Arthroplasty: US and Global Perspectives 147
David A. Crawford, Keith R. Berend, and Emmanuel Thienpont

Unicompartmental knee arthroplasty (UKA) is a treatment option for anteromedial osteoarthritis. Compared with total knee arthroplasty (TKA), UKA offers improved knee range of motion, functional recovery and decreased medical complications. Revision rates continue to be higher with UKA compared with TKA. With current UKA implants, there is no significant difference in mobile bearing or fixed bearing, or between cemented and cementless implants. Enabling technology, such as robotic-assisted surgery, has demonstrated improvements in component positioning, but no long-term difference in survival compared with traditional manual instruments.

International Collaboration in Total Joint Arthroplasty: A Framework for Establishing Meaningful International Alliances 161
Elizabeth B. Gausden, Ajay Premkumar, and Mathias P. Bostrom

Despite the increase in utilization of total joint arthroplasty (TJA) throughout high-income countries, there is a lack of access to basic surgical care, including TJA, in low- and middle-income countries (LMICs). Multiple strategies, including short-term surgical trips, establishment of local TJA centers, and education-based international academic collaborations, have been used to

from premature death and life not lived at 100% health. Surgery has long been neglected in the distribution of resources for global health. Because of years of life lived with a disability and the large proportion of children in a population, pediatric musculoskeletal conditions early in life can contribute to the GBD. Fortunately, the World Health Organization has recently promoted essential surgical services through its Emergency and Essential Surgical Care Project and Global Initiative.

Development of a Global Pediatric Orthopedic Outreach Program in Ecuador Through Project Perfect World: Past, Present, and Future Directions **219**
Eric Fornari, Richard M. Schwend, Jacob Schulz, Christopher Bray, and Matthew R. Schmitz

Global health delivery is a complex initiative requiring dedicated personnel to achieve a successful program. To be most beneficial, global health delivery should focus on cultural competence, bidirectional education, and capacity building through direct and purposeful means. The authors present the expansion of their global health delivery program in Ecuador focusing on the evolution of the program from a medical mission trip to a multilayered program that helps foster engagement, education, and learning while helping children who might not otherwise have access to care, along with future directions and potential methods to decrease the need for such initiatives in Ecuador.

Hand and Wrist

Benjamin M. Mauck and James H. Calandruccio

Ulnar Abutment Syndrome in the Athlete **227**
Thomas R. Acott and Jeffrey A. Greenberg

Ulnar abutment (ulnocarpal impaction) syndrome may be a source of ulnar-sided wrist pain in the athlete. This condition results from excessive load transfer across the triangular fibrocartilage complex and ulnocarpal joints with characteristic degenerative changes. It frequently occurs in patients with either static or dynamic ulnar positive variance. Treatment is tailored to the athlete and their sporting demands. Surgical treatment focuses on addressing ulnar variance to unload the ulnocarpal joint, with multiple surgical options, including the metaphyseal closing wedge osteotomy achieving this goal. This review focuses on the presentation, biomechanics, and treatment options for ulnar abutment syndrome in the athlete.

Operative Distal Radial Fractures: A Comparison of Time to Surgery After Evaluation by Surgical and Nonsurgical Providers in a Walk-in Clinic **235**
Matthew N. Fournier, Joseph T. Cline, Adam Seal, Richard A. Smith, Thomas W. Throckmorton, and Benjamin M. Mauck

To determine if orthopedic surgeons are more efficient than nonsurgical providers at care of operative injuries in walk-in clinics, patients in a walk-in clinic for evaluation of acute injury who subsequently had surgical treatment of isolated distal radial fracture were compared based on whether the initial visit was with a surgical or nonsurgical provider. Initial evaluation in a walk-in orthopedic clinic setting versus a conventional hand surgeon's clinic was associated with longer delay between initial evaluation and surgical treatment, but this difference may not be significant. Evaluation by a nonsurgical provider was not associated with increased duration to definitive treatment.

Shoulder and Elbow

Tyler J. Brolin

Global Perspectives on Management of Shoulder Instability: Decision Making and Treatment 241

Lisa G.M. Friedman, Laurent Lafosse, and Grant E. Garrigues

The glenohumeral joint is prone to instability. Patients with instability should have a physical examination. Imaging studies can provide additional information. Classification schemes that into account soft tissue pathology, neuromuscular control, bone loss, and activity level. An arthroscopic Bankart repair is the mainstay for unidirectional instability. Bone block procedures are indicated for patients with bone loss or a failed attempt at stabilization surgery. The arthroscopic Latarjet is a promising option for these patients. For patients with multidirectional instability, prolonged rehabilitation is indicated, followed by capsular plication or inferior capsular shift if instability is unresponsive to physical therapy.

Obesity is Associated with an Increased Prevalence of Glenohumeral Osteoarthritis and Arthroplasty: A Cohort Study 259

Kevin C. Wall, Cary S. Politzer, Jorge Chahla, and Grant E. Garrigues

The relationship between obesity and glenohumeral osteoarthritis is relatively understudied. The purpose of this study was to better define this relationship by age- and gender-matching 596,874 patients across six body mass index (BMI) cohorts and determining the prevalence of glenohumeral osteoarthritis and the standardized rate of glenohumeral arthroplasty in each cohort. Individuals with a BMI over 24 were found to be at increased odds for developing glenohumeral osteoarthritis, compared to the normal BMI cohort, and individuals with a BMI over 30 were additionally found to be at increased odds for undergoing glenohumeral arthroplasty.

Elbow Hemiarthroplasty for the Treatment of Distal Humerus Fractures 265

Nicholas Chang and Graham J.W. King

Distal humerus hemiarthroplasty is a good surgical option for nonreconstructable intraarticular distal humerus fractures in selected lower-demand patients. The lifetime activity restrictions have not been determined, but are likely less than a total elbow arthroplasty. From a technical standpoint, distal humeral prostheses should be implanted at the correct depth and rotation. The collateral ligaments, condyles, and epicondyles should be preserved and/or repaired to maintain joint stability. Short- to midterm retrospective studies have shown promising results.

Food and Ankle

Clayton C. Bettin and Benjamin J. Grear

Orthopedic Surgical Foot Management in Hansen Disease 279

Jose Carlos Cohen and Silvana Teixeira de Miranda

Hansen disease remains a common problem worldwide with 750,000 new cases diagnosed each year. Nerve injury is a central feature of the pathogenesis because of the unique tendency of Mycobacterium leprae to invade Schwann cells and the peripheral nervous system, that can be permanent and develop into disabilities. The orthopedic surgeon has an important role in the management of neuropathy, performing surgical release of the tibial and common peroneal nerves in potentially constricting areas, thus providing a better environment for nerve function. In cases of permanent loss of nerve function with drop foot, specific tendon transfers can be used.

Brazilian Total Ankle Replacement Experience 293
Caio Nery, André Vitor Kerber C. Lemos, Cesar Eduardo Castro Ferreira Martins, and Daniel Baumfeld

Brazil experiences a late participation in total ankle arthroplasty, which could have positive and negative aspects. The positive view argues about the modern implants that Brazil has received in the past years, skipping the early total ankle replacement generation who present more complications and low survival rate in the literature. The negative aspects are related to gap of experience with Brazilian surgeons unable to participate in the development of the technique and implant designs during these years. This article discusses the aspects of the Brazilian experience with total ankle replacement since the earliest procedures performed.

GLOBAL PERSPECTIVES IN ORTHOPEDIC SURGERY

PREFACE

Global Perspectives in Orthopedic Surgery

In his 1954 American Academy of Orthopedic Surgeons Presidential Address, Dr Harold Boyd made this observation: *Modern transportation and communication have contracted the world until all nations are neighbors. To promote peace and to live to the best advantage of all, we should know and understand each other. . . . This is particularly true of those engaged in the practice of medicine and surgery. We speak an international language as no other group can. Anatomy, physiological response to trauma or disease, and psychological reactions of patients are little influenced by race or place of residence.* This observation is as true today as it was then, and is nowhere more applicable than the world of orthopedics. This issue of *Orthopedic Clinics of North America* covering global perspectives of orthopedic surgery reminds us of how interconnected and interdependent we are as fellow surgeons. Discoveries and innovations made in parts of the world other than ours inspire us and, perhaps, offer us new ways to provide better patient care.

The challenges facing developing countries in establishing total joint arthroplasty programs are finely detailed by Drs Pedneault et al, Gaudsen et al, and Abdelaal et al, as are their suggestions for how the global orthopedic community can assist in the maintenance of meaningful international collaborations. Dr Crawford and colleagues describe the use of unicompartmental knee arthroplasty in the United States and globally, while Dr Ahmed et al point out the universality of prosthetic joint infection as a complication of total joint arthroplasty. This article summarizes recent developments in the diagnosis and management of this increasingly prevalent issue.

Orthopedic trauma is one of the most common and most devastating orthopedic conditions seen globally. Dr Chang et al point out that, as the geriatric population continues to increase rapidly, hip fractures are increasingly of interest worldwide. They offer 20 concepts in hip fracture management developed over the past 20 years. Dr von Kaeppler and colleagues describe an unmet need for locally relevant and sustainable orthopedic research in low- and middle-income countries. They note that partnerships between high-income and low-income countries can bridge gaps in resources, knowledge, infrastructure, and skill and present a select list of models for research partnerships.

Drs Schwend and Fornari et al describe efforts to improve pediatric orthopedic care in underserved areas, including the World Health Organization Emergency and Essential Surgical Care Project and Global Initiative and the expansion of a global health delivery program in Ecuador that helps foster engagement, education, and learning while helping children who might not otherwise have access to care.

In an effort to provide more efficient and more cost-effective care, many orthopedic practices are employing nonsurgeon providers. Dr Fournier et al compared patients seen in a walk-in clinic for evaluation of an acute injury who subsequently had surgical treatment of an isolated distal radial fracture based on whether the initial clinic visit was with a surgical or nonsurgical provider. Initial evaluation in a walk-in orthopedic clinic setting was associated with a longer delay between initial evaluation and surgical treatment than a conventional hand surgeon's clinic, but this difference may not be clinically significant. Evaluation by a nonsurgical provider was not associated with an increased duration to definitive treatment. Treatment of ulnar abutment syndrome (Acott and Greenberg), shoulder instability (Friedman et al), glenohumeral osteoarthritis (Wall et al), and distal humeral fractures (Chang and King) round out the discussions on upper-extremity trauma.

Orthop Clin N Am 51 (2020) xv–xvi
https://doi.org/10.1016/j.ocl.2020.01.001

Although rare in most developed countries, Hansen disease remains a common problem worldwide, with 750,000 new cases diagnosed each year. Dr Cohen notes that the orthopedic surgeon has an important role in the management of neuropathy involving the lower limb in both the subacute and chronic stages of disease. Dr Nery and colleagues relate their experience with total ankle replacement in Brazil, describing both positive and negative aspects.

Overall, these reports from all over the globe should inspire us to work harder to make connections with our fellow surgeons through international organizations, study groups, research efforts, and reciprocal educational missions to ensure that all patients receive the best care possible.

Frederick M. Azar, MD
Department of Orthopaedic Surgery
University of Tennessee–
Campbell Clinic
1211 Union Avenue, Suite 510
Memphis, TN 38104, USA

E-mail address:
fazar@campbellclinic.com

Knee and Hip Reconstruction

Challenges to Implementing Total Joint Replacement Programs in Developing Countries

Christopher Pedneault, MDCM, FRCSC[a,*],
Stefan St George, MD[b], Bassam A. Masri, MD, FRCSC[b]

KEYWORDS

- Global health • Arthroplasty • Developing countries • Total hip replacement
- Total knee replacement

KEY POINTS

- Implementing an arthroplasty program in a developing country is a very challenging endeavor.
- Developing countries often lack the financial resources, experienced staff, operating room facilities, and adequate perioperative patient care. The unique patient demographics also make the index arthroplasty procedure more challenging with a higher chance of needing revision surgery.
- Despite the challenges, there is early clinical data reporting success in the developing world for hip and knee replacement surgery although the results are difficult to generalize.
- Arthroplasty surgery must be performed in optimal conditions to achieve acceptable clinical outcomes.

INTRODUCTION

Osteoarthritis is a prevalent and disabling musculoskeletal condition. Globally, it is estimated that approximately 10% of men and 18% of women older than 60 years suffer from osteoarthritis.[1] The United Nations have estimated that the proportion of people older than 60 years will triple by 2050, and this age demographic will account for 20% of the world population.[1] With this expected increase in the proportion of elderly patients, osteoarthritis will continue to be a major burden for health care systems worldwide. In developing countries, the prevalence of osteoarthritis is also attributable to an increase in obesity, posttraumatic arthritis, and improvements in life expectancy.[2,3] Consequently, the demand for hip and knee arthroplasty surgery has also been steadily increasing. In the United States, Kurtz and colleagues[4] have predicted an increase in the demand for total knee surgery by 673% and by 174% for total hip replacement from 2005 to 2030. In Australia, by 2030, the incidence of total knee and total hip replacement surgeries is estimated to increase by 276% and 208%, respectively.[5] Despite its proven success, joint replacement surgery is resource intensive and requires a hospital setting with modern operating room facilities that are well-suited for arthroplasty surgery. Unfortunately, many countries in the developing world do not have the necessary resources to offer such surgeries to the general public. Many developing countries are also faced with more urgent public health concerns while treating and eradicating diseases

[a] Department of Adult Hip and Knee Reconstruction, University of British Columbia, Room 11295 – 2775, Laurel Street, Vancouver, British Columbia V5Z1M9, Canada; [b] Department of Orthopedic Surgery, University of British Columbia, Room 11295 – 2775, Laurel Street, Vancouver, British Columbia V5Z1M9, Canada
* Corresponding author.
E-mail address: Christopher.pedneault@mail.mcgill.ca

Orthop Clin N Am 51 (2020) 131–139
https://doi.org/10.1016/j.ocl.2019.11.001
0030-5898/20/

such as malaria, gastrointestinal diseases of childhood, and pneumonia such that joint replacement surgery is expectedly not a top priority for local health officials.[6] Despite these burdens, total joint replacement surgeries do take place in many developing countries and there is a growing body of literature reporting encouraging outcomes in several small case series.[7–10] The objective of this review article is to expose the difficult challenges that developing countries face in implementing a successful arthroplasty program.

COST

Total hip and knee replacement (THR/TKR) surgeries are expensive operations. In the United States, joint replacement surgeries constitute the largest hospital expenditure category of Medicare.[11] The implant costs alone represent a significant portion of these expenditures, whereas hip and knee implant costs range anywhere from US$2392 to US$12,651 and US$1797 to US$12,093, respectively.[11] In Canada, the average cost per primary total hip arthroplasty procedure in 2017 to 18 was approximately CAD$11,500 and the average cost of a primary total knee arthroplasty was CAD$7800.[12] Meanwhile in Europe, Stargardt[13] demonstrated that the total cost of treatment ranged from €1290 in Hungary to €8739 in the Netherlands with a mean cost of €5043 between 9 European Union member states. Interestingly, despite the elevated cost of implants and total treatment costs for hip and knee arthroplasties, cost-effective analyses have deemed these surgeries beneficial when considering the cost of long-term medications and lost productivity.[14] Unfortunately, these analyses do not always apply to many patients in developing countries, as most do not receive nonoperative treatment despite having advanced osteoarthritis.[7] Patients with advanced disease thus endure severe disability, which places an enormous burden on their families and communities.[15]

When patients do elect to undergo surgery, they are often performed in private or mission hospitals. In both settings, the surgeries are unaffordable for most of the local population. For example, in Kenya, the cost of a total hip replacement was US$1650 in a mission hospital and US$4000 in a private hospital.[6]

To limit surgery-related costs, some hospitals borrow the surgical equipment and only pay the manufacturer for every implant used.[6] Also, the limited number of surgeries being performed have made many implant companies reluctant to offer competitive prices for implants. It is therefore important for surgeons to select the fewest implants possible while insuring their versatility. Cemented hip implants are also much cheaper than cementless implants and should be the implant of choice when budget constraints are a major issue.[6] Nonetheless, the resources required to run a modern operating room facility with proper sterile instruments and modern implants as well as staffing experienced medical personnel remain the biggest impediment to implementing a successful arthroplasty program.

PATIENT DEMOGRAPHICS

The patient population undergoing arthroplasty surgery in the developing world has notable differences that can either complicate the index surgery or make the possibility of revision surgery more likely. Some of these differences include age at time of surgery, indication for surgery, and medical comorbidities.[6] The average age for total hip and knee arthroplasty in North America is between 65 and 70 years.[12,16] This is in agreement with registry data from Sweden, Australia, and England and Wales, which have also reported the average age for hip and knee replacement surgery to be between 65 and 70 years.[17–20] In the developed world, primary osteoarthritis is the main indication for surgery with registry data citing osteoarthritis as the indication for THR in more than 80% of patients and as the indication for TKR in more than 95% of patients.[12,17–20] There is also an increasing trend in performing total hip replacements for acute hip fractures rather than the traditional hemiarthroplasty surgery. Total hip arthroplasty has been shown to offer better pain relief and functional outcomes as compared with hemiarthroplasty, as well as a reduced reoperation rate despite the known higher dislocation rate.[12,16,21] Registry data from developed nations also reveal a female preponderance for both THR and TKR, which is consistent with osteoarthritis being more prevalent in women than men.[22]

In contrast, demographic data from the available literature in developing countries reveal a much younger population with a larger variety of indications. Many of the existing case series for total hip replacements in Africa have a mean age of 50 years at the time of surgery, ranging anywhere from 41 years in Benin[23] to 58 years in Zambia.[24] A similar trend of younger patients undergoing THR is seen in studies from Asia where the average age varies from 41 years in Cambodia[25] to 52 years in India.[26] This directly correlates with the higher proportion of patients undergoing THR for avascular necrosis (AVN) in these regions, which accounted for 40% to 50% of patients in case series from India, Nigeria, Malawi, and Burkina Faso.[9,10,26,27] The causes of AVN in these series were attributed to the higher rates of human immunodeficiency virus (HIV) and sickle cell disease, untreated femoral neck fractures, and the common practice of chronic steroid use for pain relief.[9,23,25–28] Alcohol was also determined to be the major cause of AVN in a subset of patients in Hong Kong.[29] Tuberculosis of the hip and unreduced hip dislocations were also indications reported in multiple series.[8,10,25,29–31] Despite the prevalence of these other indications, osteoarthritis remains the most common indication for THA across the literature in the developing world.[2,7,22]

On the other hand, the demographics of patients undergoing total knee replacements in developing countries are more similar to those in developed countries. Although slightly younger, the mean age of patients undergoing TKR is comparable at 60 to 65 year.[26,32–35] As in developed nations, total knee arthroplasty patients were predominantly women in studies from countries in Asia, Africa, South America, and the Caribbean.[26,34,36,37] This corresponds with osteoarthritis being the indication formost of TKRs and the known higher prevalence of osteoarthritis in women.[22,38]

The increased rate of HIV and sickle cell disease in combination with the reliance on traditional healers or bone setters and the limited public awareness surrounding the available treatment options all contribute to the delayed presentation and complex nature of primary arthroplasty in the developing world.[39] The soft tissue scarring, fibrosis, and bone loss associated with old femoral neck fractures can make the surgeries technically challenging.[9] Similarly, AVN secondary to sickle cell disease causes significant sclerosis and canal narrowing of the proximal femur.[9,40] The high HIV rate and prevalence of patients receiving antiretroviral therapy also contribute to decreasing the mean age of patients undergoing surgery, as these have both been shown to be independent risk factors for the development of AVN.[41] The combination of younger patients and more complex primary surgeries make it more likely that revision arthroplasty will be required in the future.[42] Ideally, orthopedic surgeons should have additional training in hip and knee reconstructive surgery in order to tackle complex primary cases and revision surgery cases in order to limit complications and improve the longevity of the index procedure. It is therefore imperative that arthroplasty centers in developing countries simultaneously develop skills in revision surgery.

STERILITY

Operating room sterility is of paramount importance when it comes to implanting foreign material during a surgical procedure. Surgical site infections (SSI) are a substantial burden to patients and health care systems worldwide due to their morbidity, mortality, and significant cost.[43,44] SSIs disproportionately affect low- and middle-income countries.[45,46] Although many of these infections are preventable, guidelines and recommendations for the prevention of SSIs have been developed by organizations such as the Center for Disease Control and the World Health Organization (WHO).[47,48] Among these guidelines are the recommendations for alcohol-based and chlorhexidine-based antiseptic solutions for surgical site skin preparation and the use of alcohol-based hand rub. Unfortunately, the availability and cost of such products in resource-scarce low- and middle-income countries can be prohibitive. Programs for local production of these products as developed by the WHO in 5 African hospitals offer a creative and successful solution.[49]

Many improvements with regard to sterility have contributed to reducing the infection rates to very low percentages.[43] Although laminar air flow and space suits are used in some centers, their utility remains controversial.[50,51] Understandably, most hospitals in developing countries cannot afford such ventilation devices.[7] However, other factors are easily modifiable even in the most rudimentary operating room setting, such as operating room traffic and personnel. Limiting the amount of entrances and exits during the operation limits the particle count in the room. Ensuring appropriate ventilation and operating room temperature also helps reduce the rate of infection.[44] Solutions to these problemsinclude keeping a small number of implants in the room based on templating, restricting the number of observers, and avoiding surgery in the warmer summer months.[8] In addition, having access to a well-functioning sterilizing facility is absolutely mandatory for keeping infection rates low. As developing countries become more experienced with arthroplasty, the rate of prosthetic infections should also decrease, as hospital and surgeon volume have been shown to be inversely related to the infection rate.[52]

The hospital ward must also be clean and free of communicable diseases. Certain centers in developing nations such as Nigeria have decided to bundle the arthroplasty surgeries together in order to clear the ward of patients with communicable disease and appropriately clean the facilities before surgery.[34] Other centers use private wards for their arthroplasty patients.[53] Isolating patients to a dedicated arthroplasty ward has been shown to reduce the levels of infection.[54] The ultimate goal of such strategies is to limit the number of superficial and deep infections in order to decrease the need for revision surgery and ensure the cost-effectiveness of arthroplastyprograms.[55]

MEDICAL MISSIONS

In an attempt to decrease the local burden of disease in developing countries, many health care professionals including orthopedic surgeons embark on short-term medical mission trips. They provide a unique opportunity to build local capacity through education and training of local medical professionals.[56] From the United States alone, roughly 6000 short-term medical mission trips, representing approximately US$250 million dollars in donations, occur on an annual basis.[57]

Although many orthopedic medical missions exist, very few are well equipped to perform arthroplasty surgery safely. Nonetheless, well-established organizations such as Operation Walk Canada have been sending teams to Ecuador since 2009 and have performed 253 hip surgeries on patients with developmental dysplasia of the hip.[58] They also have teams that travel to Guatemala, and since 2006 they have performed nearly 1000 THR/TKRs.[59] Another arthroplasty-focused mission is Operation Walk Boston, which has provided total joint replacements to nearly 300 residents of the Dominican Republic. They have also created a robust research program that tracks patient outcomes via pre- and postoperative pain and functional scores, which affords insights into the quality and outcomes of their surgeries in resource-poor countries.[60]

While providing treatment to a relatively small group of patients, these medical missions provide a unique training opportunity for local orthopedic surgeons and residents while they are exposed to rare and uncommon operations performed by highly qualified orthopedic surgeons from high-volume centers. Oftentimes these groups will cover the cost of the implants being used. Their success also relies on the recurring nature of their trips to ensure adequate patient follow-up and continuity of care.

Another way to ensure follow-up is to maintain close communication with expert arthroplasty surgeons via Internet. Telecommunications provide an excellent opportunity for remote teams in developing countries to seek expert opinion in an expedited manner. Such is the case in a district hospital in Burkina Faso who has partnered with a team of Belgian orthopedic surgeons from Medics Without Vacations who are available via email or telephone to address any patient concerns once they have returned home from their medical mission.[9]

Surgeons on medical missions should always balance the unique risks and benefits of each case and should always aim to do no harm. Eager and valiant efforts can sometimes result in catastrophic outcomes for patients, as the local hospitals are not always well equipped to deal with surgical complications because they lack the expertise or necessary equipment.[56] With resection arthroplasty being the only viable bailout surgery for many late-presenting complications, surgeons should make every effort to communicate clearly the possible risks and benefits of surgery in a language their patients understand.

REGISTRIES

The first country to develop an arthroplasty registry was Sweden in 1975.[19] Currently, countries with active national registries include Sweden, Finland, Norway, Denmark, Australia, England and Wales, Scotland, Canada, the United States, Australia, New Zealand, India, and Malawi.[26] The benefits of registries include minimizing reporting bias and the ability to make outcomes comparisons between different implants and techniques.[61] The pooling of outcomes data in registries also allows for better assessment of longevity and detection of early failures, thus permitting timely intervention, preventing harm to patients, and reducing revision rates.[62,63] One such case was the detection of the high early revision rates in metal-on-metal total hip replacements in the Australian registry that lead to an eventual global recall.[64]

Quoting the success and utility of national registry data, Malawi set out to create the first national joint registry in a developing country in 2005.[10] Since then, multiple groups in low- to middle-income countries have set out to establish regional registries in an effort to contribute to outcomes data in these unique populations.[24–26,31] The role of registries in low-income countries differs slightly from that of Western registries. There is less of a focus on different implants and techniques, rather an increased focus on the influence of different health, social, and economic settings on arthroplasty surgeries, such as the impact of HIV.[10] Unfortunately, many regional registries are often missing such data points, and therefore synchronization of data is necessary to allow for accurate comparisons between registries.[24,25] The success of registries also depends on the voluntary reporting of results and is therefore inherently prone to reporting bias, where centers with good results are more likely to report their outcomes.[7]

Despite these challenges, registries in developing countries have had a positive contribution to the arthroplasty literature. The introduction of antiretroviral therapy in 1997 has resulted in a significant decrease in HIV-related infection, morbidity, and mortality.[65] This increased survival in combination with the aging population means that the number of HIV-positive patients who are considered candidates for total joint replacement surgery is increasing.[66] Although it was previously thought that HIV was an independent risk factor for infection and other perioperative complications in total joint replacement, more recent studies have shown this not to be true.[66–69] Data from the Malawi registry support this finding and have shown excellent short-term results for both total knee and total hip arthroplasty in HIV-positive patients with no increase in complications.[30,35] Long-term results remain to be seen, but the data to date are promising.

EARLY OUTCOMES

Although there exist many challenges to the implementation of total joint replacement programs in developing countries, early outcomes have been positive.[7,35,70] A big challenge to the assessment of early outcomes in these regions is the accessibility to points of care.[31] Patients often have to travel long distances with limited resources, making follow-up difficult and inconsistent.[8] This has been demonstrated in many studies where loss to follow-up has been reported as high as 34% in the first 6 months.[71] In contrast, certain groups have reported success in maintaining 100% follow-up by establishing weekly dedicated arthroplasty clinics and outreach clinics to district hospitals with transport arranged with local facilities ahead of time.[8,72] The increased use and access to mobile phones, even in remote communities, has been previously used to improve compliance with HIV treatments in this population by sending text message reminders and could be similarly used to prevent loss to follow-up after arthroplasty.[24,73]

Data from the available literature would suggest that, although slightly higher, the complication rates in developing countries are certainly within acceptable limits.[6,7] Evidence shows that with proper training and experience these complication rates only stand to improve, as complication rate is inversely proportional to volume.[52,74] Complications related to inexperienced assistants and surgeons such as intraoperative fractures and increased blood loss improve with case load.[6,9,71] Reductions in overall complications were seen in a series from Sub-Saharan Africa and rural Australia as programs matured.[8,9,72] As in developed nations, the most common major complications include dislocations and infections. Dislocation rates in studies from Sub-Saharan Africa ranged from 1.3% in Burkina Faso to 6.8% in Zambia.[8,9,24] Although similar rates were seen in Asia ranging from 1.1% in Cambodia to 3.5% in Singapore,[25,70] compared with dislocation rates seen in early series from the western world ranging from 2.1% to 3.2% it is slightly higher than newer western studies showing dislocation rates as low as 0.43% to 1.01%.[75–77]

Part of the challenge in the developing world is educating patients surrounding postoperative restrictions. Low literacy rates combined with cultural activities such as deep squatting, kneeling, subsistence farming, and the use of squat toilets make patients especially prone to dislocation and make prevention difficult.[7,24,31] Many centers have tried to counter this by extending their length of stay to allow for appropriate rehabilitation before discharge, as few rehabilitation facilities exist in the developing world.[70] Thus, the average length of stay for arthroplasty patients in developing nations is more than a week.[7,25] Similarly, many centers have made a point of discharging patients with custom seat raises for installation over squat toilets.[8,10,31] In Cambodia, for example, a postoperative rehabilitation protocol was adapted from western protocols and created using plain language and culture-specific imaging to increase understanding of postoperative restrictions.[31]

Other common complications seen were related to the complex nature of these primary arthroplasties. In more than one series, high rates of intraoperative fracture or the need for osteotomy and cabling were seen. These rates were as high as 25.9% in a series from Ghana, which was attributed to the sclerotic nature of the proximal femoral canal in AVN.[40,78] Many studies also reported neuropraxias to either the sciatic nerve from limb lengthening in severe coxavalga or foot drop secondary to correction of severely valgus knees.[34,53,71] Foot drop was in fact the most common complication reported in a series examining total knee replacements in Nigeria, with an incidence of 8.9%.[34] Spinal anesthesia was used in most of the cases and is known to be beneficial in low-resource environments where sufficient trained personnel, general anesthesia drugs, and oxygen are often in short supply.[79] However, this led to a high incidence of postspinal headaches in certain centers, with rates as high as 18.5% in one study from Nigeria.[40] Fortunately, deep vein thromboses (DVTs) were noted to be rare in most studies, likely attributable to the widespread use and availability of DVT prophylaxis, in the form of both compression stockings and anticoagulant medications.[6,8]

With the increasing demand for arthroplasty surgery in the resource-limited context of the developing world, there comes a need to determine which patients will benefit the most from surgery. It has been shown through a variety of outcomes measures that arthroplasty surgery in developing countries results in dramatic increases in function and that the mean observed improvement in this population is higher than typically seen in high-income countries.[7,32,33] In the developed world, studies have shown that although patients with lower preoperative scores improve the most on average, these patients have lower final functional outcome scores at 12 months.[80] This has led certain investigators to suggest earlier intervention.[81] Although it was found that the preoperative functional scores were on average lower in low- to middle-income countries as compared with higher income countries, there was in fact no difference in the final functional outcome scores seen at 1-year follow-up when comparing the patients with low and high preoperative scores in this population.[32,33] This suggests that in a resource-constrained environment focusing on the most affected patients may optimize improvement following TJA.

SUMMARY

Although the global demand for hip and knee arthroplasty surgery continues to grow, many countries in the developing world have started offering these surgeries to select patients. These nascent joint replacement programs, although burdened by substantial health care costs and equipped with limited resources, should continue to strive for improved patient outcomes and safety. With an aging population and an increasing awareness about these types of surgeries, the demand for such life-changing surgeries will continue to increase globally. It is up to the orthopedic surgeons and allied medical professionals to continue to negotiate with their local governments and district hospitals to develop such programs in the safest way possible.

DISCLOSURE

The authors have nothing to disclose.

REFERENCES

1. World Health Organization. Chronic Rheumatic Conditions. Chronic diseases and health promotion 2012.
2. Brooks PM. The burden of musculoskeletal disease—a global perspective. ClinRheumatol 2006; 25(6):778–81.
3. Nugent R. Chronic diseases in developing countries: health and economic burdens. Ann N Y Acad Sci 2008;1136:70–9.
4. Kurtz S, Ong K, Lau E, et al. Projections of primary and revision hip and knee arthroplasty in the United States from 2005 to 2030. JBone Joint Surg Am 2007;89(4):780–5.
5. Ackerman IN, Bohensky MA, Zomer E, et al. The projected burden of primary total knee and hip replacement for osteoarthritis in Australia to the year 2030. BMCMusculoskeletDisord 2019;20(1):90.
6. Mulimba J. Is hip arthroplasty viable in a developing African country? East Cent Afr J Surg 2007; 12(1):30–2.
7. Davies PS, Graham SM, Maqungo S, et al. Total joint replacement in sub-Saharan Africa: a systematic review. Trop Doct 2019;49(2):120–8.
8. Lisenda L, Mokete L, Nwokeyi K, et al. Development of a lower limb arthroplasty service in a developing country: lessons learned after the first 100 cases (joints). ActaOrthopBelg 2016;82:2016.
9. Dossche L, Noyez J, Ouedraogo W, et al. Establishment of a hip replacement project in a district hospital in Burkina Faso: analysis of technical problems and peri-operative complications. Bone Joint J 2014;96(2):177–80.
10. Lubega N, Mkandawire N, Sibande G, et al. Joint replacement in Malawi: establishment of a National Joint Registry. J Bone JtSurg Br 2009;91(3):341–3.
11. Robinson JC, Pozen A, Tseng S, et al. Variability in costs associated with total hip and knee

replacement implants. J Bone Joint Surg Am 2012; 94(18):1693–8.
12. Canadian Institute for Health Information. Hip and knee replacements in Canada CJRRARO, Ontario. CIHI; 2019.
13. Stargardt T. Health service costs in Europe: ccost and reimbursement of primary hip replacement in nine countries. Health Econ 2008;17:9–20.
14. Hunter DJ, Felson DT. Osteoarthritis. BMJ (ClinRes Ed) 2006;332(7542):639–42.
15. Arnold W, Fullerton DS, Holder S, et al. Viscosupplementation: managed care issues for osteoarthritis of the knee. J Manag Care Pharm 2007;13(4 Suppl):S3–19 [quiz:S20–12].
16. Surgeons AAoO. Fifth AJRR annual report on hip and knee arthroplasty data 2018.
17. Registry NJ. 15th annual report, 2018 2018.
18. Register SHA. Annual report 2017 2018.
19. Robertsson OL, Lars, Sundberg, et al. The Swedish knee arthroplasty register - annual report 2018 2018.
20. AOANJRR. Hip, knee & shoulder arthroplasty: 2018 annual report. Adelaide (Australia): 2018.
21. Yu L, Wang Y, Chen J. Total hip arthroplasty versus hemiarthroplasty for displaced femoral neck fractures: meta-analysis of randomized trials. ClinOrthopRelat Res 2012;470(8):2235–43.
22. Cross M, Smith E, Hoy D, et al. The global burden of hip and knee osteoarthritis: estimates from the global burden of disease 2010 study. Ann Rheum Dis 2014;73(7):1323–30.
23. Sambo BT, Allode SA, Ouorou GYJ, et al. Total hip arthroplasty in a developing country: epidemiological, clinical and etiological aspects and indications. J Surg 2017;5(6):130–3.
24. Mulla Y, Munthali J, Makasa E, et al. Joint replacement in Zambia: a review of hip & knee replacement surgery done at the Zambian-Italian Orthopaedic Hospital. Med J Zambia 2010;37(3): 153–9.
25. Holt JA, Aird JJ, Gollogly JG, et al. Developing a sustainable hip service in Cambodia. Hip Int 2014; 24(5):480–4.
26. Pachore JA, Vaidya SV, Thakkar CJ, et al. ISHKS joint registry: a preliminary report. Indian J Orthop 2013;47(5):505.
27. Katchy AU, Katchy SC, Ekwedigwe H, et al. Total hip replacement for management of severe osteoarthritis in a developing country: A 5-year assessment of functional outcome in 72 consecutive hip. Niger J OrthopTrauma 2018;17(2):46.
28. Singh G, Krishna L, De SD. The ten-year pattern of hip diseases in Singapore. J Orthop Surg 2010; 18(3):276–8.
29. Chan V, Chan P, Chiu P, et al. Why do Hong Kong patients need total hip arthroplasty? An. Hong Kong Med J 2015;21:21.
30. Graham S, Lubega N, Mkandawire N, et al. Total hip replacement in HIV-positive patients. Bone Joint J 2014;96(4):462–6.
31. Peek KN, Noor S, Thormodsson HS, et al. Total hip arthroplasty rehabilitation in Cambodia. Disability, CBR & Inclusive Development 2013;24(4):116–21.
32. Dempsey KE, Collins JE, Ghazinouri R, et al. Associations between preoperative functional status and functional outcomes of total joint replacement in the Dominican Republic. Rheumatology 2013; 52(10):1802–8.
33. Niu NN, Collins JE, Thornhill TS, et al. Pre-operative status and quality of life following total joint replacement in a developing country: a prospective pilot study. Open OrthopJ 2011;5:307.
34. Anyaehie U, Eyichukwu G, Nwadinigwe C. Total knee replacement in a resource constrained environment: A preliminary report. Niger J ClinPract 2017;20(3):369–75.
35. Graham SM, Moffat C, Lubega N, et al. Total knee arthroplasty in a low-income country: short-term outcomes from a National Joint Registry. JBJS Open Access 2018;3(1).
36. Bido J, Yang YH, Collins JE, et al. Predictors of patient-reported outcomes of total joint arthroplasty in a developing country. J Arthroplasty 2017;32(6):1756–62.
37. Carvalho RTd, Canté JCL, Lima JHS, et al. Prevalence of knee arthroplasty in the state of São Paulo between 2003 and 2010. Sao Paulo Med J 2016; 134(5):417–22.
38. Wittenauer R, Smith L, Aden K. Background paper 6.12 osteoarthritis. World Health Organisation; 2013.
39. Dada A, Yinusa W, Giwa S. Review of the practice of traditional bone setting in Nigeria. Afr Health Sci 2011;11(2).
40. Uwatoronye NC, Ego AU, Amaechi KU. Total hip replacement in Nigeria: a preliminary report. Kuwait Med J 2012;44(4):291–6.
41. Mary-Krause M, Billaud E, Poizot-Martin I, et al. Risk factors for osteonecrosis in HIV-infected patients: impact of treatment with combination antiretroviral therapy. AIDS 2006;20(12):1627–35.
42. Wainwright C, Theis J-C, Garneti N, et al. Age at hip or knee joint replacement surgery predicts likelihood of revision surgery. J Bone Joint Surg Br 2011;93(10):1411–5.
43. Bullock MW, Brown ML, Bracey DN, et al. A bundle protocol to reduce the incidence of periprosthetic joint infections after total joint arthroplasty: A single-center experience. J Arthroplasty 2017; 32(4):1067–73.
44. Rezapoor M, Parvizi J. Prevention of periprosthetic joint infection. J Arthroplasty 2015;30(6):902–7.
45. Allegranzi B, Nejad SB, Combescure C, et al. Burden of endemic health-care-associated

infection in developing countries: systematic review and meta-analysis. Lancet 2011;377(9761):228–41.
46. Nejad SB, Allegranzi B, Syed SB, et al. Health-care-associated infection in Africa: a systematic review. Bull WorldHealth Organ 2011;89:757–65.
47. Berríos-Torres SI, Umscheid CA, Bratzler DW, et al. Centers for Disease Control and Prevention guideline for the prevention of surgical site infection, 2017. JAMA Surg 2017;152(8):784–91.
48. Allegranzi B, Bischoff P, de Jonge S, et al. New WHO recommendations on preoperative measures for surgical site infection prevention: an evidence-based global perspective. Lancet Infect Dis 2016;16(12):e276–87.
49. Allegranzi B, Aiken AM, Kubilay NZ, et al. A multimodal infection control and patient safety intervention to reduce surgical site infections in Africa: a multicentre, before–after, cohort study. Lancet Infect Dis 2018;18(5):507–15.
50. James M, Khan W, Nannaparaju M, et al. Suppl 2: M7: current evidence for the use of laminar flow in reducing infection rates in total joint arthroplasty. Open Orthop J 2015;9:495.
51. Hooper G, Rothwell A, Frampton C, et al. Does the use of laminar flow and space suits reduce early deep infection after total hip and knee replacement? The ten-year results of the New Zealand Joint Registry. J Bone Joint Surg Br 2011;93(1):85–90.
52. Katz JN, Losina E, Barrett J, et al. Association between hospital and surgeon procedure volume and outcomes of total hip replacement in the United States Medicare population. J Bone Joint Surg Am 2001;83(11):1622–9.
53. Gokcen EC, Wamisho BL. Total hip replacement surgery in Ethiopia. East Cent Afr J Surg 2017;22(2):35–48.
54. Barlow D, Masud S, Rhee S, et al. The effect of the creation of a ring-fenced orthopaedic ward on length of stay for elective arthroplasty patients. Surgeon 2013;11(2):82–6.
55. Alp E, Cevahir F, Ersoy S, et al. Incidence and economic burden of prosthetic joint infections in a university hospital: a report from a middle-income country. J Infect Public Health 2016;9(4):494–8.
56. Sheth NP, Donegan DJ, Foran JRH, et al. Global health and orthopaedic surgery—A call for international morbidity and mortality conferences. Int J Surg Case Rep 2015;6:63–7.
57. Maki J, Qualls M, White B, et al. Health impact assessment and short-term medical missions: a methods study to evaluate quality of care. BMC Health Serv Res 2008;8:121.
58. Canada OW. Operation Walk Canada: Ecuador Mission. 2019. Available at: https://www.operationwalk.ca/ecuador. Accessed September 2019.
59. Canada OW. Operation Walk Canada: Guatemala Mission. 2019. Available at: https://www.operationwalk.ca/guatemala. Accessed September 2019.
60. Katz JN, TST. Operation Walk Boston:outcomes research informs surgery, education, and sustainable care. 2019. Available at: https://www.brighamandwomens.org/orthopaedic-surgery/advances-newsletter/operation-walk-boston. Accessed September 2019.
61. Delaunay C. Registries in orthopaedics. OrthopTraumatolSurg Res 2015;101(1):S69–75.
62. Herberts P, Malchau H. Long-term registration has improved the quality of hip replacement: a review of the Swedish THR Register comparing 160,000 cases. ActaOrthop Scand 2000;71(2):111–21.
63. Hughes RE, Batra A, Hallstrom BR. Arthroplasty registries around the world: valuable sources of hip implant revision risk data. Curr Rev Musculoskelet Med 2017;10(2):240–52.
64. Bernthal NM, Celestre PC, Stavrakis AI, et al. Disappointing short-term results with the DePuy ASR XL metal-on-metal total hip arthroplasty. J Arthroplasty 2012;27(4):539–44.
65. Chen LF, Hoy J, Lewin SR. Ten years of highly active antiretroviral therapy for HIV infection. Med J Aust 2007;186(3):146–51.
66. Lin CA, Kuo AC, Takemoto S. Comorbidities and perioperative complications in HIV-positive patients undergoing primary total hip and knee arthroplasty. J Bone Joint Surg Am 2013;95(11):1028–36.
67. Hicks J, Ribbans WJ, Buzzard B, et al. Infected joint replacements in HIV-positive patients with haemophilia. J Bone Joint Surg Br 2001;83(7):1050–4.
68. Govender S, Harrison W, Lukhele M. Impact of HIV on bone and joint surgery. Best Pract Res ClinRheumatol 2008;22(4):605–19.
69. Brijlall S. Hip arthroplasty in HIV-infected patients. SA Orthopaedic Journal 2008;7(1):10–7.
70. Liu Y, Hu S, Chan S, et al. The epidemiology and surgical outcomes of patients undergoing primary total hip replacement: an Asian perspective. Singapore Med J 2009;50(1):15.
71. Kingori J, Gakuu L. Total hip replacements at Kikuyu Hospital, Kenya. East AfrOrthop J 2010;4(2).
72. Stewart GD, Stewart PC, Nott ML, et al. Total joint replacement surgery in a rural centre. Aust J RuralHealth 2006;14(6):253–7.
73. Mayer JE, Fontelo P. Meta-analysis on the effect of text message reminders for HIV-related compliance. AIDS Care 2017;29(4):409–17.
74. Sharkey PF, Shastri S, Teloken MA, et al. Relationship between surgical volume and early outcomes of total hip arthroplasty: do results continue to get better? J Arthroplasty 2004;19(6):694–9.

75. Woo RY, Morrey BF. Dislocations after total hip arthroplasty. J Bone Joint Surg Am 1982;64(9):1295–306.
76. Ali Khan M, Brakenbury P, Reynolds I. Dislocation following total hip replacement. J Bone JointSurg Br 1981;63(2):214–8.
77. Kwon MS, Kuskowski M, Mulhall KJ, et al. Does Surgical Approach Affect Total Hip Arthroplasty Dislocation Rates? ClinOrthopRelat Res 2006;447:34–8.
78. George A, Ofori-Atta P. Joint replacement surgery in Ghana (West Africa)—an observational study. IntOrthop 2019;43(5):1041–7.
79. Newton M, Bird P. Impact of parallel anesthesia and surgical provider training in sub-Saharan Africa: a model for a resource-poor setting. World J Surg 2010;34(3):445–52.
80. Fortin PR, Penrod JR, Clarke AE, et al. Timing of total joint replacement affects clinical outcomes among patients with osteoarthritis of the hip or knee. Arthritis Rheum 2002;46(12):3327–30.
81. Lingard EA, Katz JN, Wright EA, et al. Predicting the outcome of total knee arthroplasty. J Bone Joint Surg Am 2004;86(10):2179–86.

The Changing Face of Infection, Diagnosis, and Management in the United Kingdom

Syed S. Ahmed, MBChB, LLM, MSc, FRCS (Tr & Orth)[a,*],
Khaled M. Yaghmour, MBBS[b],
Fares S. Haddad, BSc, MD(Res), MCh(Orth), FRCS(Orth), FFSEM[b]

KEYWORDS

• Prosthetic joint infection • Dair • Diagnosis • One stage • Two stage

KEY POINTS

- The diagnosis of PJI should be based on a combination of clinical and laboratory findings. One must be cautious to not diminish the role of a positive growth in periprosthetic tissue and fluid culture.
- There is an established role for DAIR and one-stage revision in appropriately selected patients with excellent results. The authors also recommend using a one-stage exchange procedure in early PJI in uncemented implants.
- A favorable success rate for DAIR is reported when performed within 1 week from onset of symptoms, 4 to 6 weeks from index surgery, and when modular component exchange is implemented.
- The criteria for a one-stage revision at our institution is that: the organism is identified preoperatively, the organism is susceptible to an antibiotic, and there are good soft tissues around the implant.

INTRODUCTION

Prosthetic joint infection (PJI) is a rare but devastating complication following total hip arthroplasty (THA) and total knee arthroplasty (TKA). The incidence of PJI ranges from 2% to 4% in primary procedures as opposed to nearly 20% in revisions. The UK National Joint Registry is in its 15th year. There are 3872 patients that underwent first-stage revision out of 992,090 records of primary THA, and 5982 underwent first-stage revision out of 1,087,611 records of primary total knee arthroplasty for infection.[1]

Highly cross-linked polyethylene has shown wear rates 40 times lower than conventional polyethylene.[2–5] Improvement in implant machinery and surgical technique will result in a decline of revisions associated with these reasons. This will possibly see PJIs becoming the leading cause of revision procedures. PJIs are notoriously difficult to manage, resulting in the need for multiple revision procedures and prolonged courses of systemic antibiotics. The impact on the patient's life is burdensome, and involves long periods of immobility, recurrent hospital admissions, and psychological agony. There is also a significant economic burden for PJI with an average cost of £50,000 for a revision procedure for an infected total hip in the United Kingdom. Hence, recognizing trends aids in the suitable identification and management to preserve function and prevent morbidity.

[a] Lower Limb Arthroplasty, University College London Hospital, 250 Euston Road, Bloomsbury, London NW1 2BU, UK; [b] University College London Hospital, 250 Euston Road, Bloomsbury, London NW1 2BU, UK
* Corresponding author.
E-mail address: syedahmed@doctors.org.uk

Orthop Clin N Am 51 (2020) 141–146
https://doi.org/10.1016/j.ocl.2019.12.003
0030-5898/20/

The challenges that arise, including diagnostic uncertainty, management in immunocompromised patients, recurrent infection, infection around a well-fixed implant, and substantial bone loss, require careful preoperative assessment and well-defined management plans. This article summarizes the recent developments in the diagnosis and management of this increasingly prevalent issue in the United Kingdom, specifically focusing on outcomes following debridement, antibiotics, and implants retention (DAIR) and one-stage revision procedures.

DIAGNOSIS OF PROSTHETIC JOINT INFECTION

Diagnostic Criteria

There has been a great deal of interest recently in the diagnosis of PJI. An attempt has been made to change the widely used Musculoskeletal Infection Society criteria with a score-based system in the consensus meeting in 2018. However, the significance attached to new biomarkers, such as α-defensin and D dimer, should make one question its validity. There are several studies that investigate the sensitivity and specificity of α-defensin using the lateral flow test and not all of them report consistent results,[6–13] and the data supporting D dimer as a key test are much less robust.[14]

This leads to an increase in the number of culture negative infections that are reported. Changing the diagnostic criteria for PJI will also lead to inconsistencies in literature on the subject.

The diagnosis of PJI should be based on a combination of clinical and laboratory findings. One must be cautious not to diminish the role of a positive growth in periprosthetic tissue and fluid culture. The National Health Service certainly lacks the new industry-driven bedside tests for PJI and this may well be a positive thing considering their reliability.

Therefore, the 2012 Musculoskeletal Infection Society criteria[15] should for now, still be considered the standard definition of PJI. Based on that, definite PJI exists when:

1. There is a sinus tract communicating with prosthesis; or
2. A pathogen is isolated by culture from at least two separate tissue or fluid samples obtained from the affected prosthetic joint; or
3. Four of the following six (minor) criteria exist:
   I. Elevated C-reactive protein (CRP) and erythrocyte sedimentation rate (ESR)
   II. Elevated synovial fluid white blood cell or ++ change on leukocyte esterase test strip
   III. Elevated synovial fluid polymorphonuclear neutrophil (PMN) percentage
   IV. Presence of purulence in the affected joint
   V. Isolation of a microorganism in one culture of periprosthetic tissue or fluid, or
   VI. Greater than five neutrophils per high-power field in five high-power fields observed from histologic analysis of periprosthetic tissue at ×400 magnification.

Inflammatory Markers

CRP and ESR are still the most widely used blood markers, mainly because of their quick turnaround time and ease of availability. These are also extremely useful in the early postoperative period. It has been found that the serum CRP is the least invasive test that maximizes sensitivity and specificity. A value of 93 mg/L should trigger performing an aspiration of the joint. Synovial white cell count is the single best predictor of PJI in the early postoperative period. The optimal value being 12,800 cell/μL with a PMN of 89%.[16]

Other Markers

Recently there has been much emphasis on synovial white cell count; D dimer; and new biomarkers, such as α-defensin. This has to an extent been driven by new tests available in the market for the same. D dimer is a nonspecific hematologic marker and its validity in detecting PJI is questionable.[14] There are several studies that have investigated the sensitivity and specificity of α-defensin, using the lateral flow test to detect PJI. It has been found that the results are inferior when compared with the enzyme-linked immunosorbent assay method.[6,11–13,17,18]

Synovial Fluid and Tissue Culture

The next step in the evaluation, following suspicious clinical findings and blood work, should be the assessment of a synovial fluid analysis. The aspirate should be analyzed for cell count, PMN cells, and culture. Although antibiotic therapy is likely to impact culture results, it is unlikely to have an impact on the cell count. A high percentage (>80%) of PMN cells is likely to represent delayed-onset or late PJI. In the early postoperative stage there is a normal inflammatory response and therefore the same numbers are not reliable.

Intraoperative tissue specimens for microbiology are more accurate for detecting an infective microorganism (sensitivity, 45%–78%; specificity, 91%–96%). The current recommendations for microbiologic diagnosis of PJI includes taking five samples from visibly inflamed regions.

MANAGEMENT OF PROSTHETIC JOINT INFECTION

Debridement, Antibiotic Therapy, Irrigation, and Retention

A lot of emphasis has been placed on the definition of early PJI and the optimum time to use DAIR. This is caused by the formation of a biofilm. The biofilm is composed of a matrix of polypeptides, polysaccharides, and nucleic acids, forming a microenvironment enabling the bacteria to flourish and become inaccessible to the patient's immune system and to systemic antibiotics.[19] A biofilm has been reported to be produced by microorganisms from a few hours to 6 weeks following bacterial invasion. Early intervention with a DAIR procedure could therefore prevent the formation of this biofilm on the implant surface.[20–22]

A meta-analysis focusing on PJI following THA reported a substantial difference in success rates of DAIR before and after 2004, going from 43.3% to 67.2%. A review of the recent literature does show that success rates now vary between 60% and 89.3%. The primary reason behind this improvement is the awareness that time since onset of symptoms improves results. Success rates in DAIR performed within 1 week of symptom onset ranged from 72% to 83%, compared with a success rate of 51.8% to 66% when DAIR is performed after 1 week since onset of symptoms.

An analysis of 39 studies that included 1296 patients revealed that less success was noted in studies that had a median time from the onset of symptoms to debridement of greater than 7 days. In these studies, when the median time from the onset of symptoms to debridement was greater than 7 days, the pooled proportion of success was 51.8%. In comparison, in those where the median time from the onset of symptoms to debridement was less than 7 days, the pooled proportion of success was 72.0%.[23]

Functional outcomes following a DAIR procedure have also been shown to be superior to a two-stage revision with similar eradication rates.[24] Hence, not disturbing a sound implant bone interface leads to superior functional outcomes. The presence of a stable implant without a breach in the bone implant interface can therefore be used as an indicator to perform a DAIR procedure.

Exchange of modular component has been reported to be a significant factor in a successful DAIR and is recommended by several studies. In our review, the success rate following modular component exchange ranged from 73.9% to 90%, whereas in those without modular component exchange the success rate was only 60.7% to 63%. The exchanging of components reduces the residual biofilm.[25]

A lower rate of success has been reported with polymicrobial infection ranging from 14% to 40%. Evaluating the difference in success rates with regards to antibiotic duration reveals a higher nonsignificant success rate in patients with antibiotic therapy for greater than 12 weeks in comparison with those receiving antibiotics for less than 12 weeks (**Figs. 1–3**).

Host factors that predict an increased risk of failure include immunosuppression, rheumatoid arthritis, body mass index greater than 30, presence of more than two comorbidities, diabetes, previous infection in the same joint, and presence of a sinus tract.[26,27]

A favorable success rate for DAIR is reported when performed within 1 week from onset of symptoms, 4 to 6 weeks from index surgery, and when modular component exchange is implemented. Additionally, polymicrobial infections, immunosuppressed host, previous joint infections, and revision arthroplasty are poor prognostic factors.

One-Stage and Two-Stage Revision

The debate between a one-stage or two-stage revision is no longer relevant. It is now recognized that the indications for these procedures are different.

The criteria for a one-stage revision at our institution is that:

1. The organism is identified preoperatively,
2. The organism is susceptible to an antibiotic, and
3. There are good soft tissues around the implant.

If these criteria are met, we can proceed to a one-stage revision arthroplasty and the rate of recurrence is also lower.[28] The senior author's technique for one-stage revisions has been described previously.[29] Broadly, this involves preparation, initial debridement, timeout, and reimplantation.

The success of a one-stage revision previously was mainly because antibiotic-loaded cement and powder were used.[7] However, meticulous

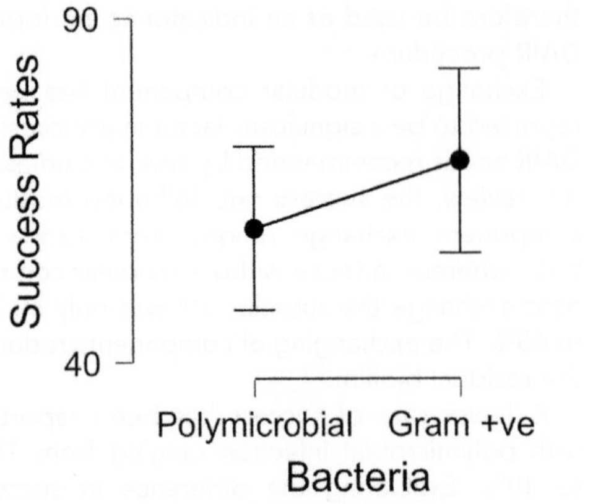

Fig. 1. A higher success rate is noted in studies reporting infections with gram-positive bacteria.

attention to detail in each of the steps of the procedure does improve outcomes even in an uncemented setting. Local antibiotics are added in other ways using calcium sulfate substrates.

The obvious advantage of a single stage is that implant removal and reimplantation are performed in the same setting. This has a significant reduction in overall cost and operative time when compared with a two-stage procedure. There are suggestions that it reduces overall blood loss.[30] However, no recent comparative studies analyze these parameters specifically.

In early PJI involving uncemented implants a one-stage exchange arthroplasty is a good option. In uncemented THA when we see an acute infection, it is much easier to use this time-limited opportunity to remove the implants and the associated biofilm and do a single-stage revision instead of just doing a debridement and a change of insert.

The senior author has previously presented a series of 39 patients between 2004 and 2014 who underwent a one-stage exchange arthroplasty. Infection control at 5 years was obtained in 90% of these patients. This is clearly experience and prosthesis-dependent but if the cementless implant is easy to remove, then it should be explanted. One critical aspect of this procedure is to use one set of instruments and drapes for the debridement and to reprepare and use fresh drapes to implant the new components. Units that have gained expertise in single-stage revision find this easier to do. Patients are then continued on broad-spectrum intravenous antibiotics until culture results are available. Culture-sensitive antibiotics are then continued for a period of 3 months following discussions with a multidisciplinary team, which includes a microbiologist.

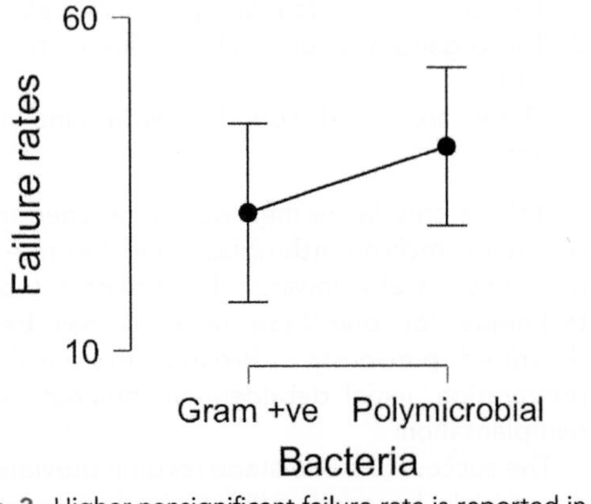

Fig. 2. Higher nonsignificant failure rate is reported in patients with polymicrobial infection rates.

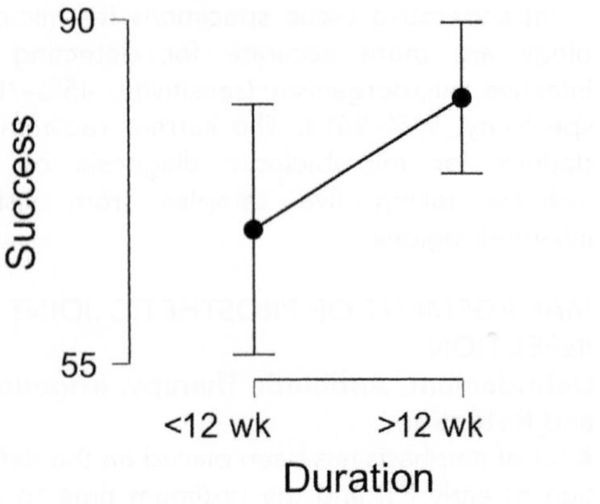

Fig. 3. A higher nonsignificant success rate in patients receiving antibiotics for greater than 12 weeks when compared with those receiving antibiotics for less than 12 weeks.

The two-stage revision arthroplasty involves the removal of the infected implant and a delayed reimplantation of the second prosthesis. A 2- to 4-week interval is recommended for patients with a known and treatable organism, soft tissue compromise, or sinus tracts. A longer interval of around 8 weeks is suggested for cases that are more difficult to manage because of compromised tissue or unknown organisms. The success rate is greater than 90%; however, reinfection rates are higher when patients have greater than three comorbidities and a raised ESR/CRP before the second implantation.

Surgical Salvage and Antibiotic Suppression

The Girdlestone procedure was described in the 1920s and was mainly used to deal with pyogenic infections as a result of tuberculosis. It has been found that, on mobilizing, the energy consumed in resection arthroplasty patients was greater than that in patients with above-knee amputation.[31] For these reasons, it is only performed in patients unfit for multiple surgeries and general anesthetic. Other indications include poor bone and soft tissue, recurrent infections, multiresistant organisms, and multiple previous surgery failures. The total success rate varies from 60% to 100%.

Long-term antibiotic suppression is only recommended in patients who are unfit for surgical intervention. Bacterial load is suppressed with sensitive antibiotics. Increasingly, fungal causes of infection require an antifungal to be added to the regime.

SUMMARY

There has been recent development in PJI. Interest in the accurate and early diagnosis has led to several tests being developed. However, one must be vigilant of the commercial drivers behind them before accepting their routine clinical application.

There is an established role for DAIR and one-stage revision in appropriately selected patients with excellent results reported in the literature. We also recommend using a one-stage exchange procedure in early PJI in uncemented implants.

Despite recent attempts, there is yet to be agreement on an internationally accepted diagnostic and treatment algorithm.[32] The registries reflect the growing epidemic of PJI, and one must therefore focus on prevention and management strategies to control the infection burden.

DISCLOSURE

The authors have nothing to disclose.

REFERENCES

1. NJR Annual reports. Available at: http://www.njrcentre.org.uk/njrcentre/Reports-Publications-and-Minutes/Annual-reports. Accessed April 29, 2019.
2. Glyn-Jones S, McLardy-Smith P, Gill HS, et al. The creep and wear of highly cross-linked polyethylene. J Bone Joint Surg Br 2008;90-B(5):556–61.
3. Hanna SA, Somerville L, McCalden RW, et al. Highly cross-linked polyethylene decreases the rate of revision of total hip arthroplasty compared with conventional polyethylene at 13 years' follow-up. Bone Joint J 2016;98-B(1):28–32.
4. Kuzyk PRT, Saccone M, Sprague S, et al. Cross-linked *versus* conventional polyethylene for total hip replacement. J Bone Joint Surg Br 2011;93-B(5):593–600.
5. Langlois J, Atlan F, Scemama C, et al. A randomised controlled trial comparing highly cross-linked and contemporary annealed polyethylene after a minimal eight-year follow-up in total hip arthroplasty using cemented acetabular components. Bone Joint J 2015;97-B(11):1458–62.
6. Suen K, Keeka M, Ailabouni R, et al. Synovasure "quick test" is not as accurate as the laboratory-based α-defensin immunoassay: a systematic review and meta-analysis. Bone Joint J 2018. https://doi.org/10.1302/0301-620X.100B1.BJJ-2017-0630.R1.
7. Kendoff D, GT. One stage exchange arthroplasty: the devil is in the detail. J Bone Jt Surg 2012;1–6.
8. Gehrke T, Lausmann C, Citak M, et al. The accuracy of the alpha defensin lateral flow device for diagnosis of periprosthetic joint infection. J Bone Joint Surg Am 2018;100(1):42–8.
9. Bonanzinga T, Zahar A, Dütsch M, et al. How reliable is the alpha-defensin immunoassay test for diagnosing periprosthetic joint infection? a prospective study. Clin Orthop Relat Res 2017;475(2):408–15.
10. Deirmengian C, Kardos K, Kilmartin P, et al. The alpha-defensin test for periprosthetic joint infection responds to a wide spectrum of organisms. Clin Orthop Relat Res 2015;473(7):2229–35.
11. Berger P, Van Cauter M, Driesen R, et al. Diagnosis of prosthetic joint infection with alpha-defensin using a lateral flow device: a multicentre study. Bone Joint J 2017;99-B(9):1176–82.
12. Marson BA, Deshmukh SR, Grindlay DJC, et al. Alpha-defensin and the Synovasure lateral flow device for the diagnosis of prosthetic joint infection: a systematic review and meta-analysis. Bone Joint J 2018. https://doi.org/10.1302/0301-620X.100B6.BJJ-2017-1563.R1.
13. Sigmund IK, Holinka J, Gamper J, et al. Qualitative α-defensin test (Synovasure) for the diagnosis of periprosthetic infection in revision total joint arthroplasty. Bone Joint J 2017;99-B(1):66–72.
14. Li R, Shao H-Y, Hao L-B, et al. Plasma fibrinogen exhibits better performance than plasma D-dimer in the diagnosis of periprosthetic joint infection. J Bone Joint Surg Am 2019;101(7):613–9.
15. Parvizi J, Zmistowski B, Berbari EF, et al. New definition for periprosthetic joint infection: from the Workgroup of the Musculoskeletal Infection Society. Clin Orthop Relat Res 2011;469(11):2992–4.
16. Yi PH, Cross MB, Moric M, et al. The 2013 Frank Stinchfield Award: diagnosis of infection in the early postoperative period after total hip arthroplasty. Clin Orthop Relat Res 2014. https://doi.org/10.1007/s11999-013-3089-1.
17. Suda AJ, Tinelli M, Beisemann ND, et al. Diagnosis of periprosthetic joint infection using alpha-defensin test or multiplex-PCR: ideal diagnostic test still not found. Int Orthop 2017. https://doi.org/10.1007/s00264-017-3412-7.

18. Kasparek MF, Kasparek M, Boettner F, et al. Intraoperative diagnosis of periprosthetic joint infection using a novel alpha-defensin lateral flow assay. J Arthroplasty 2016. https://doi.org/10.1016/j.arth.2016.05.033.
19. La Tourette Prosser B, Taylor D, Dix BA, et al. Method of evaluating effects of antibiotics on bacterial biofilm. Antimicrob Agents Chemother 1987;31(10):1502–6.
20. Ramage G, Tunney MM, Patrick S, et al. Formation of *Propionibacterium acnes* biofilms on orthopaedic biomaterials and their susceptibility to antimicrobials. Biomaterials 2003. https://doi.org/10.1016/S0142-9612(03)00173-X.
21. Costerton JW, Stewart PS, Greenberg EP. Bacterial biofilms: a common cause of persistent infections. Science 1999. https://doi.org/10.1126/science.284.5418.1318.
22. Donlan RM, Costerton JW. Biofilms: survival mechanisms of clinically relevant microorganisms. Clin Microbiol Rev 2002. https://doi.org/10.1128/CMR.15.2.167-193.2002.
23. Tsang STJ, Ting J, Simpson AHRW, et al. Outcomes following debridement, antibiotics and implant retention in the management of periprosthetic infections of the hip: a review of cohort studies. Bone Joint J 2017;99B(11):1458–66.
24. Grammatopoulos G, Bolduc ME, Atkins BL, et al. Functional outcome of debridement, antibiotics and implant retention in periprosthetic joint infection involving the hip. Bone Joint J 2017;99B(5):614–22.
25. Sendi P, Lötscher PO, Kessler B, et al. Debridement and implant retention in the management of hip periprosthetic joint infection outcomes following guided and rapid treatment at a single centre. Bone Joint J 2017. https://doi.org/10.1302/0301-620X.99B3.
26. Buller LT, Sabry FY, Easton RW, et al. The preoperative prediction of success following irrigation and debridement with polyethylene exchange for hip and knee prosthetic joint infections. J Arthroplasty 2012. https://doi.org/10.1016/j.arth.2012.01.003.
27. Kuiper JWP, Vos SJC, Saouti R, et al. Prosthetic joint-associated infections treated with DAIR (debridement, antibiotics, irrigation, and retention): analysis of risk factors and local antibiotic carriers in 91 patients. Acta Orthop 2013;84(4):380–6.
28. Thakrar RR, Horriat S, Kayani B, et al. Indications for a single-stage exchange arthroplasty for chronic prosthetic joint infection. Bone Joint J 2019;101-B(1_Supple_A):19–24.
29. George DA, Haddad FS. One-stage exchange arthroplasty: a surgical technique update. J Arthroplasty 2017;32(9):S59–62.
30. Hansen E, Tetreault M, Zmistowski B, et al. Outcome of one-stage cementless exchange for acute postoperative periprosthetic hip infection. Clin Orthop Relat Res 2013;471(10):3214–22.
31. Kantor GS, Osterkamp JA, Dorr LD, et al. Resection arthroplasty following infected total hip replacement arthroplasty. J Arthroplasty 1986;1(2):83–9. Available at: http://www.ncbi.nlm.nih.gov/pubmed/3559585. Accessed June 16, 2019.
32. Ahmed SS, Haddad FS. Prosthetic joint infection: an epidemic. Bone Joint Res 2019;8(12). https://doi.org/10.1302/2046-3758.812.BJR-2019-0340.

Unicompartmental Knee Arthroplasty

US and Global Perspectives

David A. Crawford, MD[a,*], Keith R. Berend, MD[a],
Emmanuel Thienpont, MD, MBA, PhD[b]

KEYWORDS

• Unicondylar • Unicompartmental • Knee arthroplasty • Global • Survival

KEY POINTS

- With expanded indications, UKA can be considered in young, active, and obese patients.
- UKA has shown to have improved knee range of motion, kinematics, functional recovery, and decreased medical complications compared with TKA.
- UKA has higher rates of revision and decreased survivorship compared with TKA, which may be due to a lower surgeon threshold for revision of a painful UKA than TKA.
- With current implants, there is no significant difference in function or survival between mobile or fixed-bearing implants, nor between cemented and cementless.
- Aseptic loosening is the most common early indication for revision of UKA, whereas arthritic progression is the most common mid- to late-term indication.

INTRODUCTION

Debate continues regarding the optimal surgical treatment for isolated medial compartment osteoarthritis (OA) of the knee. Although high tibial osteotomy is an option, most patients are treated with either a unicompartmental knee arthroplasty (UKA) or total knee arthroplasty (TKA). UKA has been around since the 1950s; however, initial designs were fraught with complications.[1] As component designs and instrumentation have evolved, the survivorship of UKA improved greatly.[2–5] UKA has many advantages over TKA, including improved knee kinematics, range of motions, and functional outcomes.[6–10] Furthermore, medical complications with UKA are significantly less than TKA.[11–13]

US and global use of UKA has varied over the years. In the United States, there was a steady increase in UKA use from 2002 to 2008, after which there has been a decline.[14] Data from the 2018 Australian National Joint Replacement Registry demonstrate that partial knee replacement represented 8.6% of primary knee arthroplasties in 2017, which was down from 16.9% in 2003.[15] A similar incidence of use of UKA in 2017 was reported from the National Joint Registry of England and Wales (NJREW) at 8.9%, which has remained consistent over the past decade.[16] UKA is not performed by all arthroplasty surgeons, and a small percentage of surgeons perform most procedures.[17] Surgeons tend to be pretty rigid on their impression of UKA, with a handful of zealots as well as vocal detractors. This article presents US and global perspective on UKA.

INDICATIONS FOR MEDIAL UNICOMPARTMENTAL KNEE ARTHROPLASTY

The classic restrictive inclusion criteria of Kozinn and Soctt[18] have been greatly expanded with modern research demonstrating successful outcomes with UKA in younger patients,[19] obese patients,[12] patients with patellofemoral

[a] JIS Orthopedics, 7277 Smith's Mill Road, Suite 200, New Albany, OH 43054, USA; [b] Cliniques universitaires Saint Luc, Avenue Hippocrate 10, Brussels 1200, Belgium
* Corresponding author.
E-mail address: crawfordda@joint-surgeons.com

Orthop Clin N Am 51 (2020) 147–159
https://doi.org/10.1016/j.ocl.2019.11.010

disease,[20] and those who are very active.[21] However, proper patient selection is still vital to ensuring a successful outcome with UKA. Medial UKA could be considered in all patients with anteromedial OA (Fig. 1) with correctable deformity (Fig. 2), intact knee ligaments, and preserved knee range of motion with less than 15° flexion contracture.

UKA should be avoided in patients with inflammatory arthropathy and used cautiously in those who have previously undergone a high tibial osteotomy. Patients should have full thickness cartilage loss and/or avascular necrosis, because those with partial thickness loss have inconsistent pain relief and 6 times higher revision rate.[22] Studies have estimated that between 25% and 48% of patients presenting with knee OA are candidates for UKA.[23,24]

UNICOMPARTMENTAL KNEE ARTHROPLASTY VERSUS TOTAL KNEE ARTHROPLASTY: FUNCTION

Although TKA achieves excellent outcomes on a range of measures, there remains a portion of patients who are not completely satisfied with their outcome and suffer continued impaired functional activity[25] and persistent postsurgical pain.[26,27] In a multicenter study, Nam and colleagues[26] reported that, although 90% of patients after TKA had overall satisfaction with the functioning of their knee, only 66% felt that their knee was "normal," with nearly half conveying residual symptoms and functional problems. The persistence of symptoms lends itself for other implant concepts that can improve functional outcomes with a more normal feeling knee.

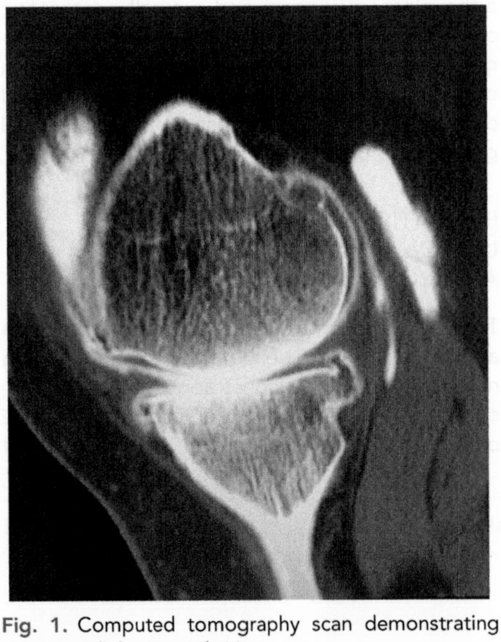

Fig. 1. Computed tomography scan demonstrating anteromedial osteoarthritis.

UKA allows for more closely matched knee kinematics of the native knee due to its cruciate-preserving nature, and its intact contralateral compartment and patellofemoral anatomy.[6–8] This results in a more normal gait, as well as reduced perioperative trauma, greater range of motion, and faster rehabilitation.[9,10] In a series of 23 patients with a UKA in 1 knee and a TKA in the contralateral knee, patients more often reported the UKA as feeling normal.[28] In a 10-year minimum propensity matched analysis of 519 UKA to 519 TKA, Burn and colleagues[29] found that UKA was associated with better Oxford Knee Scores and EQ-5D. UKA was also associated with an increased likelihood of successful outcome and chance of obtaining minimally clinically important improvements in Oxford Knee Scores and EQ-5D.

UNICOMPARTMENTAL KNEE ARTHROPLASTY VERSUS TOTAL KNEE ARTHROPLASTY: PERIOPERATIVE COMPLICATIONS

UKA is a less-invasive procedure than TKA, and as such the risk profiles of these surgeries differ as shown in both US and global research publications. In a 2:1 matched cohort study of obese patients undergoing TKA versus UKA in the United States, the UKA cohort had significantly less blood loss ($P = .004$) as well as a lower infection rate (0% vs 0.5%, $P = .016$). Furthermore, the risk of manipulation was significantly higher in the TKA group (6.5%) compared with the UKA group (0.5%) ($P<.001$).[12] Another US study by Hansen and colleagues[13] compared complications and outcomes between UKA and TKA by analyzing a 5% Medicare sample from 2004 to 2012. Compared with TKA, UKA was found to have significantly lower wound complications, pulmonary embolisms, infection, myocardial infarction, readmission, and death.

In analysis of the NJREW, Liddle and colleagues[30] found that the average length of stay, rate of medical complications, such as thromboembolism, myocardial infarction, stroke, and rate of readmission, were all higher for TKA than for UKA. Furthermore, 30-day and 8-year mortality was lower with UKA than with TKA, at hazard ratios of 0.23 and 0.85. Hunt and colleagues,[31] in an analysis of 467,779 primary knee replacements from the same registry, found that UKA was associated with substantially lower 45-day mortality than

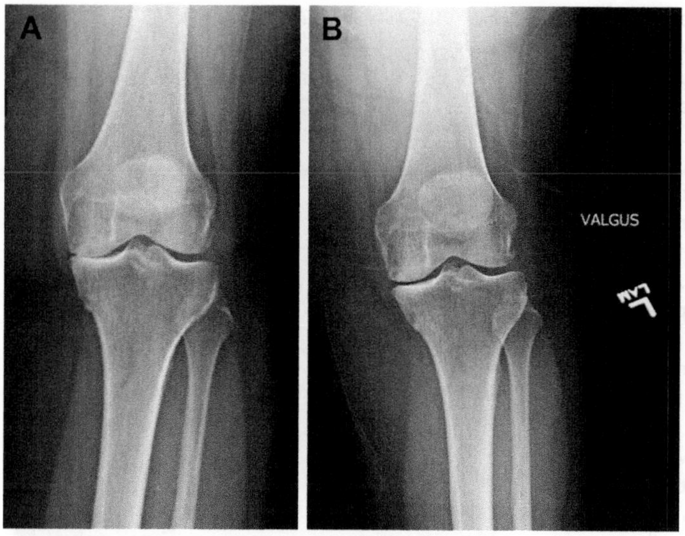

Fig. 2. (*A*) Standing anteroposterior radiograph demonstrating medial joint space loss. (*B*) Valgus stress radiograph demonstrating correctable alignment and preservation of lateral joint space.

TKA, at a hazard ratio 0.32 (*P*<.0005). There is global consensus, by way of studies out of India, England, Canada, and the United States, that UKA has a shorter length of stay and decreased rate of readmission compared with TKA.[13,31–33]

UNICOMPARTMENTAL KNEE ARTHROPLASTY VERSUS TOTAL KNEE ARTHROPLASTY: SURVIVAL

Surgeons must balance the improved function and lower medical complications of UKA with the consistently reported lower survival compared with TKA. For example, the Australian Orthopedic Association National Joint Replacement Registry report found the 10-year survival rates with TKA and UKA in primary OA were 94.4% and 84.7%, respectively.[15] This disparity is also reflected in the NJREW and Swedish Knee Arthroplasty Register annual reports.[16,34] The 15th annual NJR report noted that the 14-year cumulative revision rate for TKA was 6%, whereas that for UKA was 16.9%.[16] In a study evaluating the survivorship of UKA versus TKA over an 8-year period in US Medicare patients, Hansen and colleagues[13] reported the 7-year survivorship of UKA to be 80.9% versus 95.7% for TKA. A systematic review of cumulative data from 6 national registries and clinical studies found that the overall 10-year revision rate for TKA was 6.2% compared with 16.5% for UKA.[35] Liddle and colleagues[36] used propensity matching to adjust for confounding baseline patient demographics to compare 25,334 UKAs and 75,996 TKAs from the NJREW. At 8-year follow-up they found that UKA had worse implant survival in terms of both revision and revision/reoperation than TKA.

Some have suggested that the discrepancy in revision rates between UKA and TKA may be due a lower surgeon threshold to revise a painful UKA. In their analysis of the New Zealand Joint Registry, which includes outcome data, Goodfellow and colleagues[37] found a significantly greater percentage of patients reporting good or excellent results after UKA than TKA and fewer patients reporting poor or fair outcomes. Although both groups had an increase in revision rates with lower outcome scores, patients with UKA had a 6 times greater revision rate than those with TKA for the same score category of Oxford Knee Score of less than 20. Analysis of the Norwegian Arthroplasty Register found that UKA is more than 11 times more likely to be revised for pain than TKA, at a relative risk of 11.3 (*P*<.001).[38]

Ultimately, the choice between UKA and TKA according to available literature is still a choice between function and survivorship.[39] Better preoperative analysis of the patient's disease process leading to arthritis progression,[39] and better understanding of pain after knee arthroplasty[40] could reduce the number of necessary revisions to TKA.

CEMENTED VERSUS CEMENTLESS UNICOMPARTMENTAL KNEE ARTHROPLASTY

Although most UKA designs use cemented fixation,[41] the minimally invasive nature of the procedure can make the insertion and extrusion of cement challenging.[41–43] Cementation errors can lead to failure of fixation and aseptic loosening, which is the leading cause of revisions in UKA.[2,42,44,45] Extruded cement can break off and become a loose body creating third body wear on both the replaced surface as well as normal articular cartilage in the unresurfaced portions of the knee. Cementless UKA could be a way of reducing these failures and achieving more durable long-term fixation. Cementless UKA has consequently become increasingly popular in recent years.[42]

Early data from the Finish Arthroplasty Registry found that the 5-year survival of the cementless Oxford UKA was 92.3% compared with 88.9% for the cemented Oxford UKA.[46] In the 2018 NJREW report, cementless UKA knees had a slightly higher 10-year survival at 87.3% comparted with cemented knees at 85.1%.[16] In a comparison of cemented versus cementless Oxford Partial Knee, Pandit and colleagues[44] found significantly more radiolucencies in the cemented group at 20/30 knees versus 2/27 knees in the cementless ($P < .001$). Furthermore, there were 9 complete radiolucencies in cemented knees, as opposed to none in the cementless group ($P = .01$) [Pandit].[44] These findings were further supported by Kendrick and colleagues,[47] who noted significantly less tibial radiolucencies in cementless UKA compared with cemented UKA at 2 years ($P = .02$).

Some rare complications have been reported for cementless UKA, including early subsidence of the tibial component into a valgus position.[48] A cadaveric study has also suggested that cementless implants may be more susceptible to periprosthetic tibial plateau fracture (PTPF) [Seeger],[49] although this may be due to implantation errors known to dispose toward PTPF, such as a deep posterior cortical cut in the tibia and perforating the posterior cortex perforation during keel preparation.[42] Overall, cementless UKA is a promising technology, although more research is required and cemented fixation remains the gold standard.

FIXED VERSUS MOBILE UNICOMPARTMENTAL KNEE ARTHROPLASTY

Fixed bearing (FB) (Fig. 3) and mobile bearing (MB) (Fig. 4) are the 2 main design concepts in UKA.[50–52] Although the theoretic advantages of MB prostheses over FB designs have made it increasingly popular,[53] advances in polyethene manufacturing have significantly decreased the wear in the FB design.[54] With polyethene wear no longer a major issue with FB designs, the

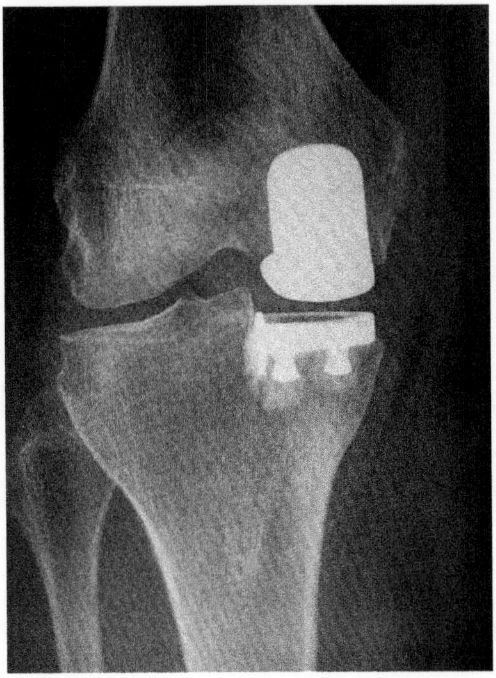

Fig. 3. Radiograph of a fixed-bearing medial UKA.

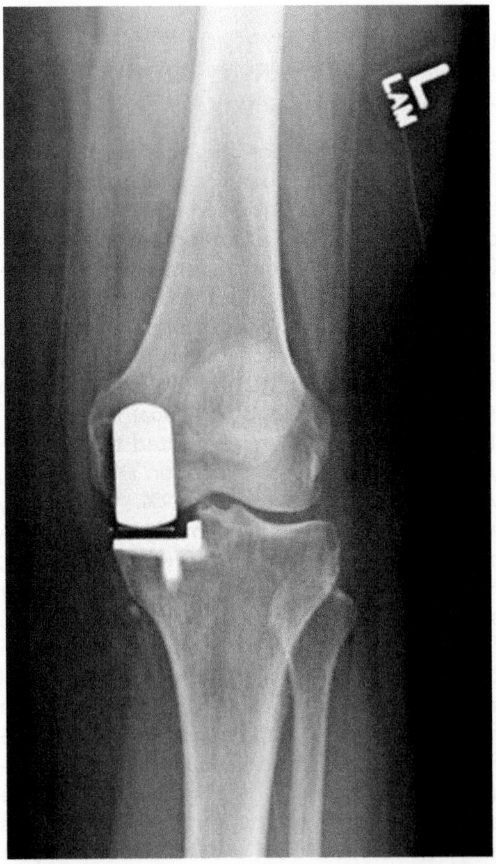

Fig. 4. Radiograph of a mobile-bearing medial UKA.

choice of design for UKA therefore remains controversial.[55]

Several meta-analyses have compared FB with MB designs. Peersman and colleagues[56] reviewed 44 comparative and noncomparative studies, involving 9463 knees. After stratification by age and follow-up time, there were no major differences in survival rates between FB and MB implants. However, the mean time to revision was shorter for MB knees, at 2.5 ± 1.8 years and 6.7 ± 2.5 years, respectively ($P<.001$).[56] In another meta-analysis comparing FB and MB UKA, Cheng and colleagues[53] examined 9 studies, involving 915 knees. They also found no significant differences between the implants in terms of clinical outcome scores, range of motion, or revision rates. Similar to Peersman and colleagues,[56] they found the time to revision was significantly sooner in MB (5.0 vs 6.3 years for FB implants, $P = .016$), with early failures in MB patients due to bearing dislocations; later failures in the FB group were more commonly due to polyethylene wear. Smith and colleagues[52] identified 5 studies comparing FB and MB implants for medial and lateral UKA, involving a total of 165 and 159 knees, respectively. There were no significant differences between the implant types in medical UKA in terms of clinical outcome, and no differences in complication rates.

In summary, any decision between FB and MB designs in UKA is hampered by a lack of robust and well-designed studies, and an evidence base limited to observational studies and small, randomized controlled trials. Nevertheless, it seems that there are no major differences between the 2 implant types.

FAILURE ANALYSIS OF UNICOMPARTMENTAL KNEE ARTHROPLASTY

Aseptic Loosening

The most common cause of early UKA failure is aseptic loosening, representing 28% to 59.2% of all UKA revisions.[2,57–59] This trend has been shown in multiple international registries, including Sweden, England/Wales, Australia, and Italy,[57–59] along with US institutional case series.[60–62] However, the overall incidence of aseptic loosening in large reports is low with rates reported between 1.5% and 2.7% in mid-term follow-up.[57,63] There are specific UKA designs that have much higher reported incidences of aseptic loosening. In a randomized trial between all-polyethylene and metal-backed tibial trays, the all-polyethylene design had a 37% incidence of aseptic loosening.[64] This may be attributed to the more focal tibial loading seen in these designs.[65] Surgeons must be cautious of interpreting all radiolucencies as aseptic loosening, which is discussed below.

Arthritic Progression

With appropriately selected patients and proper surgical technique, the risk of arthritic progression following UKA (Fig. 5) is low. At minimum 10-year follow-up, Emerson and colleagues[66] found an incidence of 4.2% for revision due to lateral progression. Progression of arthritis, however, is the most common reason for mid-term (5–10 year) and long-term (>10 year) failure in UKA.[2] In a meta-analysis Van der List and colleagues[2] showed that 40% of revisions at greater

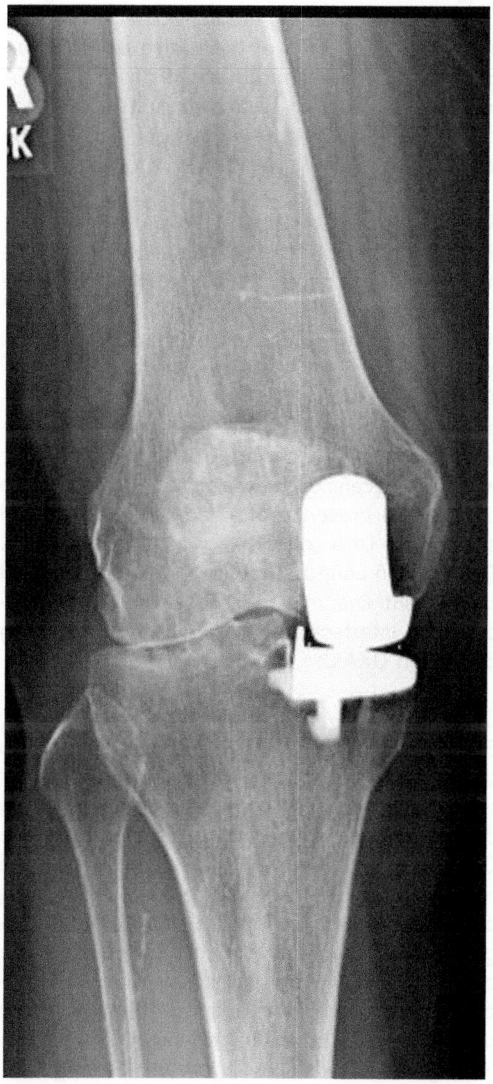

Fig. 5. Radiograph demonstrating lateral arthritic disease progression.

than 10 years were for progression of arthritis. In the Australian Orthopedic Association National Joint Replacement Registry, 43.7% of UKA failures were for disease progression.[15] The NJREW 2018 report noted that 32.3% of UKA revisions were for arthritic progression.[16] The most significant predictor of progression of OA is the arthritic grade of the lateral compartment at the time of surgery.[44] This emphasizes the importance of proper patient selection. If full thickness lateral disease is identified intraoperatively, TKA should be performed instead of UKA.

Pain

Residual medial tibial pain can persist for up to 1-year after UKA. More chronic persistent pain is the cause of 8% of early failures and 10% of late failures after UKA.[2] Even in well-aligned UKA, the proximal medial tibial stress is increased up to 50% of the native bone.[67] Surgeons should be cautious about revising a UKA for unexplained pain because results are significantly worse than when a cause of pain can be identified.[68]

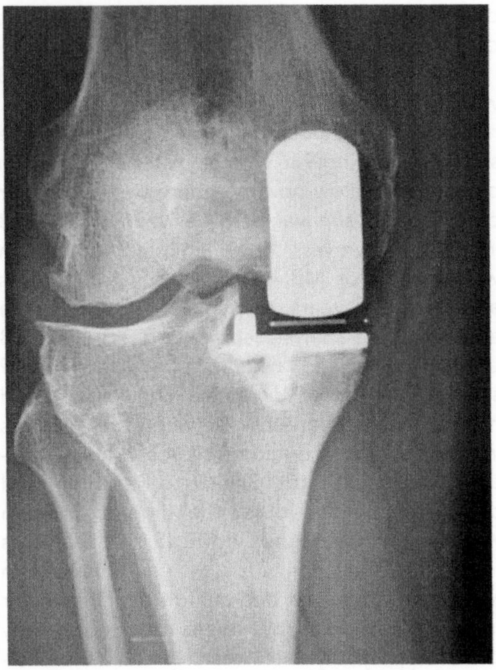

Fig. 6. Radiograph demonstrating physiologic tibial radiolucencies.

Radiolucent Lines

Radiolucencies can be an indication of component loosening; however, "physiologic" tibial radiolucencies (Fig. 6) are well-defined, nonprogressive radiolucencies that can be seen in up to 62% of UKA with the Oxford UKA.[69,70] These physiologic radiolucencies do not correlate with clinical outcome or component failure.[70] Surgeons who are relatively unfamiliar with radiolucencies may attribute medial knee pain to the presence of a radiolucent line, and convert the UKA to a TKA for aseptic loosening. This is often unnecessary, as a fine, well-defined radiolucent line may be present at the bone-cement interface even in well-functioning cemented UKAs.[71]

Other Failure Modes

Bearing dislocation is a unique complication to the MB designs, with incidence reported between 2% and 3%.[37,72] The cause of bearing dislocation is multifactorial, but advances in the Oxford instrumentation have reduced the risk.[73] It is critical to ensure there is no remaining posterior femoral osteophyte at the time of surgery, which can lead to impingement of the bearing resulting in anterior dislocation. If components are properly aligned, bearing often dislocation can be managed by removing any impingement and replacing a new bearing.

Medial tibia collapse (Fig. 7) or fracture is a rare complication after UKA, representing only

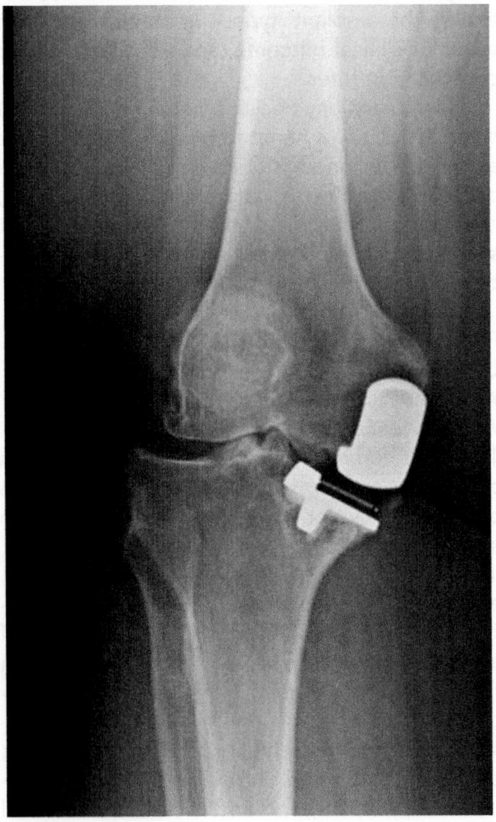

Fig. 7. Radiograph demonstrating medial tibial collapse.

2% of revisions for failed UKA.[2] These fractures can be related to component alignment as well as surgical technique. Coronal alignment in greater than 6° of varus or any valgus alignment significantly increases the load to the proximal medial tibia.[74] Treatment of these fractures can include open reduction internal fixation or revision to a TKA depending on the stability of component and size of the fracture.

Periprosthetic joint infection (PJI) after UKA is quite uncommon, with incidence reported between 0% and 1%.[5,57,75] Furthermore, PJI after UKA is significantly lower than TKA.[76] Unlike in a TKA, however, with a PJI in an UKA there is native cartilage remaining. Therefore, in these cases of chronic PJI after UKA, a 1- or 2-stage revision to a TKA should be performed to remove the damaged native cartilage from the infection.

REVISION OF UNICOMPARTMENTAL KNEE ARTHROPLASTY TO TOTAL KNEE ARTHROPLASTY

Revision of UKA to TKA (Uni to Total) has been stated to be a relatively easy procedure and might offer advantages over revision of primary TKA.[77,78] However, revision of UKA to TKA are typically more challenging than a primary TKA and approximately 50% of patients will have significant bone defects, and stemmed implants and/or augments are required in 33% of cases.[77–81] The mode by which the UKA fails influences the complexity of the revision,[60] but most UKA revisions can be successfully completed using primary components (**Fig. 8**).[82] Revision for tibial collapse poses the highest complexity (**Fig. 9**) as these cases will more frequently require augments and constraint.[60,82]

Using data from the New Zealand Joint Registry from 1999 to 2008, Pearse and colleagues[83] examined 4284 UKAs, of which 236 required revision, and compared those revisions with 34,369 primary TKAs. The authors found that the revision rate for Uni to Total was 4 times higher than that for primary TKA, at rates of 1.97 and 0.48 per 100 component years, respectively ($P<.05$). The mean Oxford Knee Score was also significantly worse in the Uni to Total group than in the primary TKA group, at 30.02 versus 37.16 ($P<.01$).[83] Contrary to these findings, Lombardi and colleagues[78] reported on 184 UKA to TKA revisions. At 6-year minimum follow-up, 4.1% of knees required re-revision. This rate was similar to the institution's revision rate of primary TKA's and much lower than their re-revision rate of failed TKA. The mean Knee Society Clinical score in the UKA to TKA revision group was 83.4.

UNICOMPARTMENTAL KNEE ARTHROPLASTY OUTCOME RELATED TO HOSPITAL AND SURGEON VOLUME

If surgeons choose to perform UKA, this should be a dedicated portion of their practice because surgeon experience influences the risk of failures. Liddle and colleagues[84] found that the revision rate following UKA dropped steeply until the annual volume reached 10 cases and plateaued at 30 cases per year. Furthermore, they found that case load more strongly affected risk of revision in UKA than TKA, indicating that UKA is possibly a more technically demanding surgery. Baker and colleagues[17] suggested that 13 surgeries per year should be the minimum threshold for performing UKA in their registry analysis of 23,400 UKAs from the New Zealand Registry and NJREW. Data from the Norwegian Arthroplasty Register suggest that the risk of UKA revision is lower in hospitals that perform more than 40 procedures a year than in those that carry out less than 10 per year, at a risk ratio adjusted for age, diagnosis, and sex of 0.59 (P = .01). The main reasons for

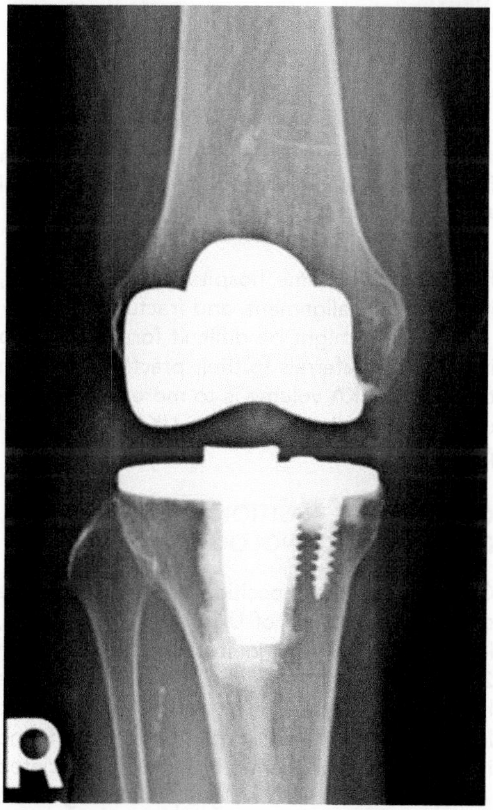

Fig. 8. Postoperative radiograph with primary components after a revision to a TKA from a previous UKA.

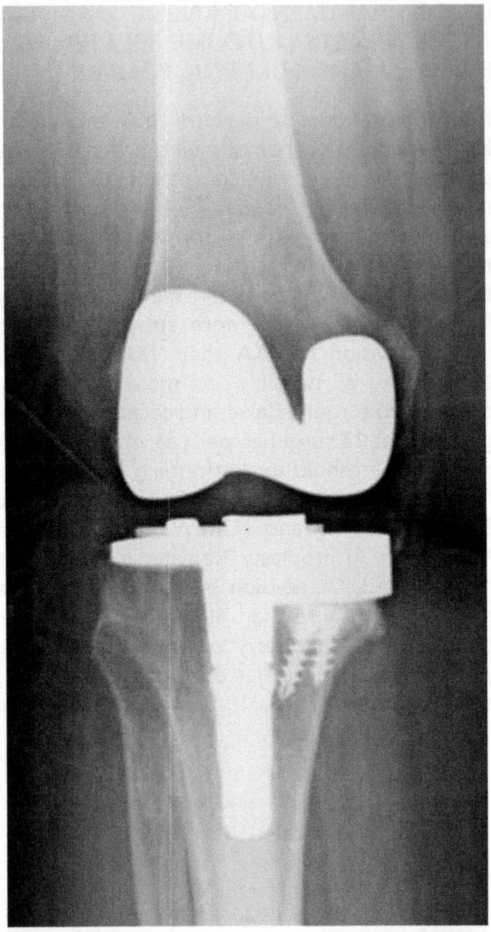

Fig. 9. Postoperative radiograph after revision for a failed UKA due to medial collapse that required a tibial augment and stem.

failure in low-volume hospitals are dislocation, instability, malalignment, and fractures.[85]

Because it might be difficult for surgeons to increase the referrals to their practice, 1 option to increase UKA volume is to more closely evaluate the indications for UKA as noted previously.[36]

COMPONENT POSITIONING AND ENABLING TECHNOLOGY

Correct component positioning is critical to the success and survival of UKA.[74,86] For example, lowering the medial joint space greater than 2 mm compared with the lateral joint space has been associated with more tibial aseptic loosening.[86] In MB designs, studies have found increased rates of bearing dislocation associated with excessive varus or valgus positioning of the tibial component, elevation of the medial joint, inadequate posterior slope, and internal rotation of the tibial component.[87] Excessive varus alignment decreases the contact area of the femoral component on the tibia, thus increasing contact stress and potentially leading to increased wear.[88] Malpositioning errors are more commonly seen in low-volume surgeons[85,89] and during the learning curve of the procedure.[90] Technologies to improve alignment accuracy may therefore benefit UKA even more than they have done for TKA.[91] Current enabling technologies for UKA include patient-specific instruments (PSI), computer navigation and robotic-assisted surgery.

PSI involves the manufacturing of instruments based on computed tomography or MRI to match the individual patient's anatomy. PSI has been shown in some studies to enhance implant alignment,[92,93] which should, theoretically, improve surgical outcomes and reduce the risk of revision. In a sawbones model, PSI technology allowed inexperienced trainee surgeons to have equivalent tibial saw cuts as high-volume experienced surgeons.[94]

Computer navigation can further enhance the accuracy of component positioning with a significant reduction in outliers.[95–98] Suda and colleagues[95] found 100% accuracy within 3° of target alignment with the use of an accelerometer-based portable navigation system, compared with 76.5% coronal and 88.2% sagittal accuracy with conventional instruments. At 5-year minimum follow-up, Chowdhry and colleagues[99] reported a 97.6% survival rate of 252 UKA performed with computer navigation. This survival rate rivals that of TKA.

Robotic technology has been at the forefront of debate in arthroplasty for the past few years. One challenge with interpreting the literature on robotic-assisted UKA is that many of the studies are funded by industry with design surgeons writing the articles.[100] Although there is little argument whether robotics improves component positioning,[92,101–103] the question remains whether this technology improves patient outcomes to justify the cost. As discussed throughout this paper, component positioning is likely more critical to the survival of UKA compared with TKA, and thus this procedure may benefit more greatly from the increased accuracy. With robotics, the surgeon receives continuous, real-time feedback on knee kinematics, range of motion, and implant placement during the procedure with extremely accurate bony resection. In a matched prospective cohort study of robotic assisted versus conventional instrumentation, Kayani and colleagues[104] found that the robotic-arm assisted group had significantly reduced postoperative pain, decreased opiate requirements, shorter time to straight leg raise, decreased therapy sessions, and reduced hospital stay. These early clinical improvements may be related to decreased periarticular soft tissue damage from confines of the stereotactic boundaries with robotic-assisted UKA. At present, however, there have been no studies to show that robotic-assisted improves UKA mid- to long-term UKA survivorship.[103,105] However, robotic technology offers lower-volume surgeons to achieve high levels of accuracy with implant positioning.

DISCLOSURES

Dr K.R. Berend is a paid consultant for Zimmer Biomet, has minority interest in SPR Therapeutics, Elutibone, Joint Development Corporation. Dr E. Thienpont is a paid consultant for ConvaTec, KCI, Lima, Medacta, and Zimmer Biomet, and receives royalties from Zimmer Biomet.

REFERENCES

1. Kurtz SM. The origins and adaptations of UHMWPE for knee replacement, biomaterials handbook. New York: Marcel Dekker; 1995. Chapter 7.
2. Van der List JP, McDonald LS, Pearle AD. Systematic review of medial versus lateral survivorship in unicompartmental knee arthroplasty. Knee 2015; 22(6):454–60.
3. Svard UC, Price AJ. Oxford medial unicompartmental knee arthroplasty. A survival analysis of an independent series. J Bone Joint Surg Br 2001;83(2):191–4.
4. Murray DW, Goodfellow JW, O'Connor JJ. The Oxford medial unicompartmental arthroplasty: a ten-year survival study. J Bone Joint Surg Br 1998;80(6):983–9.
5. Berger RA, Meneghini RM, Jacobs JJ, et al. Results of unicompartmental knee arthroplasty at a minimum of ten years of follow-up. J Bone Joint Surg Am 2005;87(5):999–1006.
6. Akizuki S, Mueller JK, Horiuchi H, et al. In vivo determination of kinematics for subjects having a Zimmer unicompartmental high flex knee system. J Arthroplasty 2009;24:963–71.
7. Heyse TJ, El-Zayat BF, De Corte R, et al. UKA closely preserves natural knee kinematics in vitro. Knee Surg Sports Traumatol Arthrosc 2014;22:1902–10.
8. Jenny JY, Boeri C. Unicompartmental knee prosthesis implantation with a non-image-based navigation system: rationale, technique, case-control comparative study with a conventional instrumented implantation. Knee Surg Sports Traumatol Arthrosc 2003;11:40–5.
9. Engh GA. Orthopaedic crossfire—can we justify unicondylar arthroplasty as a temporizing procedure? in the affirmative. J Arthroplasty 2002;17:54–5.
10. Robertsson O, Borgquist L, Knutson K, et al. Use of unicompartmental instead of tricompartmental prostheses for unicompartmental arthrosis in the knee is a cost-effective alternative. 15,437 primary tricompartmental prostheses were compared with 10,624 primary medial or lateral unicompartmental prostheses. Acta Orthop Scand 1999;70:170–5.
11. Finkelstein EA, Khavjou OA, Thompson H, et al. Obesity and severe obesity forecasts through 2030. Am J Prev Med 2012;42(6):563–70.
12. Lum ZC, Crawford DA, Lombardi AV Jr, et al. Early comparative outcomes of unicompartmental and total knee arthroplasty in severely obese patients. Knee 2018;25(1):161–6.
13. Hansen EN, Ong KL, Lau E, et al. Unicondylar knee arthroplasty has fewer complications but higher revision rates than total knee arthroplasty in a study of large United States databases. J Arthroplasty 2019;34(8):1617–25.
14. Hansen EN, Ong KL, Lau E, et al. Unicondylar knee arthroplasty in the U.S. patient population: prevalence and epidemiology. Am J Orthop (Belle Mead NJ) 2018;47(12). https://doi.org/10.12788/ajo.2018.0113.
15. Australian Orthopaedic Association National Joint Replacement Registry, annual report. Available at: https://aoanjrr.sahmri.com/.
16. National Joint Registry for England, Wales and Northern Ireland. 15th annual report. Hemel Hempstead (England): NJR; 2018.
17. Baker P, Jameson S, Critchley R, et al. Center and surgeon volume influence the revision rate following unicondylar knee replacement: an analysis of 23,400 medial cemented unicondylar knee replacements. J Bone Joint Surg Am 2013;95(8): 702–9.
18. Kozinn SC, Scott R. Unicondylar knee arthroplasty. J Bone Joint Surg Am 1989;71:145–50.
19. Greco NJ, Lombardi AV Jr, Price AJ, et al. Medial mobile-bearing unicompartmental knee arthroplasty in young patients aged less than or equal to 50 years. J Arthroplasty 2018;33(8):2435–9.
20. Berend KR, Lombardi AV Jr, Morris MJ, et al. Does preoperative patellofemoral joint state affect medial unicompartmental arthroplasty survival? Orthopedics 2011;34(9):e494–6.
21. Crawford DA, Adams JB, Lombardi AV Jr, et al. Activity level does not affect survivorship of unicondylar knee arthroplasty at 5-year minimum follow-up. J Arthroplasty 2019;34(7):1364–8.
22. Maier MW, Kuhs F, Streit MR, et al. Unicompartmental knee arthroplasty in patients with full

versus partial thickness cartilage loss (PTCL): equal in clinical outcome but with higher reoperation rate for patients with PTCL. Arch Orthop Trauma Surg 2015;135(8):1169–75.
23. Shakespeare D, Jeffcote B. Unicondylar arthroplasty of the knee—cheap at half the price? Knee 2003;10:357–61.
24. Willis-Owen CA, Brust K, Alsop H, et al. Unicondylar knee arthroplasty in the UK National Health Service: an analysis of candidacy, outcome and cost efficacy. Knee 2009;16:473–8.
25. Noble PC, Gordon MJ, Weiss JM, et al. Does total knee replacement restore normal knee function? Clin Orthop Relat Res 2005;(431):157–65.
26. Nam D, Nunley RM, Barrack RL. Patient dissatisfaction following total knee replacement: a growing concern? Bone Joint J 2014;96-B:96–100.
27. Nashi N, Hong CC, Krishna L. Residual knee pain and functional outcome following total knee arthroplasty in osteoarthritic patients. Knee Surg Sports Traumatol Arthrosc 2015;23:1841–7.
28. Laurencin CT, Zelicof SB, Scott RD, et al. Unicompartmental versus total knee arthroplasty in the same patient: a comparative study. Clin Orthop Relat Res 1991;273:151–6.
29. Burn E, Sanchez-Santos MT, Pandit HG, et al. Ten-year patient-reported outcomes following total and minimally invasive unicompartmental knee arthroplasty: a propensity score-matched cohort analysis. Knee Surg Sports Traumatol Arthrosc 2018;26(5):1455–64.
30. Liddle AD, Judge A, Pandit H, et al. Adverse outcomes after total and unicompartmental knee replacement in 101 330 matched patients: a study of data from the National Joint Registry for England and Wales. Lancet 2014;18:1437–45.
31. Hunt LP, Ben-Shlomo Y, Clark EM, et al, National Joint Registry for England and Wales. 45-day mortality after 467,779 knee replacements for osteoarthritis from the National Joint Registry for England and Wales: an observational study. Lancet 2014; 384:1429–36.
32. Kulshrestha V, Datta B, Kumar S, et al. Outcome of unicondylar knee arthroplasty vs total knee arthroplasty for early medial compartment arthritis: a randomized study. J Arthroplasty 2017;32(5): 1460–9.
33. Drager J, Hart A, Khalil JA, et al. Shorter hospital stay and lower 30-day readmission after unicondylar knee arthroplasty compared to total knee arthroplasty. J Arthroplasty 2016;31(2):356–61.
34. Swedish knee arthroplasty register-annual report. Available at: http://www.myknee.se/en/.
35. Labek G, Thaler M, Janda W, et al. Revision rates after total joint replacement: cumulative results from worldwide joint register datasets. J Bone Joint Surg Br 2011;93:293–7.
36. Liddle AD, Pandit H, Judge A, et al. Patient-reported outcomes after total and unicompartmental knee arthroplasty: a study of 14 076 matched patients from the National Joint Registry for England and Wales. Bone Joint J 2015;97-B:793–801.
37. Goodfellow JW, O'Connor JJ, Murray DW. A critique of revision rate as an outcome measure: re-interpretation of knee joint registry data. J Bone Joint Surg Br 2010;92:1628–31.
38. Furnes O, Espehaug B, Lie S, et al. Failure mechanisms after unicompartmental and tricompartmental primary knee replacement with cement. J Bone Joint Surg Am 2007;89:519–25.
39. Thienpont E, Baldini A. Unicompartmental knee arthroplasty: function versus survivorship, do we have a clue? Knee 2014;S1:S1–2.
40. Grosu I, Lavand'homme P, Thienpont E. Pain after knee arthroplasty: an unresolved issue. Knee Surg Sports Traumatol Arthrosc 2014;22:1744–58.
41. Akan B, Karaguven D, Guclu B, et al. Cemented versus uncemented Oxford unicompartmental knee arthroplasty: is there a difference? Adv Orthop 2013;2013:245915.
42. Liddle AD, Pandit H, Murray DW, et al. Cementless unicondylar knee arthroplasty. Orthop Clin North Am 2013;44:261–9.
43. Baker P, Jameson S, Deehan D, et al. Mid-term equivalent survival of medial and lateral unicondylar knee replacement: an analysis of data from a National Joint Registry. J Bone Joint Surg Br 2012;94:1641–8.
44. Pandit H, Liddle AD, Kendrick BJ, et al. Improved fixation in cementless unicompartmental knee replacement: five-year results of a randomized controlled trial. J Bone Joint Surg Am 2013;95: 1365–72.
45. Pandit HG, Campi S, Hamilton TW, et al. Five-year experience of cementless Oxford unicompartmental knee replacement. Knee Surg Sports Traumatol Arthrosc 2017;25(3):694–702.
46. Knifsund J, Reito A, Haapakoski J, et al. Short-term survival of cementless Oxford unicondylar knee arthroplasty based on the Finnish Arthroplasty Register. Knee 2019;26(3):768–73.
47. Kendrick BJ, Kaptein BL, Valstar ER, et al. Cemented versus cementless Oxford unicompartmental knee arthroplasty using radiostereometric analysis: a randomised controlled trial. Bone Joint J 2015;97-B:185–91.
48. Liddle AD, Pandit HG, Jenkins C, et al. Valgus subsidence of the tibial component in cementless Oxford unicompartmental knee replacement. Bone Joint J 2014;96-B:345–9.
49. Seeger JB, Haas D, Jäger S, et al. Extended sagittal saw cut significantly reduces fracture load in cementless unicompartmental knee

arthroplasty compared to cemented tibia plateaus: an experimental cadaver study. Knee Surg Sports Traumatol Arthrosc 2012;20(6):1087–91.
50. Bonutti P, Dethmers D. Contemporary unicompartmental knee arthroplasty: fixed vs mobile bearing. J Arthroplasty 2008;23:24–7.
51. Emerson RJ, Hansborough T, Reitman R, et al. Comparison of a mobile with a fixed-bearing unicompartmental knee implant. Clin Orthop Relat Res 2002;404:62–70.
52. Smith T, Hing C, Davies L, et al. Fixed versus mobile bearing unicompartmental knee replacement: a meta-analysis. Orthop Traumatol Surg Res 2009;95:599–605.
53. Cheng M, Chen D, Guo Y, et al. Comparison of fixed- and mobile-bearing total knee arthroplasty with a mean five-year follow-up: a meta-analysis. Exp Ther Med 2013;6(1):45–51.
54. Winnock de Grave P, Barbier J, Luyckx T, et al. Outcomes of a fixed-bearing, medial, cemented unicondylar knee arthroplasty design: survival analysis and functional score of 460 cases. J Arthroplasty 2018;33(9):2792–9.
55. Li M, Yao F, Joss B, et al. Mobile vs. fixed bearing unicondylar knee arthroplasty: a randomized study on short term clinical outcomes and knee kinematics. Knee 2006;13:365–70.
56. Peersman G, Stuyts B, Vandenlangenbergh T, et al. Fixed- versus mobile-bearing UKA: a systematic review and meta-analysis. Knee Surg Sports Traumatol Arthrosc 2015;23(11):3296–305.
57. Bordini B, Stea S, Falcioni S, et al. Unicompartmental knee arthroplasty: 11-year experience from 3929 implants in RIPO register. Knee 2014;21:1275–9.
58. Lewold S, Robertsson O, Knutson K, et al. Revision of unicompartmental knee arthroplasty: outcome in 1,135 cases from the Swedish Knee Arthroplasty study. Acta Orthop Scand 1998;69:469–74.
59. Baker PN, Petheram T, Avery PJ, et al. Revision for unexplained pain following unicompartmental and total knee replacement. J Bone Joint Surg Am 2012;94:e126.
60. Berend KR, George J, Lombardi AV Jr. Unicompartmental knee arthroplasty to total knee arthroplasty conversion: assuring a primary outcome. Orthopedics 2009;32(9):684.
61. Sierra RJ, Kassel CA, Wetters NG, et al. Revision of unicompartmental arthroplasty to total knee arthroplasty: not always a slam dunk! J Arthroplasty 2013;28(8 Suppl):128.
62. Fehring TK, Odum SM, Masonis JL, et al. Early failures in unicondylar arthroplasty. Orthopedics 2010;33(1):11.
63. Bergeson AG, Berend KR, Lombardi AV Jr, et al. Medial mobile bearing unicompartmental knee arthroplasty: early survivorship and analysis of failures in 1000 consecutive cases. J Arthroplasty 2013;28(9 Suppl):172–5.
64. Hutt JR, Farhadnia P, Massé V, et al. A randomised trial of all-polyethylene and metal-backed tibial components in unicompartmental arthroplasty of the knee. Bone Joint J 2015;97-B(6):786–92.
65. Small SR, Berend ME, Ritter MA, et al. A comparison in proximal tibial strain between metal-backed and all-polyethylene anatomic graduated component total knee arthroplasty tibial components. J Arthroplasty 2010;25(5):820–5.
66. Emerson RH, Alnachoukati O, Barrington J, et al. The results of Oxford unicompartmental knee arthroplasty in the United States: a mean ten-year survival analysis. Bone Joint J 2016;98-B(10 Supple B):34–40.
67. Simpson DJ, Price AJ, Gulati A, et al. Elevated proximal tibial strains following unicompartmental knee replacement—a possible cause of pain. Med Eng Phys 2009;31:752–7.
68. Kerens B, Boonen B, Schotanus MG, et al. Revision from unicompartmental to total knee replacement: the clinical outcome depends on reason for revision. Bone Joint J 2013;95-B(9):1204–8.
69. Tibrewal SB, Grant KA, Goodfellow JW. The radiolucent line beneath the tibial components of the Oxford meniscal knee. J Bone Joint Surg Br 1984;66-B:523–8.
70. Voss F, Sheinkop MB, Galante JO, et al. Miller-Galante unicompartmental knee arthroplasty at 2- to 5-year follow-up evaluations. J Arthroplasty 1995;10:764–71.
71. Ecker ML, Lotke PA, Windsor RE, et al. Long-term results after total condylar knee arthroplasty. Significance of radiolucent lines. Clin Orthop Relat Res 1987;(216):151–8.
72. Kim SJ, Postigo R, Koo S, et al. Causes of revision following Oxford phase 3 unicompartmental knee arthroplasty. Knee Surg Sports Traumatol Arthrosc 2014;22:1895–901.
73. Koh IJ, Kim JH, Jang SW, et al. Are the Oxford(®) medial unicompartmental knee arthroplasty new instruments reducing the bearing dislocation risk while improving components relationships? A case control study. Orthop Traumatol Surg Res 2016;102(2):183–7.
74. Innocenti B, Pianigiani S, Ramundo G, et al. Biomechanical effects of different varus and valgus alignments in medial unicompartmental knee arthroplasty. J Arthroplasty 2016;31(12):2685–91.
75. Epinette JA, Brunschweiler B, Mertl P, et al. Unicompartmental knee arthroplasty modes of

failure: wear is not the main reason for failure: a multicentre study of 418 failed knees. Orthop Traumatol Surg Res 2012;98:S124–30.
76. Bolognesi MP, Greiner MA, Attarian DE, et al. Unicompartmental knee arthroplasty and total knee arthroplasty among Medicare beneficiaries, 2000 to 2009. J Bone Joint Surg Am 2013;95(22):e174.
77. Craik JD, El Shafie SA, Singh VK, et al. Revision of unicompartmental knee arthroplasty versus primary total knee arthroplasty. J Arthroplasty 2014; 30(4):592–4.
78. Lombardi AV Jr, Kolich MT, Berend KR, et al. Revision of unicompartmental knee arthroplasty to total knee arthroplasty: is it as good as a primary result? J Arthroplasty 2018;33(7S): S105–8.
79. Barrett WP, Scott RD. Revision of failed unicondylar unicompartmental knee arthroplasty. J Bone Joint Surg Am 1987;69:1328–35.
80. Chou DT, Swamy GN, Lewis JR, et al. Revision of failed unicompartmental knee replacement to total knee replacement. Knee 2012;19:356–9.
81. Wynn Jones H, Chan W, Harrison T, et al. Revision of medial Oxford unicompartmental knee replacement to a total knee replacement: similar to a primary? Knee 2012;19:339–43.
82. Khan Z, Nawaz SZ, Kahane S, et al. Conversion of unicompartmental knee arthroplasty to total knee arthroplasty: the challenges and need for augments. Acta Orthop Belg 2013;79(6): 699–705.
83. Pearse AJ, Hooper GJ, Rothwell A, et al. Survival and functional outcome after revision of a unicompartmental to a total knee replacement: the New Zealand National Joint Registry. J Bone Joint Surg Br 2010;92:508–12.
84. Liddle AD, Pandit H, Judge A, et al. Effect of surgical caseload on revision rate following total and unicompartmental knee replacement. J Bone Joint Surg Am 2016;98(1):1–8.
85. Badawy M, Espehaug B, Indrekvam K, et al. Higher revision risk for unicompartmental knee arthroplasty in low-volume hospitals. Acta Orthop 2014;85:342–7.
86. Chatellard R, Sauleau V, Colmar M, et al. Medial unicompartmental knee arthroplasty: does tibial component position influence clinical outcomes and arthroplasty survival? Orthop Traumatol Surg Res 2013;99:S219–25.
87. Gulati A, Weston-Simons S, Evans D, et al. Radiographic evaluation of factors affecting bearing dislocation in the domed lateral Oxford unicompartmental knee replacement. Knee 2014;21: 1254–7.
88. Diezi C, Wirth S, Meyer DC, et al. Effect of femoral to tibial varus mismatch on the contact area of unicondylar knee prostheses. Knee 2010;17(5):350–5.
89. Mercier N, Wimsey S, Saragaglia D. Long-term clinical results of the Oxford medial unicompartmental knee arthroplasty. Int Orthop 2010;34: 1137–43.
90. Hamilton WG, Ammeen D, Engh CA Jr, et al. Learning curve with minimally invasive unicompartmental knee arthroplasty. J Arthroplasty 2010;25: 735–40.
91. Robertsson O, Knutson K, Lewold S, et al. The routine of surgical management reduces failure after unicompartmental knee arthroplasty. J Bone Joint Surg Br 2001;83:45–9.
92. Bell SW, Stoddard J, Bennett C, et al. Accuracy and early outcomes in medial unicompartmental knee arthroplasty performed using patient specific instrumentation. Knee 2014;21(Suppl 1): S33–6.
93. Demange MK, Von Keudell A, Probst C, et al. Patient-specific implants for lateral unicompartmental knee arthroplasty. Int Orthop 2015;39: 1519–26.
94. Jones GG, Logishetty K, Clarke S, et al. Do patient-specific instruments (PSI) for UKA allow non-expert surgeons to achieve the same saw cut accuracy as expert surgeons? Arch Orthop Trauma Surg 2018;138(11):1601–8.
95. Suda Y, Takayama K, Ishida K, et al. Improved implant alignment accuracy with an accelerometer-based portable navigation system in medial unicompartmental knee arthroplasty. Knee Surg Sports Traumatol Arthrosc 2019. https://doi.org/10.1007/s00167-019-05669-y.
96. Weber P, Crispin A, Schmidutz F, et al. Improved accuracy in computer-assisted unicondylar knee arthroplasty: a meta-analysis. Knee Surg Sports Traumatol Arthrosc 2013;21:2453–61.
97. Nair R, Tripathy G, Deysine GR. Computer navigation systems in unicompartmental knee arthroplasty: a systematic review. Am J Orthop (Belle Mead NJ) 2014;43:256–61.
98. Cobb J, Henckel J, Gomes P, et al. Hands-on robotic unicompartmental knee replacement: a prospective, randomised controlled study of the acrobot system. J Bone Joint Surg Br 2006;88: 188–97.
99. Chowdhry M, Khakha RS, Norris M, et al. Improved survival of computer-assisted unicompartmental knee arthroplasty: 252 cases with a minimum follow-up of 5 years. J Arthroplasty 2017;32(4):1132–6.
100. Cavinatto L, Bronson MJ, Chen DD, et al. Robotic-assisted versus standard unicompartmental knee arthroplasty-evaluation of manuscript conflict of interests, funding, scientific quality and bibliometrics. Int Orthop 2019;43(8):1865–71.
101. Citak M, Suero EM, Citak M, et al. Unicompartmental knee arthroplasty: is robotic technology

more accurate than conventional technique? Knee 2013;20(4):268–71.
102. Lonner JH, John TK, Conditt MA. Robotic arm-assisted UKA improves tibial component alignment: a pilot study. Clin Orthop Relat Res 2010; 468(1):141–6.
103. Batailler C, White N, Ranaldi FM, et al. Improved implant position and lower revision rate with robotic-assisted unicompartmental knee arthroplasty. Knee Surg Sports Traumatol Arthrosc 2019;27(4):1232–40.
104. Kayani B, Konan S, Tahmassebi J, et al. An assessment of early functional rehabilitation and hospital discharge in conventional versus robotic-arm assisted unicompartmental knee arthroplasty: a prospective cohort study. Bone Joint J 2019;101-B(1):24–33.
105. Gilmour A, MacLean AD, Rowe PJ, et al. Robotic-arm-assisted vs conventional unicompartmental knee arthroplasty. The 2-year clinical outcomes of a randomized controlled trial. J Arthroplasty 2018;33(7S):S109–15.

International Collaboration in Total Joint Arthroplasty

A Framework for Establishing Meaningful International Alliances

Elizabeth B. Gausden, MD, MPH*,
Ajay Premkumar, MD, MPH, Mathias P. Bostrom, MD

KEYWORDS

- International orthopedics • Global orthopedics • Total joint arthroplasty in developed world
- TJA in LMIC • Low- and middle-income countries

KEY POINTS

- Problems of total joint arthroplasty (TJA) in low- and middle-income countries (LMICs) include lack of trained surgical personnel and material resources, such as affordable implants, functional imaging equipment, and reliable access to essential laboratory testing and perioperative medications.
- In addition, LMICs often lack systems to provide adequate postsurgical follow-up care, critical for the surveillance and management of postoperative complications after TJA.
- The 3 main strategies for bridging the gap in TJA care between LMICs and high-income countries include (1) short-term surgical trips, (2) local capacity building efforts through the creation of independent TJA centers, and (3) education-based efforts.

INTRODUCTION

Total joint arthroplasty (TJA) is widely considered one of the great medical advancements of the past half-century, consistently allowing patients with severe pain and functional limitations to regain mobility and quality of life.[1] Orthopedics is a discipline deeply rooted in international collaboration. In recent years, advances in TJA have come from all around the globe, and international collaborations have connected surgeons and facilitated education, research, and coordination of patient care. Despite the increase in utilization and progress of TJA in high-income countries (HICs), patients in low- and middle-income countries (LMICs) continue to lack access to TJA.[2] Although approximately half of the world's population lives in LMICs, only 3.5% of all surgical procedures worldwide are performed in developing countries, leading to large patient populations without access to basic surgical interventions, including primary total knee and hip arthroplasty.[3,4]

In HICs, end-stage arthritis of the hip and knee is associated with lower quality of life and losses in workplace productivity. In LMICs, however, lack of access to care may lead arthritis to pose an additional burden by initiating a vicious cycle that ultimately further deepens poverty.[5] Specifically, people in LMICs often have relatively more employment vulnerability, greater earnings instability, and are unlikely to have options for "early retirement" or guaranteed living income programs from their government if they are unable to work. These factors are compounded by the relatively higher proportion of jobs requiring mobility in LMIC.

There are 3 distinct, but potentially synergistic, strategies that have been used in order to

Hospital for Special Surgery, 535 East 70th Street, New York, NY 10021, USA
* Corresponding author.
E-mail address: gausdene@hss.edu

Orthop Clin N Am 51 (2020) 161–168
https://doi.org/10.1016/j.ocl.2019.11.002

bridge gaps in orthopedic surgical delivery between HICs and LMICs. These include short-term surgical "mission" trips, the establishment of surgical care centers to promote local capacity building, and education-based international academic collaborations. In this article, the authors review the challenges, strategies, and current status of international collaboration in TJA.

UNIQUE CHALLENGES TO PROVIDING TOTAL JOINT ARTHROPLASTY IN LOW- AND MIDDLE-INCOME COUNTRIES

Challenges unique to LMICs include a potentially prohibitive cost of care, a severe shortage of arthroplasty-trained surgeons, a lack of a steady supply of implants, as well as several patient-related factors, including a high rate of HIV, malaria, and tuberculosis in many LMICs.

Each year, 81 million individuals worldwide are driven to financial hardship from the direct and indirect costs of surgery, and an additional 3.7 billion are estimated to live at risk for catastrophic health care expenditures from surgery, should they require it.[6,7] Although potentially costly, surgical diseases have been historically overlooked by the global health community, due to a legacy misperception that high cost is associated with likely poor cost-effectiveness. Indeed, several studies have shown that orthopedic surgical interventions are very cost-effective in LMICs and even more so than other widespread public health interventions such as medical treatment of ischemic heart disease or HIV treatment with multidrug antiretroviral therapy.[8–11] These findings highlight the necessity to improve on the cost of surgical care and potentially explore innovative payment models to improve access for TJA in LMICs.

Multiple studies have demonstrated an extreme shortage of trained surgeons in LMICs. As such, the orthopedic surgeons who are available are often inundated with acute trauma care and musculoskeletal infections, and elective cases are infrequently performed.[12–14] Brouillette and colleagues reported that in Ghana there are 24 surgeons compared with 23,956 in the United States and that trauma accounts for 29% of surgeries at the teaching hospital in Ghana, compared with 12% at a teaching hospital in the United States. An essential component in improving access to TJA care in LMICs involves building surgical capacity and specialized arthroplasty training. However, arthroplasty-trained surgeons are alone insufficient. To adequately meet the demand for TJA in LMICs, it is essential to establish a reliable implant supply at a reasonable cost, along with access to essential perioperative medications and implementation of modern sterilization protocols and equipment.

Regarding patient-related risks, there has been concern that performing TJA in LMICs will create too high of a burden on the country's health care system in the form of postoperative complications, including periprosthetic joint infection (PJI). This is particularly of concern because the patient population seeking TJA in LMICs are commonly more medically and surgically complex and even under optimal conditions would have higher complication rates than the patient population in HICs. Alp and colleagues[15] identified a 4.6% incidence of PJI in a study of university hospitals in Turkey, a middle-income country, where these complications created a large economic burden for the institutions. Another difference is the higher rate of deformity and progression of disease of patients presenting for TJA in LMIC. George and colleagues[16] reported that 62% of total knee arthroplasties (TKA) in a registry from Ghana used semiconstrained implants. These investigators attributed this to the high rate of severe valgus deformity that was left untreated due to financial and logistic restraints.

Sheth and colleagues[2] explore the potential pitfalls of TJA in LMIC through a case study of a young Kenyan woman with a severe hip contracture secondary to rheumatoid arthritis who had a total hip arthroplasty (THA) performed by a US surgeon who was visiting on a teaching trip to Tanzania. Although the patient recovered well initially, she ultimately developed tuberculosis and a deep PJI several months after the visiting surgeon departed, and local providers were poorly equipped to treat this serious complication. Through the lens of this devastating example, the investigators explore the logistical and ethical concerns of performing TJA in areas without the infrastructure or capacity to manage potential complications. Other investigators have also highlighted the issue of surgical teams from HIC performing operations in LMICs with limited experience in operating in low-resource settings on patients with pathology that may be distinct from what they are accustomed to treating.[17] Dossche and colleagues[17] reported on a group of Belgian orthopedic surgeons who performed THA in Burkina Faso and encountered unexpected challenges by the high incidence of patients with sickle cell anemia and poor quality of technical equipment that likely led to higher rates of bony complications in their series.

In contrast to the concerning reports of high complication rates, there have also been numerous studies indicating that TJA can safely be performed in LMIC, and specific examples will be discussed in the next section.[18,19] Furthermore, there is an enormous potential for bidirectional transfer of knowledge between sites when international collaborations are constructed with thoughtful foresight.

Broadly, global collaboration in TJA can be separated into (1) short-term surgical trips in the form of humanitarian work, (2) building capacity and surgical infrastructure, and (3) education-based efforts. Notably, these strategies can be used in combination.[20]

Short-Term Surgical Trips

One method of addressing the lack of arthroplasty care in LMIC has been the establishment of TJA "camps" where foreign surgeons visit to provide arthroplasty services intermittently to a region. These short-term trips initially originated with medical missionaries, and now the practice of various orthopedic societies or humanitarian groups sending teams to LMICs for a short period is commonplace. In fact, there are more than 6000 medical missions organized in the United States annually[21] with approximately 200,000 surgeries performed.[22] Within orthopedics, many short-term surgical trips aim to treat the unmet burden of orthopedic trauma in LMIC.[23] However, in recent years, several groups have established recurring short-term trips focusing on TJA.[17,24] The potential pitfalls of TJA-focused trips are similar to those described for any short-term surgical mission and include lack of adequate time for preoperative workup, lack of availability for postoperative follow-up care, confusion secondary to language and/or culture, difficulty in ensuring appropriate surgical consent given language and cultural differences, lack of emergency care infrastructure in the event of an adverse event, and difficulty in documentation for an adequate medical record.[25] Although these trips may provide excellent care for several patients undergoing surgery, prior investigators have noted concerns over whether visiting teams may use culturally insensitive practices or undermine the local population's perception of the local provider's ability to deliver care. Ultimately, important questions remain over how much local providers can replicate what they have observed over a short surgical mission trip, once the visiting team departs, given the systemic constraints that persist impairing care delivery. Certainly, although surgical mission trips can be of enormous value to certain patients who otherwise would have no access to care, such trips are generally poor at promoting sustained local capacity.

Pean and colleagues[26] recently proposed an ethical framework for global orthopedic surgery efforts that can guide local and visiting participants throughout their involvement before, during, and after a visit. Their recommendations include using prescreening of patient cases before the visit, the use of shared decision-making model for surgical and nonsurgical treatment plans while respecting local cultural beliefs and resources, and ensuring appropriate transition of care to host country providers for each patient.

One of these programs, Operation(Op) Walk Boston performs TJA in the Dominican Republic (DR) annually and recently published their outcomes of 81 individuals with an average age of 61 years.[27] Although local surgeons offer TJA in the surrounding areas, this particular program offers TJA to impoverished patients who could otherwise not afford their operation in the country. They found that the average WOMAC pain score improved by more than 50 points. The same group later identified that in their patients, operations on those who had low functional scores preoperatively still achieved significant gains postoperatively, a finding that may be unique to the LMIC setting.[28] Bido and colleagues[29] proposed a framework for evaluating short-term surgical missions based on contextual factors, system management, and sustainability. Unlike many short-term surgical missions, the OpWalk Boston measures their results and collects data from patients measuring their level of disease preoperatively. They also have compared the program's quality against the Blue Cross Blue Shield criteria for designating a Center of Excellence for hip and knee replacement surgery in the United States. Furthermore, one of the missions of the OpWalk program is to provide education to local providers.[30] In this way, short-term surgical trips can become a predecessor to the establishment of an independent TJA center.

Establishing Independent Total Joint Arthroplasty Centers in Low- and Medium-Income Countries

Many of the short-term surgical trips are initiated with the intention of bridging the gap in quality of care and have the ultimate goal of implementing independently functioning arthroplasty centers in LMICs. Despite the obstacles to their success, there are several examples of independently run centers in LMICs that have published their outcomes.

Graham and colleagues[19] presented the results of 127 primary TKA in Malawi, a low-income African country with a gross national income of less than $1005 per capita. The investigators reported 0% perioperative mortality rate and 2.6% overall revision rate at 6 months. The government of Malawi has invested in an arthroplasty registry, which has already revealed substantial differences between their patient population and that of developed countries, namely the younger patient population and the higher incidence of HIV in those undergoing TKA.[31] This has helped direct financial resources and guide quality improvement initiatives.

Another hip registry was recently initiated in Cambodia, where before the initiative patients had to travel internationally for arthroplasty operations. Holt and colleagues[32] reported on a sustainable hip service that developed in 2007 after an orthopedic surgeon from the United States began training local surgeons over the course of a 2-week trip with planned biannual trips. They documented 116 total operations on 95 patients, with an average age of 41 years, with the average preoperative Harris hip score of 61 improving to an average between 81 and 85. They did report failure of one stem design in 4 patients, and that stem, manufactured in India, has since been removed from the market.[32,33] This highlights the risk of using low-cost/low-quality implants and the importance of collection and reporting on patient outcomes and complications in the setting of a developing TJA program in an LMIC.

In 1998, Dr. Ohenaba Boachie-Adjei from the Hospital for Special Surgery founded the Foundation of Orthopedics and Complex Spine (FOCOS) in Accra, Ghana with the mission of providing comprehensive, affordable orthopedic care to the population there.[34] They have completed a total of 2405 surgeries over the past 19 years and established the FOCOS Hospital, a 50-bed specialty facility. Surgeons from around the world donate their time to visit FOCOS and perform surgeries as well as educate local physicians and other health care providers. The group was created to treat spinal deformity but now has expanded and completed more than 100 joint replacements at the FOCOS Hospital with support from industry collaboration.[35] The FOCOS Spine Research Group has published numerous reports of the use of halo gravity traction in patients with severe early onset spinal deformity before surgical intervention with growing rod and guided growth techniques.[36–38]

A similar program was developed in northern Tanzania, with the intent of channeling the conviction at the core of all surgical mission trips into a collaborative solution to build long-term orthopedic surgical capacity in Northern Tanzania and more broadly, East Africa. The program involves the building of an Orthopedic Center of Excellence in Moshi, Tanzania, to be initially populated year-round by international advisors, with the singular focus to build regional orthopedic surgical capacity and transition care to a new workforce of local surgeons and clinical staff, trained at this center. This is a public-private partnership led by the University of Pennsylvania, the Kilimanjaro Christian Medical Center (KCMC), the Tanzanian Health Ministry, and various third-party local and international partners. Notably, KCMC is the tertiary care hospital for 12 million in Northern Tanzania, has one of the largest orthopedic surgical residencies in East Africa, and has resources to provide modern orthopedic treatment to most of its patients. Most patients there are treated for acute trauma definitively with skeletal traction, and currently no arthroplasty cases are performed. This partnership was designed in conjunction with local orthopedic surgeons and includes 26 major academic institutions rotating on short trips, to provide year-round support for the program over the initial 5 years. Partner institutions will not only provide care but also continuity for follow-up, management of complications, research, and enhance a rigorous educational curriculum. At its core, this initiative involves resident education in modern orthopedic techniques and equipment. To achieve this vision, this initiative has partnered with GE Healthcare for hospital infrastructure development along with several other local and international partners for hospital management and the procurement of implants at low cost.[39]

EDUCATION-BASED EFFORTS

Because of some of the aforementioned material and ethical challenges in providing care in LMICs, several international alliances have focused first on education-based efforts. These efforts in large have focused on educating future surgeon leaders, as well as other health care providers and ancillary staff vital to a thriving surgical practice.[20] Meara and colleagues[31] concluded that there is a shortage of 2.2 million surgeons, anesthesiologists, and obstetrician-gynecologists who are needed to provide adequate surgical care globally. Focusing on the dearth of educated providers of orthopedic care as well as administrative support seems to be an appropriate target for bridging gaps in delivery and quality. Furthermore, educational partnerships also obviate certain ethical concerns regarding provision of care by visiting surgeons in resource-poor regions and emphasize bidirectional teaching and symmetric relationships.

The concept of international surgical training collaboration (ISTC) is not new within orthopedics. Orthopedics Overseas (OO) was established in 1958 by members of the Association of Bone and Joint Surgeons[40] with the primary goal of transferring clinical and surgical knowledge to students, clinicians, and faculty in LMICs. One of the achievements of OO was the development of a 4-year orthopedic residency in Uganda in 1995.[40]

Fallah and colleagues[20] described several themes crucial to improving the quality of ISTCs. These include consolidation, communication and collaboration, a system of support, a scholarly approach, and the use of technology. Consolidation refers to the need to have a centralized office where global efforts can be coordinated and focused within and across institutions. Communication and collaboration refers to the dissemination of ISTC findings to the parties and interest groups and the public. The Consortium of Orthopedic Academic Center Traumatologists addresses this problem with a Website that publicizes its member institutions global programs.[41] A system of support refers to the need for funding as well as administrative staff that organizes ISTCs. A scholarly approach implies the need for global surgical efforts to be "professionalized" and the need for minimum standards for ISTCs. Secondarily, there should be greater effort made to study and publish the outcome of ISTCs. The use of technology is fundamental to the success of ISTCs, as information must traverse long distances between centers and withstand the test of time.

The International Society of Orthopedic Centers, Ltd. (ISOC) was established to provide a platform through which orthopedic institutions in the world can exchange ideas and best practices. As of 2019, there are 21 ISOC member centers from 17 centers on 5 continents.[42] ISOC holds biannual meetings and engages in cross-institutional studies, international fellowship programs at ISOC centers, as well as humanitarian trips. In order to join as a member, the institution must demonstrate a minimum case volume and quality, which upholds the "minimum standard" tenet of ISTCs as proposed by Fallah and colleagues.[20]

The Hospital for Special Surgery (HSS) in New York, an orthopedic specialty institution, has several initiatives that facilitate its collaboration with international institutions. The HSS Global Orthopedic Alliance is a network of institutions to which HSS provides consulting, education, mentorship, and professional training. Hospital Alvorada in Brazil and Bumin Hospital Group in South Korea are both part of the HSS Global Orthopedic Alliance and regularly engage with HSS by sending professional staff and trainees between the institutions for knowledge transfer and consulting.[43] Member institutions of this alliance have access to HSS educational materials, including surgical training videos, lectures, and other electronic resources year-round through the online educational platform developed by HSS: HSS e-Academy.

The HSS-China Orthopedic Education Exchange competitively selects orthopedic surgeons from qualified centers in China to participate in a structured observation program at HSS and/or a research fellowship program.[44] Alumni of the HSS-China have access to participate in HSS-China Club Events and meetings annually. HSS faculty members also participate in the annual Chinese Orthopedic Association meeting as well as the annual Chinese Association of Orthopedic Surgeons meeting in order to maintain regular in-person connections with alumni.

Another international initiative designed to foster knowledge and experience sharing is the Open Medical Institute (OMI) Seminar on Bone and Joint Surgery that takes place annually in Salzburg, Austria.[43] This was created in 1993 as a bidirectional knowledge exchange with physicians from the former Eastern bloc countries including the Soviet Union. Currently, the program is thriving and now the OMI-Salzburg selects approximately 40 physicians from Central, Eastern Europe, Central Asia, and the former Soviet Union to participate in the academic seminar. As a measure of its success, nearly half of all physicians in Armenia have participated in the program. One of its core principles is to discourage "brain drain" and has programs in place that encourage physicians to return to their country of origin to improve the care there.

DISCUSSION

Global health has made tremendous progress over the past century; however, access to surgical care including orthopedic care in the world's poorest regions remains a major public health challenge. It is estimated that at least 5 billion people lack access to basic surgical care and that more than one-third of global deaths and one-fourth of the world's disability are from conditions requiring surgical care. In terms of loss of productivity, a lack of basic surgical care is estimated to cost $21 trillion between 2015 and 2030 without major investment.[31] These trends are also reflected in the disparate access to arthroplasty between the world's prosperous and poor regions.

As noted, several initiatives across a broad spectrum of geographies, scope, and intent have demonstrated promise to help bridge this gap. Optimal international alliances are founded on mutual respect and can help promote the dissemination of discoveries and advances in orthopedic care. Pean and colleagues have created an ethical framework for prioritizing surgical capacity building in LMIC; the authors believe there are similar guiding principles for all international collaborations, including those that are mainly education based. These are similar and overlapping to many of the principles and themes also previously described by Fallah and colleagues.[20]

PRINCIPLES OF SUCCESSFUL ORTHOPEDIC INTERNATIONAL ALLIANCES

- Spirit of underlying mutual respect, fostered by collaboration, bidirectional knowledge transfer, and cultural sensitivity regarding medical care and patient expectations
- Understanding local obstacles to optimal care delivery, including limitations in surgical workforce, available equipment and technology, and barriers in access to care
- Shared decision-making in developing a strategy to meet the local challenges in orthopedic care delivery, to establish clear goals for an alliance; when care is being provided, ideally this may be formalized via a needs assessment based on host country data and incorporating host partner input
- A prioritization of local surgical capacity building in resource-poor regions
- If surgical services are being provided in LMICs, a robust evaluation of the bioethics of the alliance is essential; this should include, but is not limited to, reflection of the alliance's impact on the local burden of disease, on how surgical capacity has been improved, and whether efforts provide sustainable solutions to meet challenges as identified by local providers
- Use of regularly planned symposia for the bidirectional flow of information between the collaborative institutions
- Use of technology to facilitate continuous learning and sharing of resources between institutions
- Periodic analysis of the alliance to identify and address best practices and a joint vision for future activities
- Formal debriefing to evaluate whether previously identified goals were met
- Promotion of coauthorship between alliance members for any scholarly endeavors resulting from the alliance

DISCLOSURE

The authors have nothing to disclose.

REFERENCES

1. Bumpass DB, Nunley RM. Assessing the value of a total joint replacement. Curr Rev Musculoskelet Med 2012;5(4):274–82.
2. Sheth NP, Donegan DJ, Foran JR, et al. Global health and orthopaedic surgery-A call for international morbidity and mortality conferences. Int J Surg Case Rep 2015;6C:63–7.
3. Weiser TG, Regenbogen SE, Thompson KD, et al. An estimation of the global volume of surgery: a modelling strategy based on available data. Lancet 2008;372(9633):139–44.
4. Bickler SW, Spiegel D. Improving surgical care in low- and middle-income countries: a pivotal role for the world health organization. World J Surg 2010;34(3):386–90.
5. Mamudu HM, Yang JS, Novotny TE. UN resolution on the prevention and control of non-communicable diseases: an opportunity for global action. Glob Public Health 2011;6(4):347–53.
6. Shrime MG, Dare AJ, Alkire BC, et al. Catastrophic expenditure to pay for surgery worldwide: a modelling study. Lancet Glob Health 2015;3(Suppl 2):S38–44.
7. Farmer PE, Kim JY. Surgery and global health: a view from beyond the OR. World J Surg 2008;32(4):533–6.
8. Chao TE, Sharma K, Mandigo M, et al. Cost-effectiveness of surgery and its policy implications for global health: a systematic review and analysis. Lancet Glob Health 2014;2(6):e334–45.
9. Agarwal-Harding KJ, von Keudell A, Zirkle LG, et al. Understanding and addressing the global need for orthopaedic trauma care. J Bone Joint Surg Am 2016;98(21):1844–53.

10. Gosselin RA, Gialamas G, Atkin DM. Comparing the cost-effectiveness of short orthopedic missions in elective and relief situations in developing countries. World J Surg 2011;35(5):951–5.
11. Chen AT, Pedtke A, Kobs JK, et al. Volunteer orthopedic surgical trips in nicaragua: a cost-effectiveness evaluation. World J Surg 2012; 36(12):2802–8.
12. Rose J, Weiser TG, Hider P, et al. Estimated need for surgery worldwide based on prevalence of diseases: A modelling strategy for the WHO global health estimate. Lancet Glob Health 2015;3(Suppl 2):S13–20.
13. Ozgediz D, Jamison D, Cherian M, et al. The burden of surgical conditions and access to surgical care in low- and middle-income countries. Bull World Health Organ 2008;86(8):646–7.
14. Davey S, Bulat E, Massawe H, et al. The economic burden of non-fatal musculoskeletal injuries in northeastern tanzania. Ann Glob Health 2019; 85(1). https://doi.org/10.5334/aogh.1355.
15. Alp E, Cevahir F, Ersoy S, et al. Incidence and economic burden of prosthetic joint infections in a university hospital: A report from a middle-income country. J Infect Public Health 2016;9(4): 494–8.
16. George A, Ofori-Atta P. Joint replacement surgery in ghana (west africa)-an observational study. Int Orthop 2019;43(5):1041–7.
17. Dossche L, Noyez JF, Ouedraogo W, et al. Establishment of a hip replacement project in a district hospital in burkina faso: analysis of technical problems and peri-operative complications. Bone Joint J 2014;96-B(2):177–80.
18. Lisenda L, Mokete L, Mkubwa J, et al. Inpatient mortality after elective primary total hip and knee joint arthroplasty in botswana. Int Orthop 2016; 40(12):2453–8.
19. Graham SM, Moffat C, Lubega N, et al. Total knee arthroplasty in a low-income country: Short-term outcomes from a national joint registry. JB JS Open Access 2018;3(1):e0029.
20. Fallah PN, Bernstein M. Unifying a fragmented effort: a qualitative framework for improving international surgical teaching collaborations. Glob Health 2017;13(1):70.
21. Maki J, Qualls M, White B, et al. Health impact assessment and short-term medical missions: a methods study to evaluate quality of care. BMC Health Serv Res 2008;8:121.
22. Sykes KJ. Short-term medical service trips: a systematic review of the evidence. Am J Public Health 2014;104(7):e38–48.
23. Torchia MT, Schroder LK, Hill BW, et al. A patient follow-up program for short-term surgical mission trips to a developing country. J Bone Joint Surg Am 2016;98(3):226–32.
24. Bido J, Singer SJ, Diez Portela D, et al. Sustainability assessment of a short-term international medical mission. J Bone Joint Surg Am 2015;97(11):944–9.
25. Johnston PF, Kunac A, Gyakobo M, et al. Short-term surgical missions in resource-limited environments: Five years of early surgical outcomes. Am J Surg 2019;217(1):7–11.
26. Pean CA, Premkumar A, Pean MA, et al. Global orthopaedic surgery: an ethical framework to prioritize surgical capacity building in low and middle-income countries. J Bone Joint Surg Am 2019;101(13):e64.
27. Niu NN, Collins JE, Thornhill TS, et al. Pre-operative status and quality of life following total joint replacement in a developing country: a prospective pilot study. Open Orthop J 2011;5:307–14.
28. Dempsey KE, Ghazinouri R, Diez D, et al. Enhancing the quality of international orthopedic medical mission trips using the blue distinction criteria for knee and hip replacement centers. BMC Musculoskelet Disord 2013;14:275.
29. Bido J, Ghazinouri R, Collins JE, et al. A conceptual model for the evaluation of surgical missions. J Bone Joint Surg Am 2018;100(6):e35.
30. Dossche L, Noyez JF. Letter regarding "developing a sustainable hip service in cambodia", by holt JA et al. Hip Int 2016;26(5):e43.
31. Meara JG, Leather AJ, Hagander L, et al. Global surgery 2030: evidence and solutions for achieving health, welfare, and economic development. Lancet 2015;386(9993):569–624.
32. Holt JA, Aird JJ, Gollogly JG, et al. Developing a sustainable hip service in cambodia. Hip Int 2014; 24(5):480–4.
33. Aird JJ, Gollogly JG, Ngiep OC. Author's reply: developing a sustainable hip service in cambodia. Hip Int 2017;27(1):e1.
34. Verma K, Slattery CA, Boachie-Adjei O. What's important: Surgeon volunteerism: Experiences with FOCOS in ghana. J Bone Joint Surg Am 2019;101(9):854–5.
35. Joint Replacement. Foundation of orthopaedics and complex spine. Available at: https://www.orthofocos.org/what-we-do/joint-replacement. Accessed September 27, 2019.
36. Iyer S, Duah HO, Wulff I, et al. The use of halo gravity traction in the treatment of severe early onset spinal deformity. Spine (Phila Pa 1976) 2019; 44(14):E841–5.
37. Iyer S, Boachie-Adjei O, Duah HO, et al. Halo gravity traction can mitigate preoperative risk factors and early surgical complications in complex spine deformity. Spine (Phila Pa 1976) 2019;44(9):629–36.
38. Boachie-Adjei O, Yagi M, Sacramento-Dominguez C, et al. Surgical risk stratification based on preoperative risk factors in severe pediatric spinal deformity surgery. Spine Deform 2014; 2(5):340–9.

39. Sheth NP, Hardaker WM, Zakielarz KS, et al. Developing sustainable orthopaedic care in northern tanzania: an international collaboration. J Orthop Trauma 2018;32(Suppl 7):S25–8.
40. Coughlin RR, Kelly NA, Berry W. Nongovernmental organizations in musculoskeletal care: Orthopaedics overseas. Clin Orthop Relat Res 2008;466(10):2438–42.
41. Miclau T, MacKechnie MC, Shearer DW, COACT group. Consortium of orthopaedic academic traumatologists: a model for collaboration in orthopaedic surgery. J Orthop Trauma 2018; 32(Suppl 7):S3–7.
42. About Us "ISOC". Available at: https://www.isocweb.org/about-us/. Accessed September, 2019.
43. HSS global: transforming care through innovation. Available at: https://www.hss.edu/global.asp. Accessed September 27, 2019.
44. HSS-China orthopaedic education exchange. Available at: https://www.hss.edu/hss-china-exchange.asp. Accessed September 27, 2019.

Global Perspectives on Arthroplasty of Hip and Knee Joints

Mohammad S. Abdelaal, MD[a,*], Camilo Restrepo, MD[a], Peter F. Sharkey, MD[b]

KEYWORDS

• Joint arthroplasty • Total hip • Total knee • International perspectives • National registers
• Global burden of arthroplasty

KEY POINTS

- The increased incidence of joint arthroplasty procedures is a universal phenomenon.
- There is a broad variation in utilization trends of hip and knee arthroplasty in different countries across the globe, related to economic and social differences.
- Comparing reports of different national registers is crucial to determine variations in practices and to identify prospective topics for future analysis.
- Reported outcomes, demographics, procedure volumes, and implant utilization are suited to evaluate the international trends of total hip and knee replacement procedures.

INTRODUCTION

Total knee arthroplasty [TKA] and total hip arthroplasty [THA] currently are considered the international gold standard of treatment of refractory symptomatic degenerative and rheumatologic diseases of the knee and hip joints. Hip and knee osteoarthritis (OA) is one of the leading causes of global disability.[1] The 2010 Global Burden of Disease Study reported that the burden of musculoskeletal disorders is much larger than estimated in previous assessments and accounts for 6.8% of disability-adjusted life years worldwide.[2] An estimated 10% to 15% of all adults aged over 60 have some degree of OA, with prevalence higher among women than men. With the aging of the population and increase in obesity throughout the world, it is anticipated that the burden of OA will become a major problem for health systems globally.[1,2]

Although primary and revision total joint replacement surgeries are widely recognized as highly cost-effective procedures, few studies have compared the international pattern of utilization of joint arthroplasty. A large variation of implantation rates, indications and types of prostheses used for arthroplasty exists and is related to economic and social differences across various nations all over the globe. The utilization trend for different types of joint arthroplasty can be determined based on data published by various national and regional joint arthroplasty registers (discussed later) in addition to manufacturers' reports.[3,4]

The establishment of national joint registers has improved the knowledge and the quality of data related to joint implantation. Comparing reports of different national registers is crucial to determining potential variations in practices among surgeons and arthroplasty centers in those countries and to identify prospective topics for future analysis. The usefulness of register data as sources of epidemiologic and demographic information related to arthroplasty has been demonstrated. Data from several well

[a] Department of Orthopedic Surgery, Rothman Institute at Thomas Jefferson University, 125 South 9th Street, Suite 1000, Philadelphia, PA 19107, USA; [b] Sidney Kimmel Medical College, Rothman Institute at Thomas Jefferson University, 125 South 9th Street, Suite 1000, Philadelphia, PA 19107, USA
* Corresponding author.
E-mail address: MOHAMMAD.ABDELAAL@ROTHMANORTHO.COM

Orthop Clin N Am 51 (2020) 169–176
https://doi.org/10.1016/j.ocl.2019.11.003
0030-5898/20/

established registers were used in this investigation to explore the different perspectives of the utilization of hip and knee arthroplasty and component choices across the world.[5,6]

Data were extracted from the most recent annual reports of the following arthroplasty registers: American Joint Replacement Register (AJRR), 2018; Canadian Joint Replacement Register (2017–2018); Australian Orthopaedic Association National Joint Replacement Register (AOANJRR), 2018; New Zealand Joint Register, 2018; the National Joint Register for England, Wales, Northern Ireland and Isle of Man, 2018; Swiss National Joint Register (2012–2016); Norwegian Arthroplasty Register, 2014–2016; Japan Arthroplasty Register annual reports (2013–2016); and both the Swedish Hip Arthroplasty Register, 2018, and Swedish Knee Arthroplasty Register, 2018. Although the AJRR reports only 25% to 30% of all total joint arthroplasty procedures performed in the United States, which is far less than reporting rate in other registers, the AJRR is considered the largest total hip and knee arthroplasty register in the world, with approximately 280,000 procedures reported annually.[7–18]

Data from these registers reported outcomes, demographics, and volumes of total hip and knee replacement through 2017. Based on the data size and representativeness, data from these registers are well suited for evaluating the trends of primary and revision total joints replacement. Because the date of creation for each database as well as the data collection mechanism may vary by country, however, the same time period of arthroplasty data was not always available. In addition, data from manufacturer reports reveal information about procedure, volumes, and implant utilization in 5 European countries (United Kingdom, France, Spain, Germany, and Italy).[4]

Trends of hip and knee arthroplasty utilization across countries can be compared regarding certain topics. For the hip joint, these topics include volume of hip arthroplasty procedures, patient characteristics (eg, age and sex), type of femoral and acetabular fixation utilized for primary THA, surgical approach utilized for primary THA, bearing surface type for primary THA, usage of different femoral head sizes, use of dual-mobility articulations, hip resurfacing utilization, and THA revision burden. For knee arthroplasty, topics, such as type of fixation of the knee prothesis (cemented, hybrid, or cementless), unicondylar knee arthroplasty utilization, usage of highly cross-linked polyethylene (XLPE), use of posterior-stabilized versus cruciate-retaining implants, mobile bearing implant usage, frequency of patellar resurfacing in primary TKA, utilization of computer navigation, and TKA revision burden, have been reported.

VOLUME OF PROCEDURES

Although the number of hip arthroplasties has increased over the years, it varies among individual countries. A total estimated 630,000 hip replacement procedures were performed in the United States in 2017, which was much higher utilization volumes than most of the world.[4] Many health databases report rates in the meaning of incidence, which equals procedure per 100,000 total population.[8] The available incidence rates show a range of utilization of THA among different countries that varied from 281 hip replacement cases per 100,000 total population in Germany to 106 per 100,000 population in Spain in 2017 (**Figs. 1** and **2**; **Table 1**).

For total knee replacement, the increasing incidence of TKA is a universal phenomenon. However, large utilization ranges exist in the rates of TKA procedures within and among individual countries. In 2017, The United States had the highest incidence rate of TKA worldwide, with 280 procedures per 100,000 total population all ages and an approximate total volume of 911,000 total knee procedures performed in this year. Much lower volumes of TKA were seen in other countries. Procedure volumes and rates of utilization in different countries are illustrated in **Table 1** and in **Figs. 1** and **2**.

PATIENT CHARACTERISTICS

The proportions of male and female patients undergoing total joint replacement vary across different countries; however, women have higher rates for both THA and TKA in most registers. In 2016, Switzerland reported the lowest proportion of women undergoing primary THA at 52% compared with 67.1% of THAs identified in Norway (**Table 2**). TKA data followed a slightly different trend, with the lowest rate for women

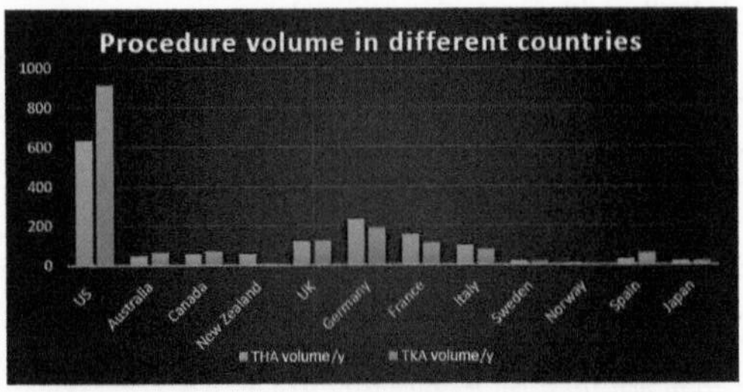

Fig. 1. Annual procedure volumes of THA and TKA reported in thousands in 2017. *Data from* Refs.[4,9–18]

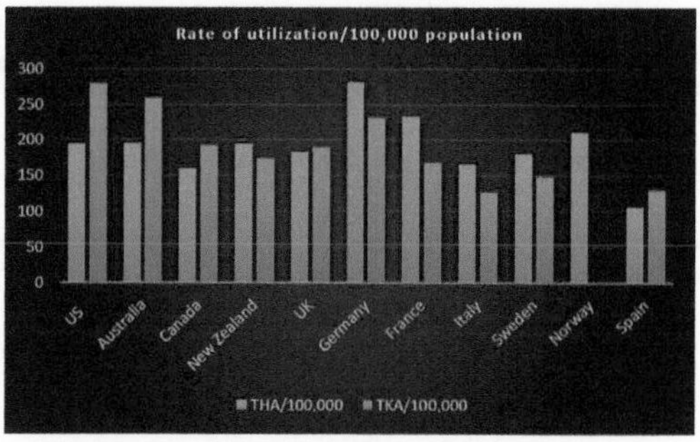

Fig. 2. Rate of utilization of total joint arthroplasty in different countries in 2017 (implants/100,000 total population, all ages). *Data from* Refs.[4,9–18]

undergoing primary TKA occurring in New Zealand, with a rate of 51.6%, whereas the highest proportion was seen in Norway and accounted for 67% (Table 3). In the United States, as documented in the most recent report of the AJRR, women accounted for 56.3% of primary THAs and 60.8% of primary TKAs.

Patient age was similar among most countries, with only small variations among the reported averages. For example, Patients who underwent primary THA in Norway were on average older than patients in other registers, with a mean age of 69 years. In contrast, the youngest average age for primary THA was reported in the United States at 66.6 years. The AJRR also reported the youngest average age for TKA patients, with a mean age of 67 years, whereas the average ages for TKA patients were highest in Germany and in the United Kingdom, at 71 years and 69 years, respectively.

Preoperative diagnoses were similar for primary THAs across most countries. OA was the most common operative diagnosis for primary THA patients in 2016, ranging from 92.2% in the United Kingdom to 76.5% in Norway. The prevalence of rheumatoid arthritis (RA) varied considerably as well, ranging from 0.2% in the United States to 2.6% in Norway. Finally, in 2016, femoral neck fractures accounted for 8.3% of hip arthroplasty procedures recorded in the United States compared with only 3.6% reported in Norway. An exception of the primary diagnosis was seen in Japan, where developmental hip dysplasia and osteonecrosis have been the main indications for prosthetic hip implantation (see Table 2). Preoperative diagnoses for primary TKAs were similar across all registers. OA was the most common diagnosis and, although it accounted for 83.4% of primary TKA patients in Norway, this percentage scaled up to 97.6% of patients in Australia. For RA, it accounted for less than 1% of the TKAs procedures performed in the United States compared with 2.3% of TKAs performed in Norway (see Table 3).

Perspectives of Primary Total Hip Arthroplasty Practice

In terms of the surgical approach, primary THA can be successfully performed using a variety

Table 1
Annual procedure volumes reported in thousands, 2017

Country	Total Hip Arthroplasty, Total Volume (N)[a]	Total Hip Arthroplasty/ 100,000[b]	Total Knee Arthroplasty, Total Volume (N)[a]	Total Knee Arthroplasty/ 100,000[b]
US	630.2	194	911.3	280.4
Australia	47.9	194.7	63.8	259.3
Canada	58.4	160	70.5	193
New Zealand	9.15	194	8.29	174
UK	120.7	182	125.4	190
Germany	232.5	281	191.8	232
France	155.5	233	113.1	169
Italy	100.6	166	77.5	128
Sweden	18 (primaries only)	180	14.9 (primaries only)	149
Norway	10.5	210	—	—
Spain	49.6	106	60.8	130.4

THA and TKA procedures, including primary total, partial, and revision arthroplasties (except for Sweden).
[a] Procedure voulme reported in thousands.
[b] Rate of utilization of THA and TKA in 2017 (implants/100,000 total population, all ages).
Data from Refs.[4,9–18]

Table 2
Total hip arthroplasty patient demographics and preoperative diagnosis

	United States	Australia	New Zealand	United Kingdom	Norway	Sweden	Switzerland
Male, %	43.7	45	46.6	40	32.9	41.2	48
Female, %	56.3	55	53.4	60	67.1	58.8	52
Mean age, y	66.6	67.7	67	68.8	69	69.5	68
OA, %	78.9	88.5	87.1	86.8	76.5	81.1	84.8
RA, %	1	1	1.3	—	1.5	—	5.8
Fracture neck of femur,%	2.4	4.3	4.9	4.7	3.7	9.3	6.1
Osteonecrosis, %	3.1	3.3	3	2.4	2.5	2.3	—

Adapted from Heckmann N, Ihn H, Stefl M, et al. Early Results From the American Joint Replacement Register: A Comparison With Other National Registries. J Arthroplasty 2019;34(7S):S127; with permission.

of surgical exposures; however, the posterior approach, direct lateral approach, and direct anterior approach are by far the most common across the globe (**Fig. 3**). Strong, convincing, high-quality studies comparing the different approaches are lacking at the present time. THA also can be done using the anterolateral approach (also known as Watson-Jones approach) as well as the 2-incision approach. In addition, recently, some surgeons have used the so-called direct superior approach for THA. The recent 3 approaches, however, are far less commonly used.[19] European registers reported different trends in surgical exposure for THA. Although the posterior approach is performed only occasionally (less than 20%) in Switzerland and in Eastern European countries, it is by contrast the most frequently used approach (more than 50%) in Sweden, Finland, Denmark, Norway, the United Kingdom, France, Netherlands, and Italy. Posterior exposure also is the most popular hip arthroplasty approach in United States, Australia, and New Zealand.[20] In comparison, approximately 60% of Canadian surgeons use a lateral hip approach, 34% use a posterior hip approach, and fewer than 5% prefer an anterior approach.[21]

Type of fixation in THA varies among different countries. Cemented fixation is used rarely for primary hip arthroplasty in the United States and only in the later decades of life; however, cement utilization increases significantly with age. In comparison, in 2017, the proportions of femoral stems that were cemented were 62.5% and 36.7% in Sweden and Australia, respectively. In other European countries, the use of cementless fixation of both cup and stem was reported in just 8% of the implants in Lithuania, but 41% in the United Kingdom, 70% in Norway, and in more than 90% of procedures in Italy[20] (**Fig. 4**).

Regarding bearing surface utilization, despite the overall trend of an increase in the usage of ceramic femoral heads, arthroplasty registers

Table 3
Total knee arthroplasty patient demographics and preoperative diagnosis

	United States	Australia	New Zealand	United Kingdom	Norway	Sweden	Switzerland
Men, %	40.2	43.9	48.5	44	36.5	43	39
Women, %	60.8	56.1	51.5	56	63.5	57	61
Mean age, y	67	68.5	68.2	69.4	68.1	68.8	69.2
OA, %	78.9	97.6	94.7	96.1	83.4	97	88
RA, %	1	1.4	2.3	—	2.2	—	1.1
Postfracture OA, %	—	—	1	0.6	2	—	2

Abbreviation: RA, rheumatoid arthritis.

Adapted from Heckmann N, Ihn H, Stefl M, et al. Early Results From the American Joint Replacement Registry: A Comparison With Other National Registries. J Arthroplasty 2019;34(7S):S127; with permission.

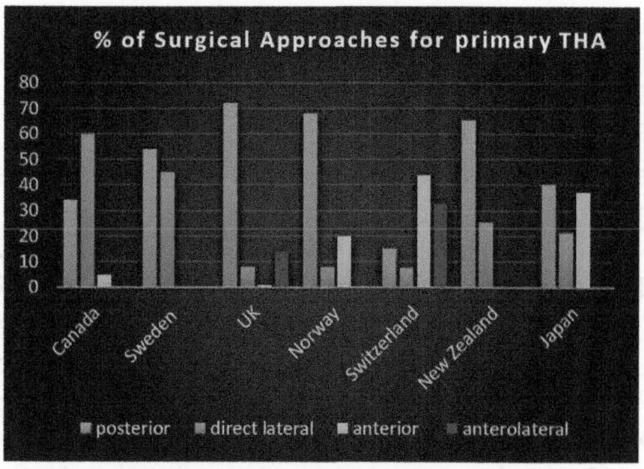

Fig. 3. Trends in surgical approaches in primary THA. *Data from* Refs.[4,9–18]

show that the utilization of metal femoral heads is the most demonstrated practice worldwide.[7] In the United Kingdom, Sweden, Australia, and New Zealand, the most commonly used combination of bearing surfaces was metal/XLPE, whereas the second most popular bearing combination was ceramic/XLPE in the United Kingdom and Sweden, ceramic/ceramic in Australia, and metal/ceramic in New Zealand. The use of a ceramic/polyethylene bearing varied greatly across Europe from less than 5% in Denmark and France to more than 50% in Norway, Switzerland, Netherlands, Germany, and Italy.[20] In Canada, the most common bearing surface combinations were metal on XPLE (80.5%), ceramic on XLPE (13.9%), ceramic on ceramic (3.3%) and metal on non-XLPE (2.3%). In the United States, the use of either XLPE or antioxidant-enhanced (vitamin E–impregnated) polyethylene has accounted for the majority of hip arthroplasty procedures since 2012. The use of conventional ultra-high-molecular-weight polyethylene (UHMWPE) has decreased each year to a negligible percentage; currently, in the United States, American surgeons prefer to use XLPE liners with both ceramic and metal heads; however, when antioxidant or enhanced

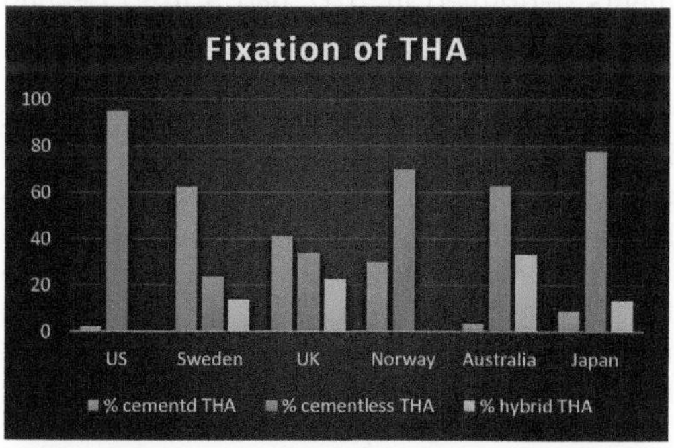

Fig. 4. Trends in cementation technique in THA. *Data from* Refs.[4,9–18]

liners are chosen, ceramic heads are favored in the vast majority (71.4% in 2017) of the time.

The increased stability afforded by larger heads coupled with diminished volumetric wear concerns when these heads are used with XLPE or enhanced polyethylene liners explains their rising popularity. There is a trend toward increasing use of femoral heads greater than 32 mm among all registers that reported femoral head sizes. In the United States, head size 36 mm is most commonly used in primary THA and it was chosen in approximately 58% of cases performed in 2017. Although the use of 32-mm heads has decreased, the utilization of 28-mm or smaller heads has increased likely secondary to the rise in the utilization of dual-mobility acetabular constructs in primary hip arthroplasty. In contrast, head size preferences showed different trends in Sweden, Norway, and New Zealand, where heads with diameter of 32 mm were most often the choice of implant in 2017.

Dual-mobility articulations continue to grow in use likely due to the enhanced hip stability and the reduced risk of dislocation they provide. In the United States, dual-mobility cups were used in approximately 9.7% of all primary hip arthroplasties and more than 28% of revision THA procedures in 2017. This represented a 10% growth rate compared with 2012. In Australia, 1.4% of primary total hip replacement procedures used dual-mobility prostheses. When all diagnoses are included, dual-mobility prostheses have a higher rate of revision compared with other acetabular prostheses in Australia. Likewise, Norway reported a 2.6% utilization rate of dual mobility for primary THA and 17.5% for revision THA.

Hip resurfacing demonstrated a decreased rate of utilization in all countries that reported on this procedure in 2017. The highest rate of resurfacing hip replacement was reported in Australia and represented 2.9% of all hip replacements performed in 2017. Hip resurfacing has declined in the United States to less than 0.5% of the THA procedures, because many surgeons have nearly abandoned metal-on-metal articulations. Hip resurfacing remains highly concentrated among a small number of hospitals and surgeons who perform this operation in the United States.

Finally, constrained acetabular prostheses use was not routinely reported across the various registers. In Australia, although often considered revision components, 0.05% of primary total hip replacement procedures reported using constrained acetabular prostheses. When all diagnoses are included, constrained acetabular prostheses have a higher rate of revision compared with other acetabular prostheses, especially if they are used in patients aged less than 70 years.

THE BURDEN OF HIP ARTHROPLASTY REVISION

This burden was similar among most countries, showing a decrease in revision rates over time. In 2016, the United Kingdom had the lowest revision burden of 8.2%, whereas the Norwegian register reported the highest revision burden at 13.8%. In the United States, there has been a yearly decline in revision burden; the revision burden declined from 13.5% in 2014 to 8.6% in 2016.[7]

The reasons for revisions also were variable across different countries. In Australia, the most common reason for revision varied with time. In the first 5 years, dislocation was the most frequent reason for revision, whereas after 7 years loosening was the predominant reason for revision. In Canada, The 5-year revision risk for total hip replacement was approximately 3% or less. Among women, instability and infection were the primary reasons for revision for those younger than 65 years, and periprosthetic fracture for those 65 and older. Among men, infection was the most common reason for revision across all age groups. In Norway, the most common reason for hip revision in 2017 was loosening of the acetabular component followed by deep infection. In Switzerland, for all revisions of hip arthroplasties, the main causes were aseptic loosening of the femoral and/or acetabular component (41%), infection (18%), periprosthetic fracture (15%), and dislocation (12%).

Perspectives of Primary Total Knee Arthroplasty Practice

The designs and types of primary knee arthroplasty implants among different countries vary slightly. In Australia, when considering all knee arthroplasty procedures, primary partial knee accounts for 7.9%, primary total knee 84%, and revision knee replacement 8.1%. In Canada, 94.8% of primary knee replacements were total knee replacements and 5.2% were partial replacements (86% of which involved the medial compartment).[22]

Unicondylar knee arthroplasty had a range of utilization among different countries, varying from 7.9% in Australia to 14% in Switzerland. In 2016, New Zealand and the United Kingdom reported that almost 1 in 10 knee arthroplasty procedures were unicondylar (9.2%). By contrast, the United States showed the lowest utilization rate of unicondylar knee arthroplasty , which accounted for 3.2% of all primary knee arthroplasties performed in 2017, down from 6.8% in 2012. Patellofemoral arthroplasty was even less performed, accounting for less than 0.5% of primary knee arthroplasty procedures in the United States.

The type of polyethylene used in a primary TKA was reported by 2 registers: the AJRR (US) and AOANJRR (Australia). In Australia, the use of XLPE in primary total knee continued to increase. The proportion of procedure using XLPE increased from 40% in 2012 to 60.9% in 2017. At the same time, conventional polyethylene use declined from 35.2% in 2012 to 25.1% in 2016. In the United States, for primary knee arthroplasty procedures performed from 2012 to 2017, usage rates of conventional polyethylene continued to decline, balanced by a steady increase in the use of antioxidant polyethylene over the same time frame from 2.5% in 2012 to more than 25% by 2017. During revision knee arthroplasty, conventional polyethylene was used in more than 50% of the procedures performed. More than one-third of revision TKA patients, however, received XLPE between 2012 and 2017, and there has been a corresponding increase in the use of antioxidant polyethylene similar to that seen in primary TKA.

Modular and nonmodular tibial implants both were utilized in knee replacement procedures. Modular prostheses have a metal baseplate and tibial insert, which may be fixed or mobile. In 2016, mobile bearing usage ranged from 8.8% in the United Kingdom to 28.4% in New Zealand. In the United States, mobile bearing designs continued to represent a small but relatively constant percentage of primary TKAs (7%–9%) performed between 2012 and 2017. Their use remained higher in revision TKA arthroplasty (19.3% of the cumulative total), where surgeons might perceive benefits to increased rotational freedom, especially when used with increasing constraint. In Canada, 98% of knee replacements performed in 2017 had a fixed bearing tibial insert.

In terms of posterior-stabilized TKA utilization, the United States reported the highest rate of 50% in 2017 compared with other countries that reported utilization rates from 8.2% in Norway to 28.7% in New Zealand. In contrast, other countries (Australia, New Zealand, the United Kingdom, Canada, Norway, and Sweden) reported that cruciate-retaining implants were the predominant type of implant used, ranging from 66.2% in Norway to 91% in Sweden. Other used designs were reported in some registers and included ultracongruent designs, varus/

valgus constrained designs, and rotating hinge implants.

Patellar resurfacing during primary TKA varied markedly across different countries. In the United States, patellar resurfacing remained the predominant practice during TKA, with more than 90% of patients receiving a patellar component each year. In Australia, patellar resurfacing at the time of the primary total knee replacement continues to increase from a low of 41.5% in 2005 to 66.6% in 2017. In comparison to other national registers, patellar resurfacing was performed in 3.2% of primary TKA in Norway and only 2.4% of procedures in Sweden.

In terms of computer navigation, its use was not routinely reported across all registers. In Australia, the proportion of primary total knee replacement procedures inserted with computer navigation has increased from 2.4% in 2003 to 33.5% in 2017.The AOANJRR reported that patients aged less than 65 years had a lower rate of revision when computer navigation was used. In Switzerland, 24% of knee arthroplasties performed in 2017 used either computer-assisted or patient-specific instrumentation.

THE BURDEN OF KNEE ARTHROPLASTY REVISION

The knee arthroplasty revision burden was similar across the registers examined, with most registers showing a decrease in the revision burden over the past several years. In 2016, the United Kingdom had the lowest revision burden of 5.7%, whereas Norway had the highest revision burden of 8.3%.[7] The reason for revision varies among countries. In Australia and Canada, loosening has been the main reason for revision followed by infection, pain, and instability. In comparison, patella problems constituted the main reason for an early revision in Switzerland whereas deep infection was the main reason for revision in New Zealand. In the United States, the main causes of revision were aseptic loosening and infection. Regarding the type of revision, the most commonly performed procedure was replacement of both tibial and femoral components and showed a wide variation from 25% of cases in Australia to 51.4% of revision cases in Canada. In almost all countries, the second most common intervention for revision was polyethylene insert exchange only.

In summary, few studies have broadly compared the trends in international variations related to how primary and revision joint arthroplasties are performed. The reasons for these variations remain poorly understood. As registers around the world continue to grow, future studies should focus on determining why international differences in THA and TKA practices exist and attempt to identify optimal strategies for performing these procedures.

DISCLOSURE

The authors have nothing to disclose.

REFERENCES

1. Singh JA. Epidemiology of knee and hip arthroplasty: a systematic review. Open Orthop J 2011;5:80–5.
2. Cross M, Smith E, Hoy D, et al. The global burden of hip and knee osteoarthritis: estimates from the global burden of disease 2010 study. Ann Rheum Dis 2014;73(7):1323–30.
3. Kurtz S, Ong K, Lau E, et al. International survey of primary and revision total knee replacement. Int Orthop 2011;35:1783–9.
4. US and European Markets for joint arthroplasty products. Medical market and technology report. Meddevicetracker; 2016.
5. Maloney WJ. The role of orthopaedic device registries in improving patient outcomes. J Bone Joint Surg Am 2011;93:2241.
6. Malchau H, Graves SE, Porter M, et al. The next critical role of orthopedic registries. Acta Orthop 2015; 86:3e4.
7. Heckmann N, Ihn H, Stefl M, et al. Early results from the american joint replacement registry: a comparison with other national registries. J Arthroplasty 2019;34(7S):125–34.e1.
8. Pabinger C, Geissler A. Utilization rates of hip arthroplasty in OECD countries. Osteoarthritis Cartilage 2014;22(6):734–41.
9. Australian Orthopaedic Association National Joint Replacement Registry (AOANJRR). Hip, knee & shoulder arthroplasty: 2018 annual report. Adelaide (Australia): AOA; 2018. Available at: https://aoanjrr.sahmri.com/annual-reports-2018.
10. The American Joint Replacement Registry (AJRR), Annual report 2018. Available at: http://www.ajrr.net/publications-data/annual-reports/597-5-2018-annual-report.
11. Canadian Institute for Health Information. Hip and knee replacements in Canada, 2017–2018: Canadian joint replacement registry annual report. Available at: https://www.cihi.ca/sites/default/files/document/cjrr-update-summer-2018-en-web.pdf.
12. The New Zealand Joint Registry Ninteen Year Report January 1999 to December 2017. Available at: https://nzoa.org.nz/system/files/DH8152_NZJR_2018_Report_v6_4Decv18.pdf.

13. The National Joint Registry [NJR] for England, Wales, Northern Ireland and the Isle of Man,15th Annual report 2018. Available at: https://reports.njrcentre.org.uk/downloads.
14. Swedish Hip arthroplasty register, Annual report 2017. Available at: https://registercentrum.blob.core.windows.net/shpr/r/Eng_Arsrapport_2017_Hoftprotes_final-Syx2fJPhMN.pdf.
15. The Swedish Knee Arthroplasty Register – Annual Report 2018. Available at: http://www.myknee.se/en/start/202-annual-report-2018-english-version.
16. Annual Report of the Swiss National Implant Registry, Hip and Knee, SIRIS 2012-2016. Available at: https://www.anq.ch/wp-content/uploads/2018/09/ANQ_Akut_SIRIS_Jahresbericht_2012-16.pdf.
17. The Norwegian Arthroplasty Register NRL, 2018 annual report. Available at: http://nrlweb.ihelse.net/eng/Rapporter/Report2018_english.pdf.
18. The Japan Arthroplasty Register Annual report 2012-2016. The Japanese Society For Replacement Arthroplasty. Available at: https://jsra.info/pdf/2013~2016(JAR2017English version).pdf.
19. Moretti V, Post Z. Surgical approaches for total hip arthroplasty. Indian J Orthop 2017;51(4):368–76.
20. Lübbeke A, Silman AJ, Barea C, et al. Mapping existing hip and knee replacement registries in Europe. Health Policy 2018;122(5):548–57.
21. Petis S, Howard J, Lanting B, et al. Comparing the anterior, posterior and lateral approach: gait analysis in total hip arthroplasty. Can J Surg 2018; 61(1):50–7.
22. Inacio M, Paxton E. Projected increase in total knee arthroplasty in the United States e an alternative projection model. Osteoarthritis Cartilage 2017; 25:1797–803.

Trauma

Impact of North American Institutions on Orthopedic Research in Low- and Middle-Income Countries

Ericka von Kaeppler, BS[a], Claire Donnelley, BS[a], Heather J. Roberts, MD[a], Nathan N. O'Hara, MHA[b], Nae Won, BA, MPH[a], David W. Shearer, MD, MPH[a], Saam Morshed, MD, PhD, MPH[a,*]

KEYWORDS

• Orthopaedics • Research • Developing countries • International cooperation
• Program development • Global health • Musculoskeletal burden • Orthopedic surgery

KEY POINTS

- Low- and middle-income countries (LMIC) face a high burden of musculoskeletal injury and disease.
- To address this burden, there exists an unmet need for locally relevant and sustainable orthopedic research.
- Partnership between high income countries (HIC) and LMIC is mutually beneficial by leveraging LMIC researchers' in-depth understanding of locally relevant needs and HIC researchers' resources and experience.
- Multiple models, each with benefits and challenges, exist for HIC-LMIC partnership including: academic partnerships, large-scale international research consortia, professional society–associated working groups, and NGO partnerships.

INTRODUCTION

Globally, the burden of orthopedic injury and disease outweighs that of human immunodeficiency virus, tuberculosis, and malaria,[1,2] yet remains undersupported by many global health funders and Ministries of Health.[3] Developing the evidence base to guide medical and surgical practice in low- and middle-income countries (LMIC) to address this unmet need demands the advancement of sustainable global orthopedic research. Currently, only 13% of the world's scientists are located in Africa, Latin America, and the Middle East,[4] necessitating partnerships between LMIC and high-income country (HIC) institutions for the improvement of global health.[5] Well-resourced HIC can provide the research skills, experience, and funding necessary to initiate and support research in LMIC. HIC-LMIC partnerships designed around the pillars of mutually beneficial relationships, training and integration of local leaders, and commitment to developing research capacity ensure the lasting sustainability of these research efforts.[6]

Nearly two decades ago, Costello and Zumla called for a move away from a semicolonial model of HIC-lead research in LMIC toward cooperative research partnerships that incorporate four main principles[7]:

[a] Department of Orthopaedic Surgery, University of California San Francisco, 2550 23rd Street, Building 9, 2nd Floor, San Francisco, CA 94110, USA; [b] Department of Orthopaedics, University of Maryland School of Medicine, Suite 300, 110 South Paca Street, Baltimore, MD 21201, USA
* Corresponding author.
E-mail address: saam.morshed@ucsf.edu

Orthop Clin N Am 51 (2020) 177–188
https://doi.org/10.1016/j.ocl.2019.11.004

1. Mutual trust and shared decision making
2. National ownership
3. Emphasis on translating research findings into policy
4. Development of national research capacity

Recently, many of these initial recommendations were echoed in an empirical study that proposed an updated framework for developing sustainable, locally led clinical trial capacity in LMIC. In this report, Franzen and colleagues[8]outlined four key strategies to developing sustainable health research capacity:

1. Fostering proresearch culture
2. Developing local trial leaders and staff
3. Providing a facilitative operational environment
4. Ensuring that trial research has local impact

Leading North American institutions in modern LMIC orthopedic research use the strategies articulated by Costello and coworkers[7] and again by Franzen and coworkers,[8] but their implementation of these strategies has differed. Several implementation models, ranging from one-to-one direct collaboration to large-scale international consortia, have been used by US institutions to promote orthopedic research in LMIC, including academic partnerships, international research consortia, professional society–associated working groups, and nongovernmental organization (NGO)-supported initiatives (**Table 1**). Although not an exhaustive list, this article introduces each aforementioned model, discusses its strengths and weaknesses, and provides examples to illustrate its impact in practice.

ACADEMIC PARTNERSHIPS

The academic partnership model (**Fig. 1**) is a one-to-one relationship in which academicians from an HIC institution partner with academicians from an LMIC institution to exchange knowledge and ideas. The initiation and maintenance of this model depends on previously existing, generally long-term relationships between members of each institution. Often these relationships stem from prior volunteerism, training, or association through professional societies. Many of the mutual benefits experienced by both partners draw on the multidisciplinary nature of the academic triad: clinical care, education, and research. Rather than focusing solely on research, this model works to benefit both partners by meeting a multiplicity of needs, including clinical care and trainee exchanges, and research training and collaboration.

In the academic partnership model, academicians from HIC work to support local LMIC investigators by providing assistance with study design, research training, labor, and funding opportunities.[9] These long-term relationships result in sustained, bidirectional mentorship and knowledge exchange wherein the HIC surgeons supplement career development of LMIC surgeons, and LMIC surgeons deepen their counterparts' expertise in orthopedic disease treatment in low-resource settings.[10]

Although this model has long been used in the United States and elsewhere, it has evolved over time to involve LMIC partners more significantly in all aspects of research efforts. Former iterations have included couriering of biologic samples from LMIC to HIC partners, short-term travel by HIC researchers to LMIC to collect biologic samples, and expatriate staff leading and managing research efforts in LMIC.[7] These types of studies typically do not involve collaboration with LMIC authors, forgoing these academicians' unique insights into locally relevant research questions and the translation of research findings into policy.[7]

In the current academic partnership model, local academic leaders manage research inspired by locally relevant clinical problems with regular correspondence and input from HIC academics. Junior HIC investigators and research fellows may work within the country under the supervision of local academic leaders. Importantly, local individuals are employed as research staff, which lowers costs and builds infrastructure and institutional memory.[7]

One example of the academic partnership model is the Uganda Sustainable Trauma Orthopedic Program (USTOP), a partnership between the University of British Columbia (UBC) Department of Orthopedics and Makerere University (MU), Uganda. This multifaceted partnership emphasizes teaching, clinical care, research, and advocacy toward achieving the overarching objective of reducing human suffering, disability, and poverty caused by traumatic injuries.[11] This partnership was initiated at the invitation of MU surgeons who aimed to reduce the unmet burden of musculoskeletal trauma in Uganda and was supported by seed funding from the Canadian Institutes of Health Research. A core aim of the project is to create a sustainable Ugandan health care system to fully meet the needs of Ugandan trauma patients.[11]

The USTOP effort incorporates clinical training of surgeons, trainees, nurses, physiotherapists, administrators, and other staff[11] via workshops, skills sessions, and trainee exchange programs developed and taught by MU and UBC participants. World Wide Web–based

Table 1
Summary of HIC-LMIC partnership models for research in LMIC

Model	Benefits	Challenges
Academic Description: one-to-one partnership between HIC academic center and LMIC academic center for research, training, and clinical care Structure: one-to-one Examples: USTOP, IGOT-MOI	Encourages proresearch culture Supports academic advancement of HIC and LMIC investigators Rigorously addresses locally relevant research questions	Fragile because of dependence on personal relationships Must navigate institutional bureaucracies Time-intensive development of memorandum of understanding to cover the breadth of clinical, teaching, and research
International Consortium Description: large multicenter collaboration with centralized coordinating center focused on a single research topic in many locations Structure: one-to-many Examples: INORMUS, ACTUAR	Robust because of large number of research sites Far reaching, scalable Diverse investigator skillsets Well-suited to evaluate epidemiologic and economic burden Generalizable results	High organizational management costs Difficulty providing individualized support to LMIC partners Requires preexisting infrastructure from participants
Professional society–associated Description: collaboration of professional societies or society members that promotes academic endeavors in LMIC Structure: many-to-many Examples: COUR, GCIS	Leverages far reaching network of individual investigators from many countries	High demand for collective commitment
NGO Description: philanthropic organization that may support research as part of broader mission to improve orthopedic care in LMIC Structure: variable Example: SIGN, AO Alliance, FOCOS	Well-resourced Innovative, agile, and adaptable to LMIC environment Leverages provision of services or resources Unique legal and political status	Dependence on continued existence and beneficence of NGO

ACTUAR, Asociación de Cirujanos Traumatólogos de las Américas; COUR, children's orthopedics in underserved regions; FOCOS, foundation of orthopedics and complex spine; GICS, global initiative for children's surgery; IGOT, institute for global orthopedics and traumatology; INORMUS, international orthopedic multicenter study in fracture care; MOI, muhimbili orthopedic institute; SIGN, surgical implant generation network; USTOP, Uganda sustainable trauma orthopedic program.

training models are used between on-site sessions. Although not directly contributing to research productivity, clinical teaching activities are important to relationship-building when such knowledge exchange is explicitly requested and can, therefore, indirectly further the research-focused elements of the program.[11]

The USTOP research initiatives, including organizing formal research training activities and prioritizing close collaboration, are key to its mission.[11] For example, USTOP organized and hosted an international clinical research course with attendees from UBC and MU to prepare local research personnel to establish self-sustaining research programs. In addition to ongoing training programs, collaborative research projects, such as economic and clinical studies into best practices for policy and resource allocation, are conducted by Ugandan partners working with Canadian investigators.[11] USTOP research efforts have led to cost-conscious solutions; one such innovation is a drill

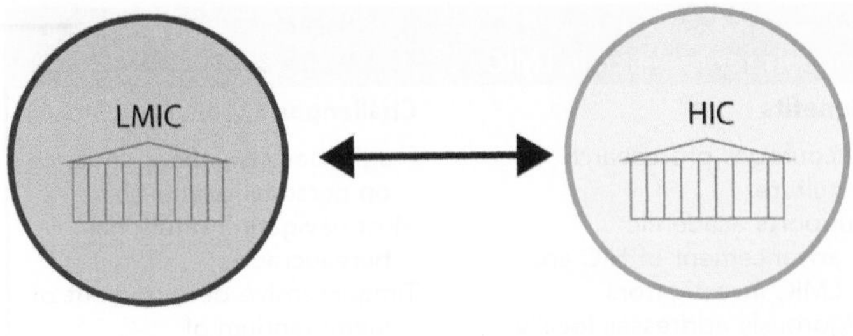

Fig. 1. Academic partnership. Schematic representation of the one-to-one relationship between HIC (*blue*) and LMIC (*purple*) institutions, which is characteristic of many academic research partnerships. IGOT, Institute for Global Orthopedics and Traumatology; MOI, Muhimbili Orthopedic Institute; USTOP, Uganda Sustainable Trauma Orthopedic Program.

cover system that allows nonsterile hardware drills to be used safely for surgical bone drilling.[12] The USTOP partnership has published multiple prospective studies on locally relevant topics[13–15] and an ongoing randomized controlled trial comparing external fixation with intramedullary nailing in the treatment of open tibial fractures.[16] The resulting publications have included Ugandan and Canadian authors, an indicator of reciprocal partnership.[11,13–16]

The partnership between the Institute for Global Orthopedics and Traumatology (IGOT) at the University of California San Francisco (UCSF) and the Muhimbili Orthopedic Institute (MOI) in Dar es Salam, Tanzania is another successful example of the academic partnership model.[17] The IGOT-MOI partnership is centered around the core values of equity, collaboration, and scholarship, and leverages elements of the academic triad outlined in their three pillars: (1) education, (2) research, and (3) leadership. The Global Research Initiative (GRI) aims to build clinical research capacity and facilitate high-quality research that addresses locally relevant clinical questions. GRI activities range from minimally intensive collaboration on research proposals to more intensive collaboration on large-scale clinical research projects including: study design, funding, personnel, and data analysis. By partnering with teaching hospitals in LMIC, IGOT's efforts establish local research leaders and address locally relevant research questions.

GRI efforts resulting from the collaboration between IGOT and local partners have produced high-quality research projects, including numerous prospective observational and randomized controlled trials and surveys and cross-sectional studies, and over time these partnerships have led to increasing independence in LMIC research.[17] The results of GRI initiatives better define the unmet burden of orthopedic trauma in LMIC, ultimately paving the way to a higher standard of care.[17]

Beyond supporting research in LMIC, the GRI contributes to global research efforts through the training of LMIC and junior HIC investigators. Every year, IGOT awards a 1-year research fellowship to a senior medical student, contributing to the pipeline of global health–oriented future orthopedic leaders who, along with their LMIC peers, are critical to the successful continuation of IGOT's overarching mission. IGOT is reciprocally involved in the training of LMIC researchers, supporting junior investigators and doctoral candidates. LMIC trainees have completed observerships at UCSF along with attending and hosting surgical education courses. Former LMIC trainees have published in peer-reviewed journals and are now partners for current IGOT projects.[9,18–27]

An extension of the academic partnership model includes the efforts of individual investigators who operate independent of a formal group. Often these relationships[28–40] stem from existing academic partnerships centered around clinical care, education, and research. These investigators may be expatriates working within an HIC academic system, but living in the LMIC during the time of the partnership. Full immersion in the local context, ability to communicate directly with research staff in-country, and constant in-person presence in the LMIC yields quality research and educational objectives. The benefit of the experienced expatriate's ultimately limited-time stay may come at the expense of not building lasting infrastructure,[7] but there are several outstanding examples of adjustments to address this shortcoming.[41–59]

Through leveraging the multipronged academic mission, academic partnerships have trained LMIC and HIC future global orthopedic researchers, produced locally relevant and high-quality clinical research, and supported sustainable long-term LMIC research programs. This model has been similarly successful in nonsurgical fields: the National Institutes of Health–funded Fogarty International Clinical Research Scholars and Fellows Program supports year-long mentored global health research training for HIC and junior LMIC investigators. This model, in which trainees collect data, prepare articles, and apply for grants under the guidance of experienced senior investigators, can serve as a roadmap for the broader implementation of academic partnership models in orthopedics.

An inevitable characteristic of the academic partnership model is the scope of inferences from its research results, which may not generalize beyond the confines of the study population. Additionally, this model is fragile: in the event of changes to the relationships between key individuals at the partner sites, continued research efforts can be threatened.

INTERNATIONAL RESEARCH CONSORTIA

In the international research consortium model (Fig. 2), a single institution or collaborative brings together investigators from HIC institutions around the world to work on a common goal. These consortia are often built around one overarching study goal to be completed by the cumulative research efforts in many LMIC sites around the world. Often the resources, institutional knowledge, and experience provided by these consortia enable large-scale studies that can broadly inform an epidemiologic understanding of orthopedic diseases and their treatment.

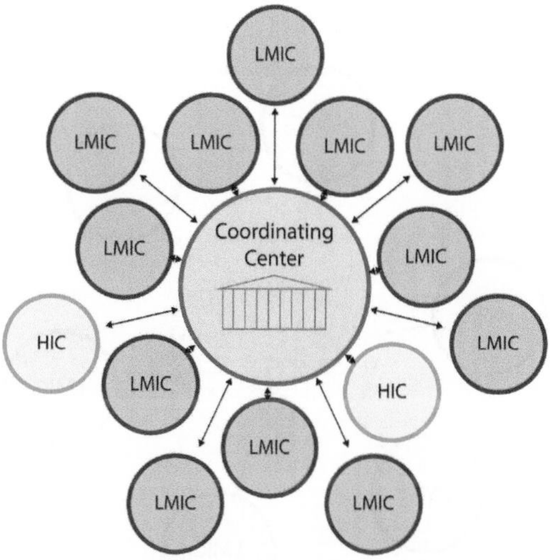

Fig. 2. International consortium. Schematic representation of the one-to-many relationship characteristic of many large-scale international research consortia in which a centralized coordinating center (*red*) organizes the efforts of many international HIC partners to conduct a focused research project in LMIC (*purple*) and sometimes HIC (*blue*). ACTUAR, Asociación de Cirujanos Traumatólogos de las Américas; INORMUS, International Orthopedic Multicenter Study in Fracture Care.

The working group for the International Orthopedic Multicenter Study in Fracture Care (INORMUS) is one example of the international research consortium model for LMIC research. Led by an international team of investigators from McMaster University, UCSF, and The George Institute of Global Health, INORMUS is a large prospective cohort study of 40,000 men and women with musculoskeletal trauma in LMIC that aims to characterize the burden of fractures and associated complications in LMIC around the world.[60] The breadth and reach of LMIC partners have enabled patient enrollment at 50 hospitals from 17 different countries around the world. Furthermore, multiple hospital types within a single country have been included, adding to the generalizability of study results. Although study headquarters are based at the Center for Evidence-Based Orthopedics at McMaster University, relationships with local researchers at study sites is key to study success.[60] One challenge in the global scale-up of this model was difficulty engaging local investigators where no previous relationships existed.[60] Without local partners, it was nearly impossible to navigate local barriers, such as resource limitations and opaque infrastructure, guidelines, policies, or research practices.[60] Ultimately, regional leaders were identified who could help traverse such hurdles by leveraging personal contacts and existing academic partnerships, and attending local meetings. These partners also serve as liaisons between local and international partners.[60] INORMUS is an example of the international research consortium model that facilitates the undertaking of large cohort studies that would be impossible with smaller working groups. Although still in early stages, this global research effort will address a major knowledge gap in orthopedic trauma burden while also establishing sustainable global research infrastructure.

Another recently formed international research consortium, the Asociación de Cirujanos Traumatólogos de las Américas (ACTUAR) aims to promote awareness of orthopedic research methodology, facilitating collaborations between HIC institutions and LMIC in Latin America. By including members from 18 countries across North, Central, and South America, ACTUAR provides access for LMIC partners to North American research training and resources. ACTUAR hosts research symposia on clinical research design and multicenter studies. At its inaugural symposium, the group selected open tibia fracture management as its first collaborative research project. With IGOT serving as the central project hub, ACTUAR members meet monthly by videoconference to discuss project aims and progress. Through the infrastructure, resources, and professional network developed by this partnership, HIC and LMIC members are enabled to conduct high-quality, locally relevant research and publish findings in high-impact journals. Ultimately, ACTUAR will establish necessary workflows for sustainable research in LMIC by enhancing research engagement and opportunities for training and publication.[61]

The international research consortia approach has unique strengths. One is its many study sites. Unlike in the academic model, the success of the overall project does not depend on relationships between one or two key individuals or institutions; rather, forward progress is possible even when some sites underperform or drop off. The model is also likely to yield more generalizable findings. Finally, the scale of the model is appropriate for answering epidemiologic and economic research questions.

The large size of the international research consortia model conversely creates unique challenges. The wide geographic distribution of the working group requires intensive management by experienced leadership to maintain direction and organization of the group. In the same vein, providing individualized support to LMIC partners is more difficult than in the academic model, because each of the multiple LMIC partners may have unique needs.

PROFESSIONAL SOCIETY–ASSOCIATED WORKING GROUPS

Several orthopedic subspecialty societies have dedicated committees and earmarked funding for international research to address the unmet needs of global musculoskeletal disease. As with other models, these working groups often use a multipronged approach that includes education and research to develop sustainable improvements in orthopedic care in LMIC. Professional societies may provide funding and a formal structure and forum for clinicians and researchers from institutions in different countries to organize around a common theme (**Fig. 3**). Such coordinated efforts leverage cumulative skill and group contributions to magnify individual impact.

One example of a professional society–associated working group is the Children's Orthopedics in Underserved Regions (COUR) working group of the Pediatric Orthopedic Society of North America (POSNA). COUR strives to address the global need for pediatric orthopedic care by fostering interaction between HIC POSNA members and LMIC surgeons thorough education, training, and patient- and system-based clinical research.[62] Several LMIC scholars in the COUR International Scholars Program report maintaining connection with their HIC sponsor through research efforts.[63] Through consolidating international efforts of individual POSNA members, COUR has provided a visible entity through which other interested POSNA members may engage in LMIC orthopedic ventures, thereby establishing LMIC-focused initiatives to support and address pediatric orthopedic research and education efforts in LMIC.[62,63]

The Global Initiative for Children's Surgery (GICS) is an international coalition of diverse stakeholders from LMIC and HIC assembled to address the unmet need for pediatric surgery in LMIC. The coalition was formed with the support of several professional pediatric surgical, anesthesiology, orthopedic, and neurosurgical associations. GICS has made great strides in establishing LMIC-centric research efforts. The GICS PaedSurg Africa Research Collaboration, a research network of surgical care providers from more than 20 countries across sub-Saharan Africa, has begun a large multicenter prospective cohort study of management and outcomes of common surgical diseases in

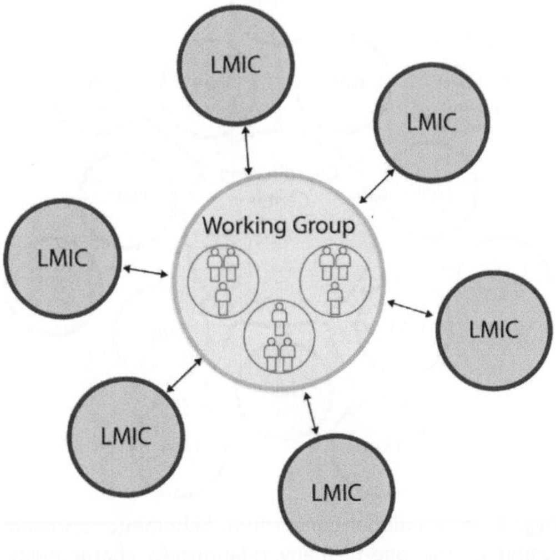

Fig. 3. Professional society working group. Schematic representation of the many-to-many relationship characteristic of many professional society–associated working groups in which individual society members or groups of society members (*yellow*) collaborate with several distinct LMIC (*purple*) partners. COUR, Children's Orthopedics in Underserved Regions; GICS, Global Initiative for Children's Surgery.

children.[64] This effort has led to local and international presentation opportunities[65] and is being expanded to incorporate additional LMIC. GICS has also partnered with Operación Sonrisa Nicaragua to evaluate local surgical capacity-increasing programs.[65] Through a well-organized international coalition that demands participation in projects and meetings rather than financial contributions from its members, GICS is enabling and enhancing research efforts in LMIC.

NONGOVERNMENTAL ORGANIZATION EFFORTS

NGO partnerships (Fig. 4) with HIC and LMIC global orthopedic researchers mirror that of private-public partnerships in public health research. NGOs provide funding, services, and infrastructure to support HIC and LMIC research collaborations. These focused efforts stimulate LMIC-targeted technological innovation by leveraging relationships in the provision of services or resources. Although not traditionally focused on developing research capacity, there are many successful examples of NGO-driven efforts promoting clinical, education, and research benefits in LMIC.

The Surgical Implant Generation Network (SIGN), a nonprofit organization, designed innovative and cost-effective intramedullary nails to be distributed in LMIC. To ensure successful implementation of the SIGN nail, SIGN created an Internet database into which LMIC surgeons were required to report demographic and case information to the database to receive the nails. Many publications[27,66–86] and ongoing studies related to disease burden and clinical outcomes have resulted from the use of the SIGN nail and associated database. The SIGN database serves as initial proof of concept and as a model for the development of future LMIC orthopedic registries and databases.[67]

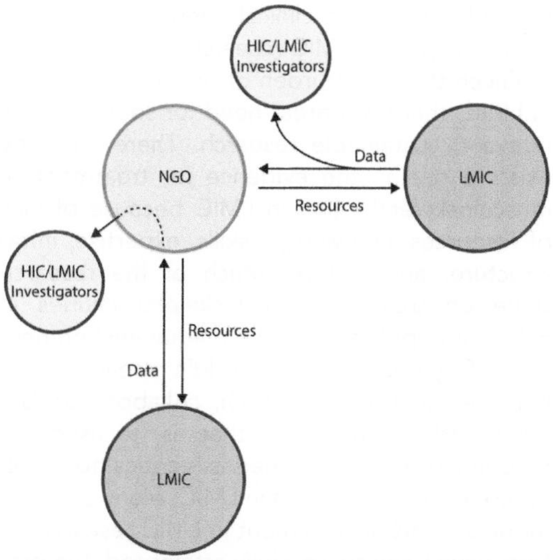

Fig. 4. Nongovernmental organization. Schematic representation of the variable relationships used by NGO research initiatives in which an NGO (*green*) provides resources to LMIC (*purple*) and the resulting data collected are provided, either directly or indirectly, to HIC-LMIC collaborating investigators (*blue-purple*). FOCOS, Foundation of Orthopedics and Complex Spine; SIGN, Surgical Implant Generation Network.

The AO Alliance is another global orthopedics-focused nonprofit committed to improving care in LMIC through advocacy, policy, and clinical care. As part of its care efforts, AO Alliance supports clinical research aiming to improving care of the injured.[87] The resulting data registries have been used to raise standards of care and publish local research in international journals.[25,88–91] Furthermore, the 2017 AO Alliance annual report highlighted the development of the AO Foundation's Program for Education and Excellence in Research (AOPEER), a clinical research course to train LMIC clinical investigators in research best practices.

Another example of NGO impact on LMIC research is the Foundation of Orthopedics and Complex Spine (FOCOS), a nonprofit organization founded in 1998 to deliver orthopedic care, education, and training to underserved communities around the world. Although primarily focused on providing clinical care and education, research from the FOCOS hospital in Accra, Ghana, has produced impactful findings and publications in spine deformity.[92,93]

Initiatives through NGOs, such as SIGN, AO Alliance, and FOCOS, can bridge resource gaps, connect global investigators and innovators, and maintain high-quality data repositories to support research. By targeting locally relevant needs, services provided and data collected can be used for rigorous and high-quality research studies. However, challenges of this model include dependency on the continued existence and beneficence of an NGO, which may limit long-term sustainability and benefits for local LMIC researchers.

DISCUSSION

HIC-LMIC partnership models have produced meaningful, locally relevant, and sustainable orthopedic research. Requisite guiding principles shared among all partnership models are as follows:

1. Development of mutually beneficial partnerships that address the needs of HIC and LMIC stakeholders and strive for equity in academic credit for the research that is produced
2. Development of sustainable research programs that include local LMIC health care providers, administrators, and other support staff

The following challenges were common to many of the partnership models:

1. Difficulty finding and maintaining funding
2. Latency in translating findings into health policy
3. Developing the human capacity and resources required for high-quality data collection
4. Need to manage the competing clinical demands of personnel in a low-resource setting

The traditional academic model has evolved from an HIC-focused, neocolonial intervention into a long-term, bidirectional collaboration with significant contributions from, and benefits for, HIC and LMIC partners. This model of partnership uses the LMIC researchers' in-depth understanding of locally relevant needs and the HIC researchers' resources and experience to develop meaningful results. Such programs as USTOP and IGOT-MOI have emerged as models for academic partnerships and efforts to replicate these initiatives at additional institutions are underway. The Consortium of Academic Traumatologists is a growing network of US and Canadian institutions, created to "support the collaboration of academic global health and orthopedic efforts through mentorship, sharing of best practices, research opportunities, and resources."[94,95] The academic relationship encourages a culture of research at LMIC partner institutions, supports academic advancement of LMIC and HIC investigators, and addresses locally relevant research questions in a rigorous manner. Although dependence on personal relationships and navigating institutional bureaucracy are challenges to this model, it remains a sustainable and widely used approach to orthopedic research in LMIC.

International research consortia have also emerged as a worthy model for undertaking research projects in LMIC. Generally focused on a circumscribed research question, these consortia leverage the far reach, diverse skillsets, and vast cumulative experience of multiple institutions around the world to conduct large-scale projects. The INORMUS study working group, a current example of this model, has the potential to produce relevant burden of disease information with generalizable results that inform best practices for fracture care in LMIC. Despite the challenges associated with managing such a large working group, this model has great power to answer large-scale epidemiologic and economic questions in LMIC.

Professional society–associated working groups bring together like-minded specialists to work toward a common goal. A few professional societies have recognized the need for improved orthopedic research in LMIC and have developed dedicated working groups committed to addressing that need. These associations often benefit LMIC partners with the transfer of knowledge on organizational operations principles that may benefit sustainability. Although potentially challenged by the political nature and demand of collective commitment, such organizations as COUR and GICS have leveraged shared networks to produce LMIC-relevant orthopedic research and establish LMIC-focused research training.

Finally, NGOs, although not always direct research partners, have facilitated LMIC orthopedic research by providing funding and resources and maintaining valuable information databases. These efforts have stimulated technologic and surgical innovation. Partnerships between NGOs and research-oriented individuals and institutions that address unmet clinical need can ultimately lead to impactful LMIC research.

Given the high burden of orthopedic disease in LMIC, there is a great need for sound, locally relevant, sustainable research. There currently exists a gap in the evidence for treatment of musculoskeletal injury in LMIC because of lack of resources, knowledge, skills, expertise, infrastructure, and culture. Much of the research done on treating musculoskeletal injuries in HIC is not applicable to the unique environment of LMIC, yet most of the world's research capability lies in HIC.[96] As such, collaboration between HIC and LMIC that is focused on meeting locally defined needs is critical to developing research pipelines in LMIC. Many different models of HIC involvement in LMIC research efforts have been successfully attempted; the programs that will have lasting legacy are those that promote mutually beneficial partnerships over individual gains. In addition to the direct benefits of high-quality research from these partnerships, LMIC-HIC collaborations can promote support from the LMIC's ministry of health and other important local stakeholders who can further advance research and clinical capacity within the LMIC.

DISCLOSURE

Dr D. Shearer serves on the board of SIGN Fracture Care International, a role for which he receives no financial compensation. All other authors have no relevant conflicts of interest pertinent to this article.

REFERENCES

1. Lozano R, Naghavi M, Foreman K, et al. Global and regional mortality from 235 causes of death for 20 age groups in 1990 and 2010: a systematic analysis for the Global Burden of Disease Study 2010. Lancet 2012;380(9859): 2095–128.
2. Gosselin RA, Spiegel DA, Coughlin R, et al. Injuries: the neglected burden in developing countries. Bull World Health Organ 2009;87(4):246-246a.
3. Farmer PE, Kim JY. Surgery and global health: a view from beyond the OR. World J Surg 2008; 32(4):533–6.
4. Nordberg E, Holmberg S, Kiugu S. Output of major surgery in developing countries. Towards a quantitative evaluation and planning tool. Trop Geogr Med 1995;47(5):206–11.
5. Meara JG, Leather AJM, Hagander L, et al. Global Surgery 2030: evidence and solutions for achieving health, welfare, and economic development. Lancet 2015;386(9993):569–624.
6. Beran D, Byass P, Gbakima A, et al. Research capacity building: obligations for global health partners. Lancet Glob Health 2017;5(6):e567–8.
7. Costello A, Zumla A. Moving to research partnerships in developing countries. BMJ 2000; 321(7264):827–9.
8. Franzen SRP, Chandler C, Siribaddana S, et al. Strategies for developing sustainable health research capacity in low and middle-income countries: a prospective, qualitative study investigating the barriers and enablers to locally led clinical trial conduct in Ethiopia, Cameroon and Sri Lanka. BMJ Open 2017;7(10):e017246.
9. Ibrahim J, Liu M, Yusi K, et al. Conducting a randomized controlled trial in Tanzania: Institute for Global Orthopaedics and Traumatology and the Muhimbili Orthopaedic Institute. J Orthop Trauma 2018;32:S47–51.
10. Morshed S, Shearer DW, Coughlin RR. Collaborative partnerships and the future of global orthopaedics. Clin Orthop 2013;471(10):3088–92.
11. O'Brien P, Kajja I, Potter JM, et al. Role of north-south partnership in trauma management: Uganda Sustainable Trauma Orthopaedic Program. J Orthop Trauma 2018;32(Suppl 7):S21–4.
12. Buchan LL, Black MS, Cancilla MA, et al. Making safe surgery affordable: design of a surgical drill cover system for scale. J Orthop Trauma 2015;29: S29–32.
13. O'Hara NN, Mugarura R, Potter J, et al. The socio-economic implications of isolated tibial and femoral fractures from road traffic injuries in Uganda. J Bone Joint Surg Am 2018;100(7):e43.
14. O'Hara NN, Mugarura R, Potter J, et al. Economic loss due to traumatic injury in Uganda: the patient's perspective. Injury 2016;47(5):1098–103.
15. Stephens T, Mezei A, O'Hara NN, et al. When surgical resources are severely constrained, who receives care? Determinants of access to orthopaedic trauma surgery in Uganda. World J Surg 2017;41(6):1415–9.
16. Kisitu DK, Stockton DJ, O'Hara NN, et al. The feasibility of a randomized controlled trial for open tibial fractures at a regional hospital in Uganda. J Bone Joint Surg Am 2019;101(10):e44.
17. Conway DJ, Coughlin R, Caldwell A, et al. The Institute for Global Orthopedics and Traumatology: a model for academic collaboration in orthopedic surgery. Front Public Health 2017;5:146.
18. Conway D, Albright P, Eliezer E, et al. The burden of femoral shaft fractures in Tanzania. Injury 2019; 50(7):1371–5.
19. Eliezer EN, Haonga BT, Morshed S, et al. Predictors of reoperation for adult femoral shaft fractures managed operatively in a sub-Saharan country. J Bone Joint Surg Am 2017;99(5):388–95.
20. Haonga BT, Areu MMM, Challa ST, et al. Early treatment of open diaphyseal tibia fracture with intramedullary nail versus external fixator in Tanzania: cost effectiveness analysis using preliminary data from Muhimbili Orthopaedic Institute. SICOT J 2019;5:20.
21. Haonga BT, Makupa JE, Muhina RI, et al. Pain management among adult patients with fractures of long bones at Muhimbili Orthopaedic Institute in Dar es Salaam, Tanzania. Tanzan J Health Res 2011;13(4):107–11.
22. Haonga BT, Zirkle LG. The SIGN nail: factors in a successful device for low-resource settings. J Orthop Trauma 2015;29(Suppl 10):S37–9.
23. Ibrahim JM, Conway D, Haonga BT, et al. Predictors of lower health-related quality of life after operative repair of diaphyseal femur fractures in a low-resource setting. Injury 2018;49(7):1330–5.
24. Kramer EJ, Shearer D, Morshed S. The use of traction for treating femoral shaft fractures in low- and middle-income countries: a systematic review. Int Orthop 2016;40(5):875–83.
25. Miclau T, Hoogervorst P, Shearer DW, et al. Current status of musculoskeletal trauma care systems worldwide. J Orthop Trauma 2018;32: S64–70.

26. Mustafa Diab M, Wu H-H, Eliezer E, et al. The impact of antegrade intramedullary nailing start site using the SIGN nail in proximal femoral fractures: a prospective cohort study. Injury 2018; 49(2):323–7.
27. Wu H-H, Liu M, Challa ST, et al. Development of squat-and-smile test as proxy for femoral shaft fracture-healing in patients in Dar es Salaam, Tanzania. J Bone Joint Surg Am 2019;101(4):353–9.
28. Alves K, Godwin CL, Chen A, et al. Gluteal fibrosis, post-injection paralysis, and related injection practices in Uganda: a qualitative analysis. BMC Health Serv Res 2018;18(1):892.
29. Alves K, Penny N, Kobusingye O, et al. Paediatric musculoskeletal disease in Kumi District, Uganda: a cross-sectional survey. Int Orthop 2018;42(8): 1967–73.
30. Banskota AK, Spiegel DA, Shrestha S, et al. Open reduction for neglected traumatic hip dislocation in children and adolescents. J Pediatr Orthop 2007;27(2):187–91.
31. Banskota B, Yadav P, Rajbhandari T, et al. Outcomes of the Ponseti method for untreated clubfeet in Nepalese patients seen between the ages of one and five years and followed for at least 10 years. J Bone Joint Surg Am 2018; 100(23):2004–14.
32. Curran PF, Albright P, Ibrahim JM, et al. Practice patterns for management of pediatric femur fractures in low- and middle-income countries. J Pediatr Orthop 2019. https://doi.org/10.1097/BPO.0000000000001435.
33. Gupta S, Groen TA, Stewart BT, et al. The spatial distribution of injuries in need of surgical intervention in Nepal. Geospat Health 2016;11(2):359.
34. Kisa P, Grabski DF, Ozgediz D, et al. Unifying children's surgery and anesthesia stakeholders across institutions and clinical disciplines: challenges and solutions from Uganda. World J Surg 2019;43(6): 1435–49.
35. LeBrun DG, Banskota B, Banskota AK, et al. Socioeconomic status influences functional severity of untreated cerebral palsy in Nepal: a prospective analysis and systematic review. Clin Orthop 2019; 477(1):10–21.
36. LeBrun DG, Talwar D, Pham TA, et al. Predictors of healthcare seeking delays among children with chronic musculoskeletal disorders in Nepal. J Epidemiol Glob Health 2017;7(4):299–304.
37. Spiegel DA, Shrestha OP, Rajbhandary T, et al. Epidemiology of surgical admissions to a children's disability hospital in Nepal. World J Surg 2010; 34(5):954–62.
38. Spiegel DA, Shrestha OP, Sitoula P, et al. Ponseti method for untreated idiopathic clubfeet in Nepalese patients from 1 to 6 years of age. Clin Orthop 2009;467(5):1164–70.
39. Spiegel D, Shrestha S, Sitoula P, et al. Atlantoaxial rotatory displacement in children. World J Orthop 2017;8(11):836–45.
40. Stewart BT, Kushner AL, Kamara TB, et al. Backlog and burden of fractures in Sierra Leone and Nepal: results from nationwide cluster randomized, population-based surveys. Int J Surg 2016;33 Pt A: 49–54.
41. Young S, Banza L, Mkandawire N. The impact of long term institutional collaboration in surgical training on trauma care in Malawi. SpringerPlus 2016;5:407.
42. Young S. Orthopaedic trauma surgery in low-income countries. Acta Orthop Suppl 2014; 85(356):1–35.
43. Young S, Banza L. Neglected traumatic anterior dislocation of the hip. Open reduction using the Bernese trochanter flip approach - a case report. Acta Orthop 2017;88(3):348–50.
44. Young S, Banza L, Munthali BS, et al. The impact of the increasing burden of trauma in Malawi on orthopedic trauma service priorities at Kamuzu Central Hospital. Acta Orthop 2016;87(6):632–6.
45. Young S, Banza LN, Hallan G, et al. Complications after intramedullary nailing of femoral fractures in a low-income country. Acta Orthop 2013;84(5):460–7.
46. Young S, Lie SA, Hallan G, et al. Risk factors for infection after 46,113 intramedullary nail operations in low- and middle-income countries. World J Surg 2013;37(2):349–55.
47. Young S, Beniyasi FJ, Munthali B, et al. Infection of the fracture hematoma from skeletal traction in an asymptomatic HIV-positive patient. Acta Orthop 2012;83(4):423–5.
48. Young S, Fevang JM, Gullaksen G, et al. Parent and patient satisfaction after treatment for supracondylar humerus fractures in 139 children: no difference between skeletal traction and crossed pin fixation at long-term followup. Adv Orthop 2012;2012: 958487.
49. Chagomerana MB, Tomlinson J, Young S, et al. High morbidity and mortality after lower extremity injuries in Malawi: a prospective cohort study of 905 patients. Int J Surg 2017;39:23–9.
50. Chokotho L, Lau BC, Conway D, et al. Validation of Chichewa Short Musculoskeletal Function Assessment (SMFA) questionnaire: a cross-sectional study. Malawi Med J 2019;31(1):65–70.
51. Chokotho L, Mkandawire N, Conway D, et al. Validation and reliability of the Chichewa translation of the EQ-5D quality of life questionnaire in adults with orthopaedic injuries in Malawi. Malawi Med J 2017;29(2):84–8.
52. Grudziak J, Gallaher J, Banza L, et al. The effect of a surgery residency program and enhanced educational activities on trauma mortality in sub-Saharan Africa. World J Surg 2017;41(12):3031–7.

53. Haug L, Wazakili M, Young S, et al. Longstanding pain and social strain: patients' and health care providers' experiences with fracture management by skeletal traction; a qualitative study from Malawi. Disabil Rehabil 2017;39(17):1714–21.
54. Kendig C, Tyson A, Young S, et al. The effect of a new surgery residency program on case volume and case complexity in a sub-Saharan African hospital. J Surg Educ 2015;72(4):e94–9.
55. Kohler RE, Tomlinson J, Chilunjika TE, et al. "Life is at a standstill" Quality of life after lower extremity trauma in Malawi. Qual Life Res 2017;26(4):1027–35.
56. Qureshi JS, Young S, Muyco AP, et al. Addressing Malawi's surgical workforce crisis: a sustainable paradigm for training and collaboration in Africa. Surgery 2013;153(2):272–81.
57. Sundet M, Grudziak J, Charles A, et al. Paediatric road traffic injuries in Lilongwe, Malawi: an analysis of 4776 consecutive cases. Trop Doct 2018;48(4): 316–22.
58. Varela C, Young S, Mkandawire N, et al. Transportation barriers to access health care for surgical conditions in Malawi: a cross sectional nationwide household survey. BMC Public Health 2019;19(1): 264.
59. Varela C, Young S, Groen R, et al. Untreated surgical conditions in Malawi: a randomised cross-sectional nationwide household survey. Malawi Med J 2017;29(3):231–6.
60. Sprague S, McKay P, Li CS, et al. International orthopaedic multicenter study in fracture care: coordinating a large-scale multicenter global prospective cohort study. J Orthop Trauma 2018; 32(Suppl 7):S58–63.
61. Miclau T, MacKechnie MC, Shearer DW. Asociación de Cirujanos Traumatólogos de las Américas: development of a Latin American research consortium. J Orthop Trauma 2018;32:S8–11.
62. Shirley ED, Sabharwal S, Schwend RM, et al. Addressing the global disparities in the delivery of pediatric orthopaedic services: opportunities for COUR and POSNA. J Pediatr Orthop 2015;1. https://doi.org/10.1097/BPO.0000000000000400.
63. Fornari ED, Sabharwal S, Schwend RM. The POSNA-COUR International Scholar Program. Results of the first 7 years. J Pediatr Orthop 2017; 37(8):570–4.
64. Children's Surgery in Sub-Saharan Africa - Full Text View - ClinicalTrials.gov. Available at: https://clinicaltrials.gov/ct2/show/NCT03185637. Accessed August 21, 2019.
65. Wright N, Jensen G, St-Louis E, et al. Global Initiative for Children's Surgery: a model of global collaboration to advance the surgical care of children. World J Surg 2019;43(6):1416–25.
66. Calafi LA, Antkowiak T, Curtiss S, et al. A biomechanical comparison of the Surgical Implant Generation Network (SIGN) tibial nail with the standard hollow nail. Injury 2010;41(7):753–7.
67. Clough JF, Zirkle LG, Schmitt RJ. The role of SIGN in the development of a global orthopaedic trauma database. Clin Orthop 2010;468(10):2592–7.
68. Ertl CW, Royal D, Arzoiey HA, et al. A retrospective case series of surgical implant generation Network (SIGN) placement at the Afghan National Police Hospital, Kabul, Afghanistan. Mil Med 2016;181(1):21–6.
69. Hansen E, Bozic KJ. The impact of disruptive innovations in orthopaedics. Clin Orthop 2009;467(10): 2512–20.
70. Ikem IC, Ogunlusi JD, Ine HR. Achieving interlocking nails without using an image intensifier. Int Orthop 2007;31(4):487–90.
71. Ikpeme I, Ngim N, Udosen A, et al. External jig-aided intramedullary interlocking nailing of diaphyseal fractures: experience from a tropical developing centre. Int Orthop 2011;35(1):107–11.
72. Khan I, Javed S, Khan GN, et al. Outcome of intramedullary interlocking SIGN nail in tibial diaphyseal fracture. J Coll Physicians Surg Pak 2013;23(3): 203–7.
73. Naeem-Ur-Razaq M, Qasim M, Khan MA, et al. Management outcome of closed femoral shaft fractures by open Surgical Implant Generation Network (SIGN) interlocking nails. J Ayub Med Coll Abbottabad 2009;21(1):21–4.
74. Nwagbara IC. Locked intramedullary nailing using the sign nailing device. Niger J Clin Pract 2019; 22(4):485–91.
75. Ogunlusi JD, St Rose RSGB, Davids T. Interlocking nailing without imaging: the challenges of locating distal slots and how to overcome them in SIGN intramedullary nailing. Int Orthop 2010;34(6):891–5.
76. Panti JPL, Geronilla M, Arada EC. Clinical outcomes of patients with isolated femoral shaft fractures treated with S.I.G.N interlock nails versus cannulated interlock intramedullary nails. J Orthop 2013;10(4):182–7.
77. Phillips J, Zirkle LG, Gosselin RA. Achieving locked intramedullary fixation of long bone fractures: technology for the developing world. Int Orthop 2012; 36(10):2007–13.
78. Sekimpi P, Okike K, Zirkle L, et al. Femoral fracture fixation in developing countries: an evaluation of the Surgical Implant Generation Network (SIGN) intramedullary nail. J Bone Joint Surg Am 2011; 93(19):1811–8.
79. Shah RK, Moehring HD, Singh RP, et al. Surgical Implant Generation Network (SIGN) intramedullary nailing of open fractures of the tibia. Int Orthop 2004;28(3):163–6.
80. Stephens KR, Shahab F, Galat D, et al. Management of distal tibial metaphyseal fractures with the SIGN intramedullary nail in 3 developing countries. J Orthop Trauma 2015;29(12):e469–75.

81. Usoro AO, Bhashyam A, Mohamadi A, et al. Clinical outcomes and complications of the Surgical Implant Generation Network (SIGN) intramedullary nail: a systematic review and meta-analysis. J Orthop Trauma 2019;33(1):42–8.
82. Whiting PS, Anderson DR, Galat DD, et al. State of pelvic and acetabular surgery in the developing world: a global survey of Orthopaedic Surgeons at Surgical Implant Generation Network (SIGN) hospitals. J Orthop Trauma 2017;31(7):e217–23.
83. Whiting PS, Galat DD, Zirkle LG, et al. Risk factors for infection after intramedullary nailing of open tibial shaft fractures in low- and middle-income countries. J Orthop Trauma 2019;33(6):e234–9.
84. Young S, Lie SA, Hallan G, et al. Low infection rates after 34,361 intramedullary nail operations in 55 low- and middle-income countries: validation of the Surgical Implant Generation Network (SIGN) online surgical database. Acta Orthop 2011;82(6): 737–43.
85. Zirkle LG. Injuries in developing countries: how can we help? The role of orthopaedic surgeons. Clin Orthop 2008;466(10):2443–50.
86. Zirkle LG, Shahab F. Shahabuddin null. Interlocked intramedullary nail without fluoroscopy. Orthop Clin North Am 2016;47(1):57–66.
87. Fracture care education and capacity building resources. AO Alliance. Available at: https://ao-alliance.org/what-we-do/care/. Accessed August 27, 2019.
88. Agarwal-Harding KJ, Chokotho LC, Mkandawire NC, et al. Risk factors for delayed presentation among patients with musculoskeletal injuries in Malawi. J Bone Joint Surg Am 2019;101(10):920–31.
89. Joshipura M, Gosselin RA. Surgical burden of musculoskeletal conditions in low- and middle-income countries. World J Surg 2018. https://doi.org/10.1007/s00268-018-4790-8.
90. Chan Y, Banza L, Martin C, et al. Essential fracture and orthopaedic equipment lists in low resource settings: consensus derived by survey of experts in Africa. BMJ Open 2018;8(9): e023473.
91. Hawkes DH, Harrison WJ. Critiquing operative fracture fixation: the development of an assessment tool. Eur J Orthop Surg Traumatol Orthop Traumatol 2017;27(8):1083–8.
92. Verma K, Slattery CA, Boachie-Adjei O. What's important: surgeon volunteerism. J Bone Joint Surg Am 2019;101(9):854–5.
93. Research and Education. FOCOS. Available at: http://www.orthofocos.org/what-we-do/research-and-education. Accessed August 21, 2019.
94. COACT. COACT mission statement. 2016. Available at: https://orthosurgery.ucsf.edu/outreach/global/COACT.html. Accessed August 31, 2019.
95. Miclau T, MacKechnie MC, Shearer DW. Consortium of orthopaedic academic traumatologists: a model for collaboration in orthopaedic surgery. J Orthop Trauma 2018;32:S3–7.
96. Aluede EE, Phillips J, Bleyer J, et al. Representation of developing countries in orthopaedic journals: a survey of four influential orthopaedic journals. Clin Orthop Relat Res 2012;470(8):2313–8.

Intertrochanteric Femur Fracture Treatment in Asia

What We Know and What the World Can Learn

Shi-Min Chang, MD, PhD[a,*], Zhi-Yong Hou, MD, PhD[b], Sun-Jun Hu, MD, PhD[a], Shou-Chao Du, MD[a]

KEYWORDS

- Hip fracture • Intertrochanteric fracture • Cephalomedullary nail • Fracture reduction
- Secondary stability

KEY POINTS

- The incidence of geriatric hip fractures in Asia continues to rise dramatically due to the larger group of old-aged population and longer life expectancy.
- The treatment of trochanteric hip fractures has undergone favorable evolution and revolution during the past 20 years, with new technical concepts, such as tip-apex distance, proximal lateral wall, cortical support reduction, and the instrumental success of intramedullary nailing.
- Anteromedial cortex-to-cortex support reduction is a key element for stability reconstruction, because it allows limited sliding to provide positive biomechanical environment for fracture contact and healing.
- Ten tips in new recognition and clinical practice were summarized to improve the overall bone-implant stability and reduce postoperative complications.

INTRODUCTION

Hip fractures are of intense interest globally.[1–3] Geriatric hip fractures represent an increasingly prevalent problem in an aging population all over the world. According to a recent systemic review, more than half of all hip fractures in the world will occur in Asia by the year 2050, mainly due to the rapidly increasing older population and longer life expectancy.[4] It is estimated that the hip fracture cases in China will increase 6-fold from 0.7 million cases in 2013 to 4.5 million cases in 2050. In Japan, a lifetime risk of hip fracture for individuals at 50 years of age was reported as 5.6% for men and 20% for women.[5]

The significant and increasing number of hip fractures that occur each year makes them a common problem to be treated among the orthopedic trauma surgeons and also has been an ever-increasing public health concern. Most hip fractures are caused by osteoporosis and fall injuries in daily life activities, with the proportion of men to women 1:4.[6] Geriatric hip fractures include femoral neck fractures and trochanteric fractures, with the incidence grossly 40% to 60%. Trochanteric fractures occur in a more aged population than femoral neck fractures. In general, older people are more seriously affected by osteoporosis and medical comorbidities, and also they are poorer ambulators.

Funding: Nature Science Foundation of China, People's Republic of China (NSFC No. 81772323).
[a] Department of Orthopedic Surgery, Yangpu Hospital, Tongji University School of Medicine, 450 Tengyue Road, Shanghai 200090, People's Republic of China; [b] Department of Orthopedic Surgery, Third Hospital of Hebei Medical University, 139 Ziqiang Road, Shijiazhuang 050051, People's Republic of China
* Corresponding author.
E-mail address: shiminchang11@aliyun.com

Orthop Clin N Am 51 (2020) 189–205
https://doi.org/10.1016/j.ocl.2019.11.011

For geriatric trochanteric hip fractures, surgical treatment is recommended for pain relief as is getting patients off bed rest as early as possible. Multidisciplinary comanagement protocols have been applied successfully for fast-track operation within 48 or even 24 hours and enhanced recovery after surgery of the patient.[7] Hip fractures can be treated with internal fixation (extramedullary side plates or intramedullary nails) or prosthetic arthroplasty.[8] Currently, more and more surgeons prefer to use cephalomedullary device for the fixation of unstable pertrochanteric/intertrochanteric fractures.[9]

FRACTURE LINE MAPPING

Trochanteric hip fractures (AO/OTA type 31A) occur at the translational area of the cervicotrochanteric junction, extending from the extracapsular basilar neck region to the region along the lesser trochanter proximal to the development of the medullary canal. Injury in this proximal metaphyseal-diaphyseal region creates a variety of fractures, with damage to the intersecting cancellous compression and tensile lamellar networks and the weak cortical bone. This results in displacement of the fracture fragments and attached muscle groups, leading to head-neck, femoral shaft, lesser trochanter-calcar, greater trochanter, lateral wall, posterior crest, and anterior cortex fragments, and even extension to the subtrochanteric region. With the complexity of neck-shaft, anteversion, and torsional angles, these broken structures are subjected to multiplanar stresses, and it is difficult to obtain satisfactory fracture reduction and stable implant fixation. More unstable pertrochanteric hip fractures (31A2) are the most frequent pattern and account for 60% to 70% trochanteric hip fractures.

Accurate fracture mapping using 3-dimensional (3-D)–computed tomographic (CT) images can display the big data of fracture line information directly on a visual template, enhance the understanding of morphologic fracture characteristics and injury mechanisms, and add more clear knowledge for surgeons during fracture diagnosis, preoperative planning, and execution of surgical strategies. Using a 3-D–CT fracture mapping technique, Zhang and colleagues[10] described the fracture characteristics of type A2 in 59 patients, with a mean age of 73 years. Apart from the head-neck and femoral shaft, which are intended to be reduced and fixed intraoperatively, all other fragments are defined as free bones, which are not reduced and fixed intentionally. The fracture lines were observed from 5 views and the features were delineated in 5 bearings (**Fig. 1**). From an anterior view, the anterior fracture line usually is simple and runs along the direction of intertrochanteric line; no free bone is identified, which means no anterior cortex comminution. From a medial view, the anterior and posterior fracture lines of the head-neck fragment converge in front of the lesser trochanter and then run posteriorly and distal. The lesser trochanter is always split as free bone (which is the principal characteristic of A2 patterns), mostly with 2 fragments. From the posterior view, the fracture line is concentrated in the middle third of the posterior crest, and 70% of cases have at least 1 free fragment. From the lateral view, the fracture line usually originates from the anterior superior great trochanter and runs obliquely ($64.6° \pm 14.5°$ to horizontal line) to the posterior inferior lesser trochanter. The lateral wall is partially injured in almost all cases in the coronal aspect in A2 fractures. From the top view, the apex of greater trochanter is most often ruptured, and 70% of cases have 1 to 2 free bone fragments.

Li and Tang's group[11] also performed a study to cluster the morphologic fracture lines in 504 cases treated with closed reduction and

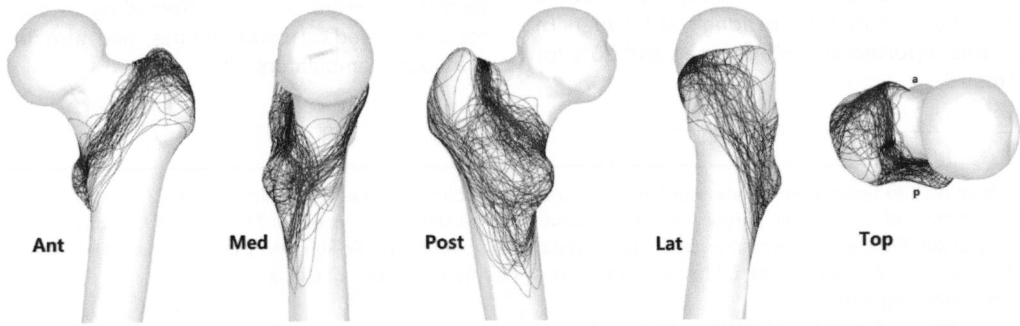

Fig. 1. Fracture line mapping of 31A2 unstable pertrochanteric hip fractures (anterior [Ant], medial [Med], posterior [Post], lateral [Lat], and top views).

intramedullary nail fixation. Based on these fracture mapping, they proposed a new classification of 5 types with comminution severity increased progressively: type I (21.4%) is simple fracture with intact femoral lateral wall and greater trochanter fragment; type II (16.9%) is simple fracture with intact lateral wall with/without lesser trochanter detachment; type III (29.2%) is a fracture with intertrochanteric crest detachment involving the lesser trochanter and greater trochanter with an intact lateral wall; type IV (22.4%) is a fracture with large intertrochanteric crest detachment and large lesser trochanter and greater trochanter detachment partially involving the lateral wall and less medial cortical support; and type V (10.1%) is a combination of pertrochanteric and lateral fracture line involving the entire lateral wall and lesser trochanter detachment.

Fracture mapping in unstable A2 pattern gives a clear recognition that only the anteromedial fracture line is simple, and only these cortices can be used for fracture reduction to get a stable support for the head-neck fragment.

PROXIMAL LATERAL WALL AND ANTERIOR CORTEX

Trochanteric lateral wall is primarily the lateral femoral cortex of the drilling site for head-neck fixation implant, as described by Gotfried[12] in 2004. This area can provide a natural buttress for the head-neck fragment and fixation.

A full description of the proximal femoral lateral wall includes height, width, thickness, area, biomechanical strength, and soft tissue attachment. The height of lateral wall is still controversial.[13–15] The authors define the lateral wall anatomically from the vastus ridge proximally to the inferior aspect of the lesser trochanter distally.[15] The real thickness of the lateral wall is the exact thickness of the lateral cortex, which is usually 2 mm to 4 mm in CT measurement.[16] Hsu and colleagues[17] defined the lateral wall thickness as the distance in millimeters from a reference point 3 cm below the innominate tubercle of the greater trochanter, angled 135° upward to the fracture line on the anteroposterior (AP) radiograph. If the thickness is less than 20.5 mm, the lateral wall is incompetent. This criterion has been accepted and included in the 2018 version of AO/OTA Fracture and Dislocation Classification Compendium and is classified as type A2.[18] This parameter is actually a mean distance between the fracture line and the lateral cortex, which contains 3 parts, the lateral femoral cortex proper and the remaining anterior and posterior cortices, that is, the sum of the remnant length of anterior and posterior cortical wall plus the true lateral cortex thickness.[15] As the fracture line in pertrochanteric fractures (A1 and A2) runs obliquely along the greater-to-lesser trochanteric direction (see **Fig. 1**. Lateral view), the distance measured in the anterior cortex is always greater than that in the posterior cortex. The width of lateral wall is the horizontal distance between the anterior and posterior cortices. The width of femoral wall can be injured by coronal fracture lines, which usually start at the trochanteric apex and exit either through posterior crest, the lesser trochanter, or the posteromedial cortex.[19] When coronal fracture line exits inferiorly through the lesser trochanter or the posteromedial cortex, the lateral femoral wall is always partially fractured and incompetent. Therefore, the authors suggest the blank space of 31A2.1 in 2018 AO/OTA classification should be filled with a multifragmentary pertrochanteric fracture with posterior coronal lateral wall rupture. The area of lateral wall (height times width) may be a more valuable parameter to estimate the risk of lateral wall rupture perioperatively.[10] The soft tissue lateral wall is a tedious aponeurotic structure formed by the attachments of gluteus medius and minus terminals and the vastus lateralis origin that get mixed and intersected with each other over the osseous.[20]

The biomechanical strength of lateral wall in osteoporotic elderly people is extremely weak, and in some patients, the preoperatively intact lateral wall (type A1) may be broken during or after operation. From this point of view, some surgeons prefer cephalomedullary nails in all pertrochanteric/intertrochanteric hip fractures, regardless of stable (A1) or unstable pattern (A2/3). Disruption of lateral femoral wall converts a pertrochanteric fracture (A1/2) into a reverse oblique fracture equivalent (A3). Complete breakage of lateral wall is always accompanied by anterior cortex fracture simultaneously, which means there is no anterior or lateral cortex that can be relied on to support the head-neck fragment.[21] In essence, the role of mechanical buttress of the lateral wall is primarily played by the anterior or anteromedial cortex, which is the first line element to sustain the head-neck.

Lateral wall fracture can be subclassified further according to its specific features, such as the course of fracture line (oblique, transverse, or reverse oblique)[22] and the presence of a free bone fragment at the junction of the greater trochanter and lateral femoral wall.[23] Whether the lateral wall fragment needs additional management remains controversial. Owing to the soft tissue lateral wall, such as the vastus lateralis muscle, a minimal displacement of lateral wall fragment (<1 cm) after nailing may not need additional reduction and fixation.[24]

POSTEROMEDIAL LESSER TROCHANTER-CALCAR FRAGMENT

The presence of a posteromedial intermediate fragment (the third lesser trochanter) is the key characteristic that differentiates simple (A1) and communited (A2) pertrochanteric fracture patterns. Previous biomechanical studies have shown that the lesser trochanter fragment plays a key role in the reconstruction of fracture stability, and the larger the size of the defect that the detached lesser trochanteric fragments create, the more unstable the fracture.[25,26]

Xiong and colleagues[27] performed a morphologic study in 58 cases of A2 fractures. The CT data (DICOM) were imported into Mimics software to form 3-D–CT reconstruction images. By simulated rotation and translation, the displaced fragments were reduced. In the results, the vertical length of the lesser trochanter was 65.5 mm in average (range 5–8 cm), and 87% of lesser trochanter fragment contained the femoral calcar, which was an intramedullary vertical cortex strut in the posteromedial region. At the midlevel of the lesser trochanter, the mean width of lesser trochanter fragments was 52.5 mm and accounted for 39% of the whole cortical circumference of the proximal femur (mean, 136.3 mm). The lesser trochanter fragment extended to the posterior cortex up to 33.5 mm in average, which disrupted 81% of the posterior wall (mean width, 41.7 mm), and to the medial cortex up to 19.0 mm in average, which disrupted 57% the medial wall (mean width, 33.5 mm) (**Fig. 2**). Sharma and colleagues[28] also measured the size of the posteromedial fragments on 3-D–CT in 50 cases of type A2 fractures and reported that the lesser trochanter fragments involved 74% of the posterior wall and 36% of the medial wall of the proximal femur.

Some investigators have advocated reduction and fixation of the lesser trochanter fragments, such as minimal invasive cerclage wiring.[29,30] The technique, however, was tedious and time consuming. Also, the technique was just to get the fragment closer to the shaft, with no rigid fixation achieved, which was less helpful for early biomechanical stability. Currently, there is no reliable and convenient method in practice to reduce and fix the posteromedial lesser trochanter-calcar fragment. This means that only the anteromedial cortex is left and can be relied on for satisfactory cortex support reduction.

ANTEROMEDIAL CORTICAL SUPPORT REDUCTION

Fracture reduction is the first step in treatment and is always of greater importance than the other factors. For trochanteric fractures, the reduction quality is assessed by fluoroscopy intraoperatively and by radiography, CT scanning, and 3-D reconstruction postoperatively.

Fracture reduction quality is evaluated by Garden alignment and fragment displacement. The most accepted criteria, proposed by Baumgaertner and colleagues,[31] categorized the reduction quality as good, acceptable, or poor. For a reduction to be considered good, there has to be normal or slight valgus alignment on the AP view, less than 20° of angulation on the lateral view, and no more than 4 mm of displacement of any fragment. To be considered acceptable, a reduction has to meet the criterion of a good reduction with respect to either alignment or displacement, but not both. A poor reduction meets neither criterion. The acceptable quality for good reduction of main fragments displacement is less than 1 cortex thickness, or 4 mm to 5 mm, regardless of its location and direction.

As a mechanical principle after fracture reduction, the head-neck fragment is permitted to telescope along the axis of the implant (lag screw/helical blade), and then a secondary stability is achieved by medial and/or anterior cortex-to-cortex contact between the femoral neck and shaft. If no cortical support is obtained at this moment, the head-neck fragment slides further until it gets buttress from the intramedullary nail, which is situated in the central canal. If a side plate is used, however, the head-neck fragment slides still further until it gets contact from the lateral wall (natural cortex or metallic plate). Otherwise, if the fracture is fixed by dynamic hip screw and the lateral wall is ruptured perioperatively, no lateral structure is left to buttress the head-neck fragment, and it is usually impossible to achieve secondary stability. Construct collapse and mechanical failure such as femoral head cutout, shaft medialization, leg shortening, or implant breakage, probably will occur.

Because the head-neck fragment has an impact obliquely to the lateral inferior direction, its position after reduction and fixation must be considered to predict the probability to achieve

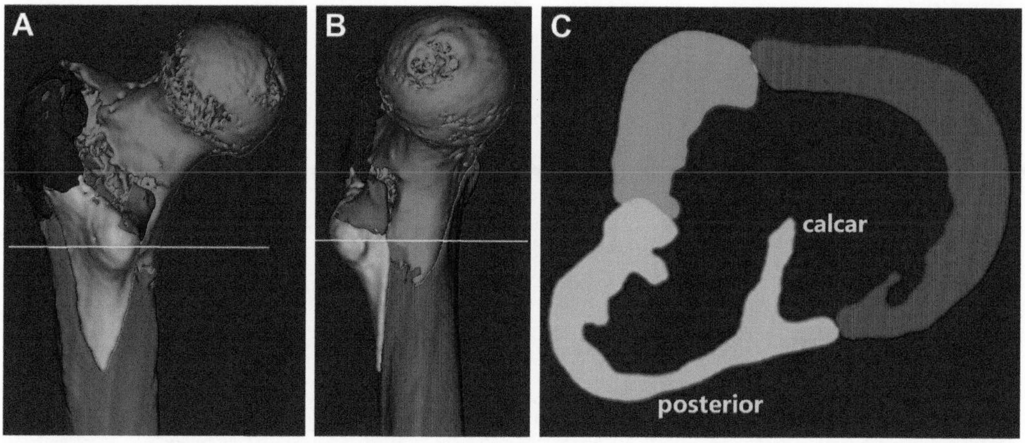

Fig. 2. Posteromedial lesser trochanter-calcar fragment. (*A*) Posterior view, (*B*) medial view, and (*C*) axial view cut at mid-lesser trochanteric level. Note the red color fragment was a free cortical bone from the posterior femoral neck. ([*A, C*] *Adapted from* Xiong WF, Zhang YQ, Chang SM, et al. Lesser trochanteric fragments in unstable pertrochanteric hip fractures: a morphological study using three-dimensional computed tomography (3-D CT) reconstruction. Med Sci Monitor 2019;25:2049-2057; with permission.)

cortical contact and mechanical buttress from the femoral shaft.

Anteromedial cortex-to-cortex support reduction was first introduced in 2015 by Chang and colleagues[32] for unstable pertrochanteric fractures. It involves a pattern of functional buttress reduction and is specific for the proximal femur as it relates to the neck-shaft angle and when various implant devices with sliding mechanisms are used for fixation. Controlled fracture impaction via limited telescoping provides secondary axial and torsional stability between the head-neck fragment and the shaft of the femur.

A full description of anteromedial cortical support reduction, or cortex-to-cortex contact, involves assessment in both the AP view (for the medial cortex) and the lateral view (for the anterior cortex), with an emphasis on the anteromedial inferior corner (oblique view). To obtain the oblique view, first the authors align the nail and blade in a straight line flouroscopically and observe the true lateral view (0°). Then the fluoroscope is gradually lowered every 10°, observing the clearer view of the anteromedial aspect. Usually at approximately 30° rotation of fluoroscope, a proper tangential view of the anteromedial portion can be seen. The relationship between the head-neck fragment and the femoral shaft, which describes the position of their cortical layers or the trend in their changes of position after sliding along the implant axis (usually 130°), is evaluated and classified into 3 categories (positive, neutral, and negative) for both medial and anterior cortical apposition (Fig. 3).

In the AP view, the relationship or the trend between the 2 medial cortices of the head-neck and shaft fragments was evaluated after oblique, lateral sliding. If the medial cortex of the head-neck fragment was located slightly (1 cortical thickness, or 4–5 mm) superomedial to the upper medial edge of the femoral shaft, it was classified as a positive position for medial cortical support. If the medial cortex of the head-neck fragment was contacted smoothly to the medial cortex of the femoral shaft, it was classified as a neutral position. If the medial cortex of the head-neck fragment was displaced laterally to the upper medial edge of the femoral shaft, it was classified as a negative position, which meant that there was a malreduction, and the medial cortical buttress from the femoral shaft had been lost.

In the lateral view, the relationship or trend between the 2 anterior cortices of the head-neck and femoral shaft was assessed after parallel sliding. If the anterior cortices made a smooth contact or if the step-off (regardless of neck cortex shifted anteriorly or posteriorly) was less than half of the cortical thickness, or 2 mm, it was classified as a neutral position for anterior cortical support. If the head-neck cortex was anteriorly displaced more than half of the cortical thickness, it was classified as positive; and if it was posteriorly displaced (posterior sag) by more than half of the cortical thickness, it was classified as negative.

Neutral positions in both the AP and lateral views on fluoroscopy are acceptable, but they do not indicate anatomic reduction. Accurate differentiation of cortical reduction quality

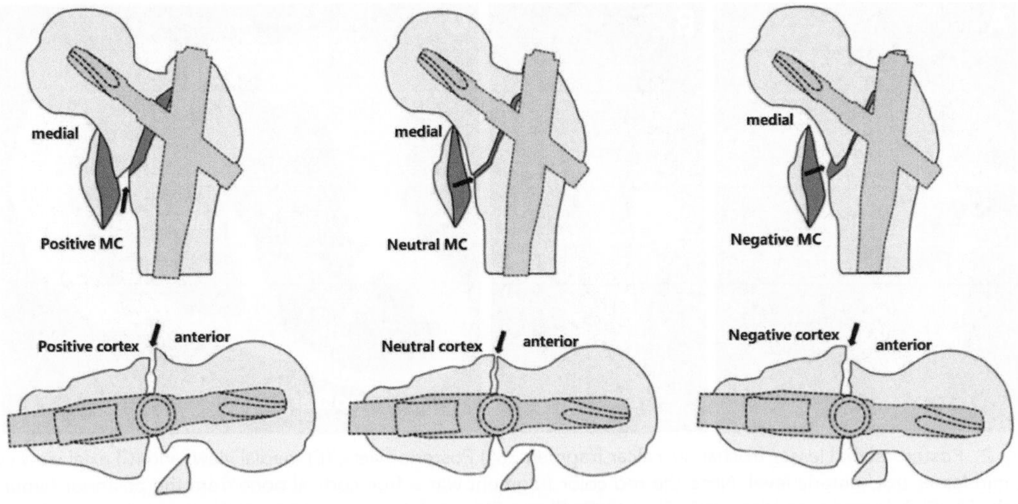

Fig. 3. Schematic diagram to show anteromedial cortical reduction. (*Upper*) AP view of medial cortex (MC). (*Lower*) Lateral view of anterior cortex.

depends on the surgeon's experience, pixel resolution, and clarity of the image intensifier. The so-called anatomic reduction shown on intraoperative fluoroscopy may actually include 3 subconditions: (1) an exact anatomic cortex-to-cortex position, (2) a slightly positive position, or (3) a slightly negative position.[32] Because intraoperative fluoroscopic image resolution is limited, however, 2-mm cortical steps may not be identifiable. Therefore, those 3 subconditions generally are not able to be clearly distinguished. The term, *neutral*, instead of *anatomic*, therefore, is used to delineate this smooth contact in fluoroscopy. After sliding and fragment impaction, a slight negative position might become a truly negative pattern in the postoperative period.[32]

Cortex-to-cortex support reduction is a nonanatomic functional buttress pattern (Table 1). A positive cortical support reduction pattern is easy to obtain in practice for unstable fractures and is used to achieve secondary stability, whereas exact anatomic reduction is difficult to obtain by closed maneuver and is used to achieve primary fracture stability. In a medial positive cortical support pattern, an end-to-side cortical contact between the 2 main fragments is achieved; meanwhile, the medial cortex of the femoral shaft can prevent further lateral sliding of the femoral head-neck fragment. Anterior cortical contact after head-neck sliding also can provide a rigid buttress for secondary stability. Considering the nature of the lateral sliding direction of the head-neck fragment, however, biomechanical study demonstrated that the medial cortical support was more important than anterior cortical contact.[33,34] In addition, obtaining both medial and anterior cortical support (anteromedial reduction) is the best option for fracture reduction (Fig. 4). Then the hip loading is distributed between the contact of cortices and the purchase of bone to implant.

Clinical case series demonstrated that patients in positive cortical support reduction group had the least loss in neck-shaft angle and neck length, and got ground-walking much earlier than negative cortex reduction group, with good functional outcomes and less hip–thigh pain presence.[35–37]

Chang's group[32] also proposed a new fracture reduction criterion for unstable pertrochanteric fractures (Table 2). Good quality of fracture reduction includes slight valgus position in alignment and positive medial cortical apposition in displacement (AP view) and central axial alignment with smooth anterior cortex contact (sagittal view).

CHANGES OF FRACTURE REDUCTION AFTER SLIDING AND SECONDARY STABILITY

Anteromedial cortical support reduction is favorable for achieving secondary stability after limited sliding. Little is known, however, about the correlation of accuracy and agreement in reduction quality between intraoperative fluoroscopy and postoperative 3-D–CT reconstruction.

The images from 3-D–CT reconstruction are considered to be accurate and the gold standard for fracture reduction assessments because

Table 1
Comparison of three patterns of cortical apposition between head-neck fragment and femoral shaft

	Positive Cortical Support	Neutral Cortical Support	Negative Cortical Support
Fluoroscopy in AP view	• Head-neck fragment located slightly superomedial to the femoral shaft (≤1 cortex thickness) • Neck-shaft angle valgus alignment	• Head-neck fragment located smoothly to the femoral shaft • Neck-shaft angle anatomic or valgus alignment	• Head-neck fragment displaced laterally to the medial edge of the femoral shaft • Neck-shaft angle varus alignment
Fluoroscopy in lateral view	• The anterior cortex of head-neck fragment located anteriorly to shaft cortex by more than half of the cortex thickness (>2 mm)	• The anterior cortices made a smooth contact or the step-off was less than half of the cortex thickness (≤2 mm)	• The anterior cortex of head-neck fragment located posteriorly by more than half of the cortical thickness (>2 mm)
Reduction quality by fluoroscopy	• Tend to get extramedullary end-to-side medial cortical contact after telescoping • Nonanatomic functional reduction, stable, adequate, satisfied, and acceptable	• Tend to get anatomic end-to-end medial cortical contact or lose contact after sliding and become negative • Ambiguous of 3 subconditions, not truthfully anatomic	• Tend to slide into intramedullary canal, no medial cortical contact • Malreduction, unstable, inadequate, unsatisfied, and unacceptable
Clinical achievability	• Easy to obtain • Secondary stability with impaction after postoperative sliding	• Exact anatomic reduction is difficult to obtain • Primary stability with intraoperative compression	• Inadequate reduction • Head-neck was buttressed by the central nail or lateral wall (cortex or plate), or collapse and failure
3-D–CT full-range view	• End-to-side cortical support at the anteromedial inferior corner	• End-to-end anatomic cortical contact at the anteromedial inferior corner, perfect • Or become negative	• No cortical contact at the anteromedial inferior corner • Head-neck slip into intramedullary canal, varus and posterior sag

they can be rotated 360° to provide a full range of view of the relationship between the head-neck fragment and the femoral shaft. Chang and colleagues[38] in 2018 performed a comparison study in 28 cases of complete intraoperative fluoroscopy and postoperative CT scanning. In the results, true anteromedial cortical contact 3-D–CT (positive and anatomic support) was observed in 18 cases (64.3%). Ten cases had no anteromedial cortical buttress. It was noted that if a positive AP cortical apposition was combined with a positive/neutral lateral cortical apposition seen on intraoperative fluoroscopy (17 cases), it was highly predictive of a reliable value, with definitive cortical support, as demonstrated by postoperative 3-D–CT (15 cases [88.2%]). On the other hand, if a negative lateral apposition was seen on intraoperative fluoroscopy (7 cases), regardless of the AP view, it was generally predictive of a final loss of cortical support, as demonstrated by 3-D–CT (6 cases [85.7%]). The study concluded that combinations of both positive/positive and positive/neutral patterns in AP and lateral fluoroscopy are reliable for predicting final and definitive cortical support, but any negative apposition, especially the anterior cortex on a lateral view (head-neck posterior sag), is highly predictive of postoperative loss of anteromedial cortical contact.

Besides the position between head-neck fragment to femoral shaft, several other factors can interfere the sliding movement and change the final cortical apposition of the anteromedial inferior corner. These may include the ability to

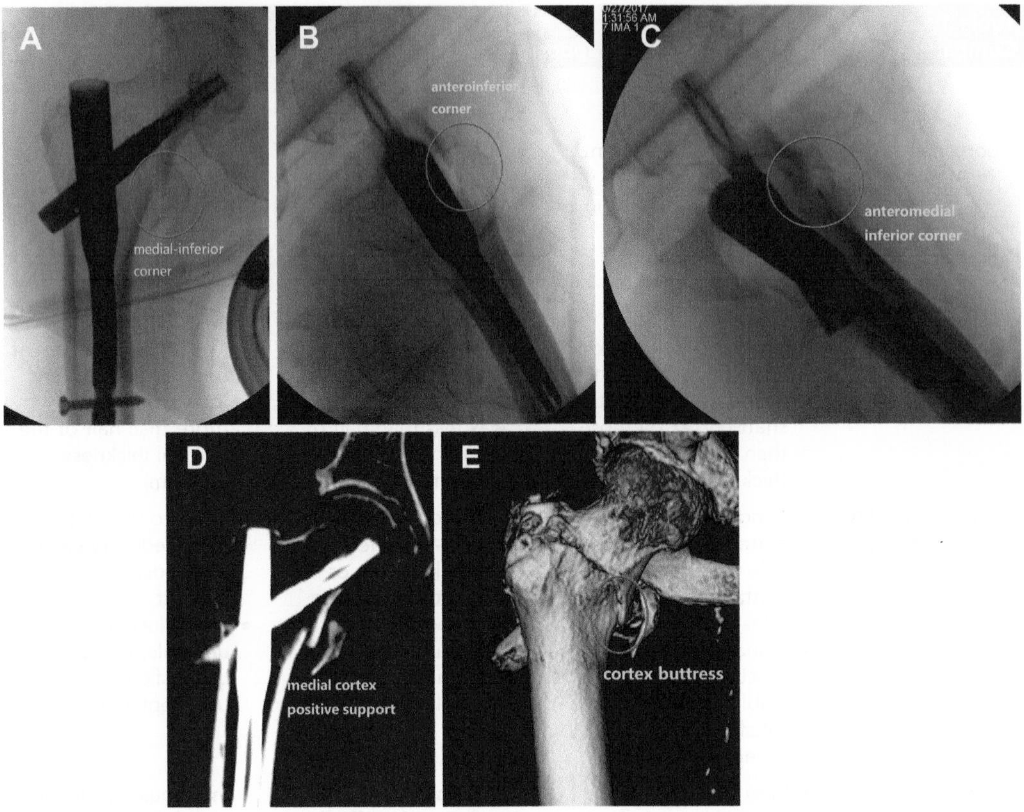

Fig. 4. Positive/neutral cortical apposition of anteromedial inferior corner. (*A*) Intraoperative AP fluoroscopy demonstrated a positive medial cortex apposition. (*B*) Lateral view shows a neutral relation of the anterior cortices. (*C*) Anteromedial oblique view shows smooth cortical apposition of the anteromedial inferior corner. (*D*) Postoperative CT scanning and coronal 2-dimensional reconstruction showed a positive end-to-side medial cortex support. (*E*) 3-D–CT demonstrated a true cortex buttress. Note a slightly flexed rotation of the head-neck fragment resulted in a minor forward shift of the inferior spike, and confirmed stable cortex-to-cortex contact of the anteromedial inferior corner.

initiate head-neck sliding, the direction of sliding, the rotation and/or tilting during sliding, the residual space between head-neck fragment and femoral shaft, and the external rotation of the femoral shaft, which opens a gap and step between the 2 anterior cortices. This unfavorable phenomenon involves more often the elderly patients with severe osteoporosis, because they have remarkably low degrees of implant-bone purchase.

Neither AP nor lateral negative apposition, which needs further corrections during the operation, should be accepted.[39,40] Instrument reduction techniques, such as passing a bone hook through the nail insertion incision proximal to the greater trochanter or a periosteal elevator through the helical blade or cephalomeduallulary screw incision distal to the greater trochanter, is very effective for digging out the posteriorly engaged head-neck fragment by rotational leverage technique.[41]

NAIL ENTRY POINT AND WEDGE-OPEN DEFORMITY

Modern cephalomedullary nails are designed with approximately 5° mediolateral angle in coronal plane, which allows it to be inserted from an easy point of the lateral trochanteric apex rather than the piriformis fossa. Insertion of a thick cephalomedullary nail between the head-neck fragment and the femoral shaft from the greater trochanteric apex makes pressure on both sides, that is, the lateral trochanteric cortex and the medial femoral neck cortex.[42]

In practice, it is ideal to ensure the instrument insertion line (guide wire, reamer, and the nail) and the femoral canal line are coaxial. There are several reasons, however, that may disturb the coaxial line and make it unachievable in some patients. These factors may include (1) the morphologic features of the fracture (some can be reduced only with the hip in abduction),

Table 2
Quality of fracture reduction in unstable pertrochanteric hip fractures

Items	Scores
Garden alignment	
AP view: normal or slight valgus[a]	1
Lateral view: angulation <20°	1
Fragment displacement of head-neck	
AP view: positive or neutral medial cortex apposition	1
Lateral view: smooth continuity of anterior cortex	1
Quality of fracture reduction	
Good	4
Acceptable	3
Poor	≤2

[a] Slight valgus means the valgus angle of no more than 10°.

Adapted from Chang SM, Zhang YQ, Ma Z, et al. Fracture reduction with positive medial cortical support: a key element in stability reconstruction for the unstable pertrochanteric hip fractures. Arch Orthop Trauma Surg 2015;135(6):817; with permission.

(2) the stiff spine in geriatric patients, (3) the soft tissue mass (fat and muscle) around the hip, (4) the operative drapes, (5) the location of skin incision and its size, and (6) the laterally oriented operating trajectory of the side-standing surgeon. Ignoring any of these factors can result in a shift of the ideal trochanteric entry point, gradual enlargement in the lateral direction, failure to remove the superolateral hard cortex crest of the femoral neck, production of an inadequate path not accommodating the large proximal diameter of the nail resulting in a wedge effect (head-neck varus rotation), an open effect (shaft lateralization), or a combination of the 2, a wedge-open effect.[43] A laterally enlarged oval hole combined with the existing trochanteric fracture line leads to more lateral placement of the intramedullary nail than intended.[44]

To avoid lateralization, a special maneuver can be taken to move the entry point slightly medial (approximately 5 mm) from the trochanteric tip, near the medial wall of the greater trochanter. Compared with anatomic measurement in intact femurs, slight medial reaming in fracture operations has several advantages: (1) it allows the desired removal of hard superolateral femoral neck bone, preventing medial abutment and thus reducing the risk of varus redisplacement of the proximal head-neck fragment or a high lag screw/helical blade position in the femoral head, both of which are undesirable[45]; (2) it provides adequate space for nail insertion, preventing a wedge-opening effect between the head-neck fragment and the shaft fragment; and (3) it provides a well-aligned tube after reaming for nail insertion, avoiding pressure on the trochanteric lateral cortex, nail-cortex impingement, or even lateral wall rupture.

Several techniques have been introduced to avoid wedge-open deformity, including temporary over-distraction of the femoral shaft before proximal reaming, protection of the softer greater trochanter by insertion of a metallic plate, using a cannulated drill or trephine reamer, and drilling a percutaneous threaded guide wire to the femoral neck as a clamp.[46–48] There usually is no space for other instruments, however, in a short stab incision (approximately 3 cm) for nail insertion. Using the best of the reamer protection sleeve is essential. In practice, a modified protection sleeve with medial deflection can effectively solve the problem (Fig. 5).

The threshold leading to implant failure may be varus malalignment greater than 5° and/or opening distance between head-neck and shaft greater than 5 mm.[49] Slight opening with 1 cortex thickness, however, is acceptable or preferable, because it provides a tendency for positive support of the medial cortex after impaction by telescoping. Minor wedge-open effect leads to minimal discrepancy compared with the contralateral intact femur and has no negative influence on fracture healing and patient recovery.

TIP-APEX DISTANCE AND CALCAR-REFERENCED TIP-APEX DISTANCE

Tip-apex distance (TAD), the distance between the screw tip and femoral head apex, was proposed by Baumgaertner and colleagues[31] in 1995 as a predictor of the risk of lag screw cutout. It was recommended that the implants should be placed central and deep both in the AP and lateral radiographs, in order to achieve a TAD of less than 25 mm. Clinical practice demonstrated, however, that positioning the lag screw inferiorly in the head and neck would also produce a stable fixation as a central–central positioning, although the TAD would be greater than 25 mm. Kuzyk and colleagues[50] in 2012 reported that TAD referenced from the calcar (Cal-TAD) also was an effective predictor of lag screw cutout.

Using mathematical simulation, Li and colleagues[51] performed a theoretic comparison of

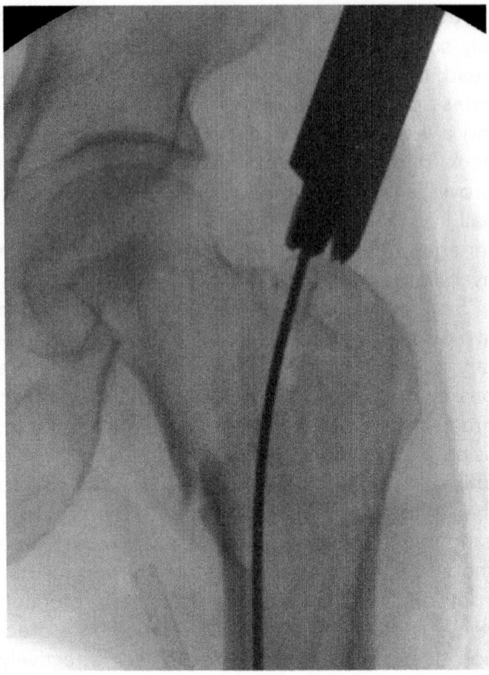

Fig. 5. Using a medial deflected reamer protection sleeve can effectively remove the hard crest of the superolateral neck cortex and produce an optimal nail entry portal.

TAD and Cal-TAD, which allowed for an accurate evaluation of the differences in plots calculated by the TAD formula and the Cal-TAD formula. The results showed there was more volume for the screw to be placed in the larger heads and the Cal-TAD provided a much larger "suitable zone" for screw positioning than the TAD. Positioning the lag screw should address geometric effects of both TAD and femoral head size, with an emphasis on measuring the position of the screw tip for the suitable zone by volume ratio. The 25-mm TAD cutoff value should be adjusted according to the individual femoral head size.

The essence of TAD is to put the implant in the dense trabecula of the femoral head to enhance its grasp. In clinical practice, the authors prefer to apply the concept of Cal-TAD to put the lag screw/helical blade in the middle-lower third of the femoral head (Table 3). This not only positions the implant in dense trabecula but also leaves more distance for the implants shift because they usually move to the upward direction. Moreover, a deeper insertion of the nail reduced the nail-tail protrusion over the greater trochanter.

FEMORAL ANTERIOR CURVATURE AND NAIL ADAPTATION

Asian people usually have a shorter stature (body height), with a smaller trochanteric area, a narrower intramedullary canal, and a larger anterior curvature of the femoral shaft. To cope with the differences in size and geometry, fixation instruments, especially the intramedullary nails, should be accordingly adapted, with modifications to reduce the presence of mismatch.[52]

While inserting a straight short nail ($\leq$24 cm in length) into the femoral canal, mismatch may occur between the nail and the anterior bow of the femur, which is manifested as impingement between the nail-tip and the anterior cortex and the over-protrusion of the proximal nail-tail outside the greater trochanter.

Table 3
Pros and cons of inferiorly implant seating in femoral head

Advantages	1. Accepts the concept of Cal-TAD 2. Favors valgus reduction of the head-neck fragment 3. Puts the implants in the dense compression trabecula of femoral head, also with a greater implant-bone grasp 4. Leaves more distance for implant shift to the upward direction to prevent cutout 5. Decreases the opportunity of iatrogenic lateral wall rupture in A1/2 pertrochanteric fractures by leaving more distance from fracture line to helical blade/lag screw entry portal 6. Reduces nail-tail protrusion over the greater trochanter by deeper nail insertion, which can be compensated by different height caps 7. Enhances fixation stability in type A3 fractures by deeper insertion of the thicker proximal nail segment
Disadvantages	1. The head-neck implant is not as deep as that in central position 2. The implant is not coaxial central with the axis of femoral head-neck 3. Possible rotation of the head-neck fragment on the implant after early weight bearing, causing head-neck rotation in flexed direction

Anterior entry point nailing has been advocated to avoid nail-tip abutment. For the most commonly used proximal femur nail antirotation (PFNA)-II of size 20 cm in length and 10 mm in distal diameter, however, Chang and colleagues[53] found the presence of distal tip-cortex impingement in 40% cases in an Asian population. In Hispanic Colombians, the anterior cortical impingement rate was reported to be as high as 70%.[54] Moreover, Hu and colleagues[55] reported proximal nail-tail protrusion in PFNA-II over the greater trochanter (>5 mm in 60.8% of cases) to cause lateral hip pain or greater trochanter syndrome.

The full-length femur has an anterior bowing with an average of $10.6° \pm 1.8°$. The radius of the full-length femur varies in different reports, ranging from 110 cm to 145 cm. Elderly Asian women usually have an even shorter radius, which means a greater femoral anterior bowing.[56–58] Chapman and colleagues[59] divided the femur into 4 segments in 3-D–CT images and found that the greatest degree of curvature was in the distal segment (mean 4.5°), followed by the proximal (mean 4.4°), proximal intermediate (mean 3.7°), and distal intermediate (mean 1.8°) segments. There also is a lateral bowing of the femur in the coronal plane, usually less than 3°, but approximately 10% of people may have a lateral curvature greater than 3°.

For better compatibility between the short cephalomedullary nail and the femur in Asians, Zhang and colleagues[60] made further adaptations in three aspects, and designed a short curved femoral intertrochanteric nail (FITN) (**Fig. 6**). (1) The proximal segment was 16.5 mm in diameter and 90 mm in length from the turning point of 4° valgus angle. (2) The distal segment was 105 mm in length and available in 9 mm and 10 mm in diameter. The distal segment was built with an anterior curvature (radius = 110 cm). (3) The distal 3 cm of nail-tip was opened in a cross-slot for further accommodations to the anterior and/or lateral bowing of the femur. Proximal nail-tail caps are available in 3 different heights: 0 mm, 5 mm, and 10 mm. The angle of helical blade was set at 130°. Compared with the short straight PFNA-II, the proximal segment of the newly adapted FITN was shortened by 5 mm in length and the oblique hole for helical blade insertion was moved 3 mm further to the proximal direction (thus, total 8 mm), to solve the problem of nail-tail over-protrusion. The distal segment was bent backward by 2.0 mm (20% of distal nail diameter) in 195-mm long nails to avoid tip impingement.

Chang and colleagues[61] reported the first 50 cases in clinical usage. For the distal nail-tip position, 32 cases (64%) were located along the central canal axis, 13 cases (26%) were located anteriorly but did not contact the anterior inner cortex, 2 cases (4%) showed less than one-third anterior cortex thickness contact, and 3 cases (6%) were located posteriorly with no cortex contact. For the proximal nail-tail level, there were no protrusions over the greater trochanter in 15 cases (30%), protrusion of less than 5 mm in 29 cases (58%), and protrusion of more than 5 mm in 6 cases (12%). The compatibility of this new adaptation was very high, because 96% cases showed no tip-cortex contact, and 88% cases showed less than 5 mm proximal tail protrusion (**Fig. 7**). This newly adapted FIT nail has been implanted more than 130 patients as of August 2019.

LONG NAILS FOR WIDE MEDULLARY CANAL AND LARGE POSTERIOR CORONAL FRAGMENT

Proximal antegrade femoral nails can be classified into short (inserted not over the femoral

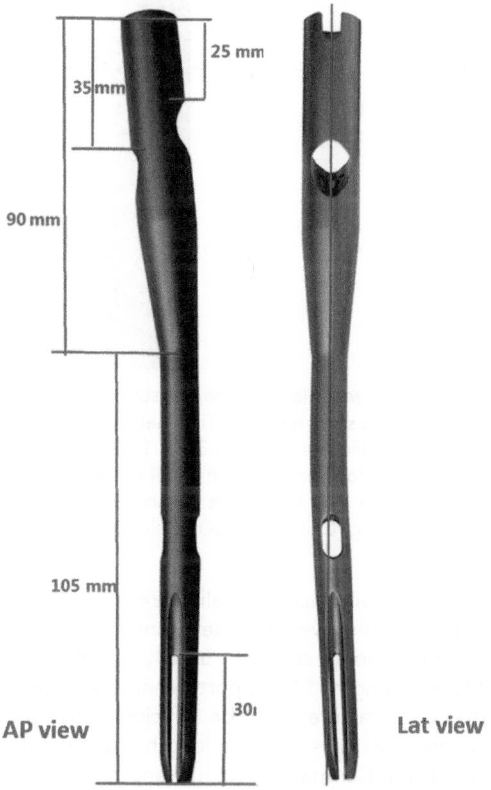

Fig. 6. The new adapted fitn, manufactured by Beijing BEST Bio-Technical Co. Ltd, China. (*Courtesy of* Beijing BEST Bio-Technical Co. Ltd, Beijing, China; with permission.)

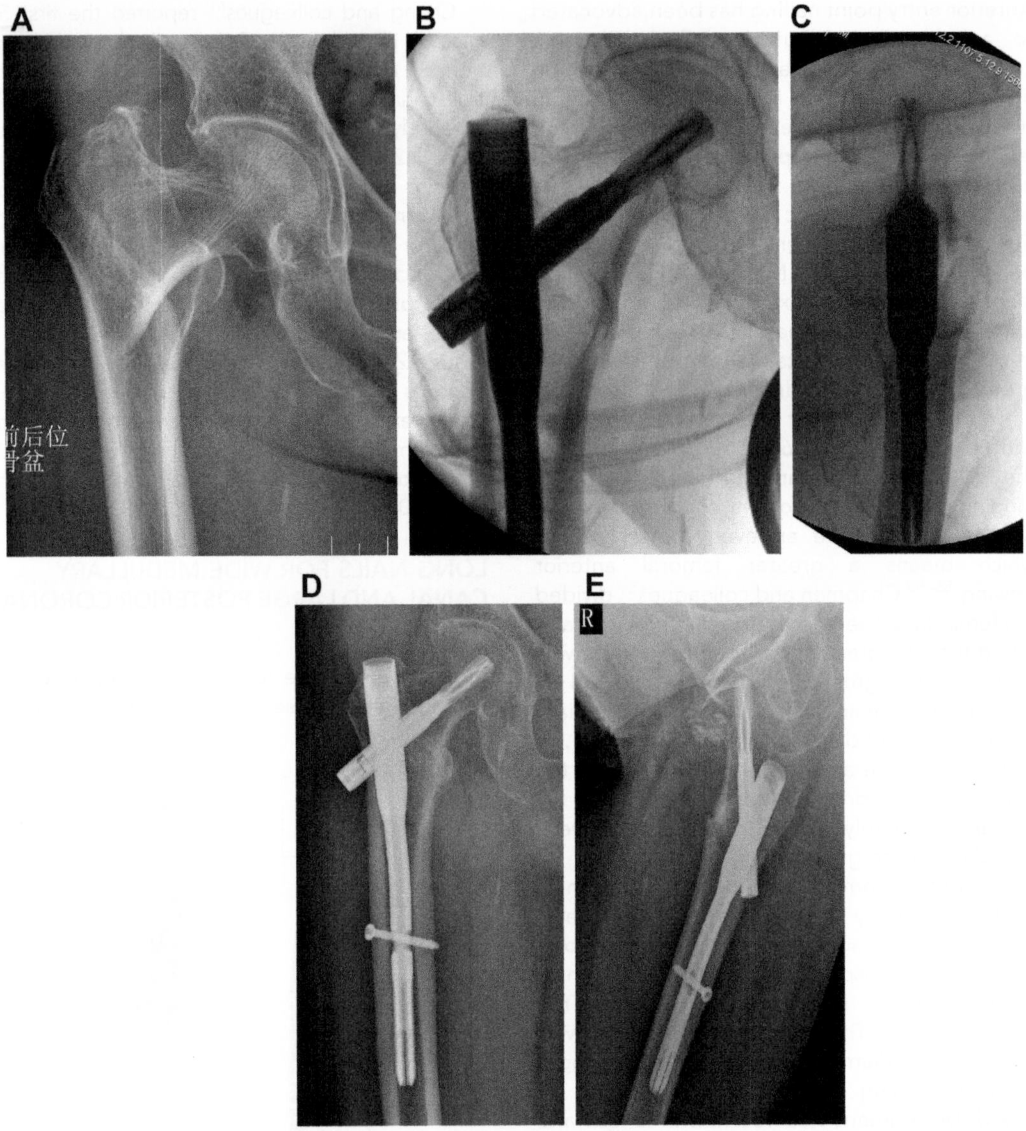

Fig. 7. An 85-year-old Asian woman suffered unstable pertrochanteric fracture of her right hip that stabilized with a novel adapted short nail, the FITN that is manufactured by Beijing BEST Bio-Technical Co. Ltd, China. (*A*) The fracture was classified as AO/OTA 31A2.1. (*B, C*) AP and lateral views in intraoperative fluoroscopy. Note, there were no proximal protrusion of the nail-tail and no distal cortex impingement of the nail-tip. (*D, E*) Postoperative radiographs 1 week after head-neck telescoping and fracture impaction. ([*B–E*] *Courtesy of* Beijing BEST Bio-Technical Co. Ltd, Beijing, China; with permission.)

anterior bowing apex, usually <24 cm), intermediate (inserted over the apex), and full (inserted to the femoral condyle, usually greater than 300 mm) length.[62] Most pertrochanteric/intertrochanteric fractures can be efficiently fixed by normal short nails (working length approximately 15–18 cm). Compared with full-length nails, short nails have a low reoperation rate while significantly decreasing operative time, radiation exposure dose, and estimated blood loss with the additional benefit of being cost effective.[63–65]

From a mechanical point of view, however, there are some specific patterns that require full-length nail. These may include the revision surgery of short nails, pathologic fractures, type A3 intertrochanteric fractures (primary lateral wall rupture), pertrochanteric fractures with subtrochanteric extension (such as A2.3), large coronal fracture of the lateral wall cortex, and wider proximal medullary canal.

In the setting of an extremely wide proximal canal diameter, adequate stability may not be

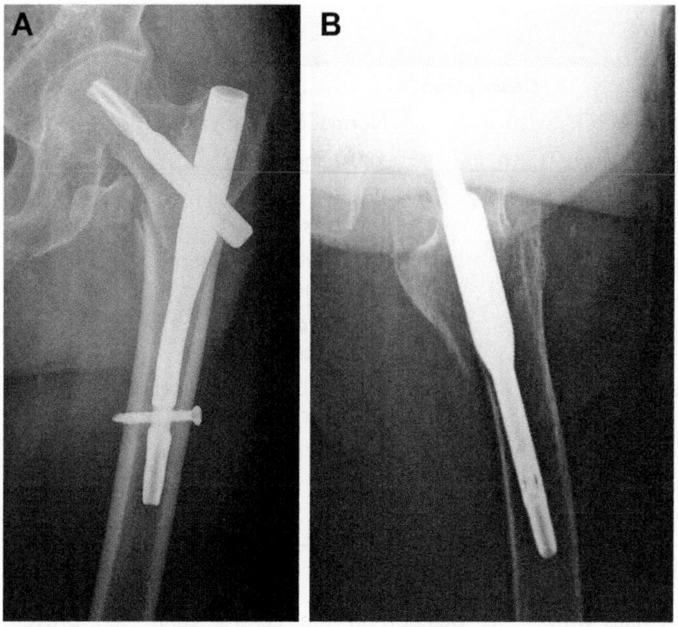

Fig. 8. An extrashort cephalomedullary nail (17 cm in length) in a wide proximal medullary canal; toggle movement resulted in negative cortex apposition in both medial and anterior aspects. (*A*) AP view. The distal nail-tip was shifted laterally by loading, thus resulted in an overall varus alignment. (*B*) Lateral view. The distal nail-tip swayed anteriorly.

achievable with a short nail fixation. There is potentially a pendulum-like movement of short nail in a capacious medullary canal. The distal interlocking screw acts as a pivot point, leading to proximal nail toggle back and forth, in both coronal and sagittal directions. This phenomenon

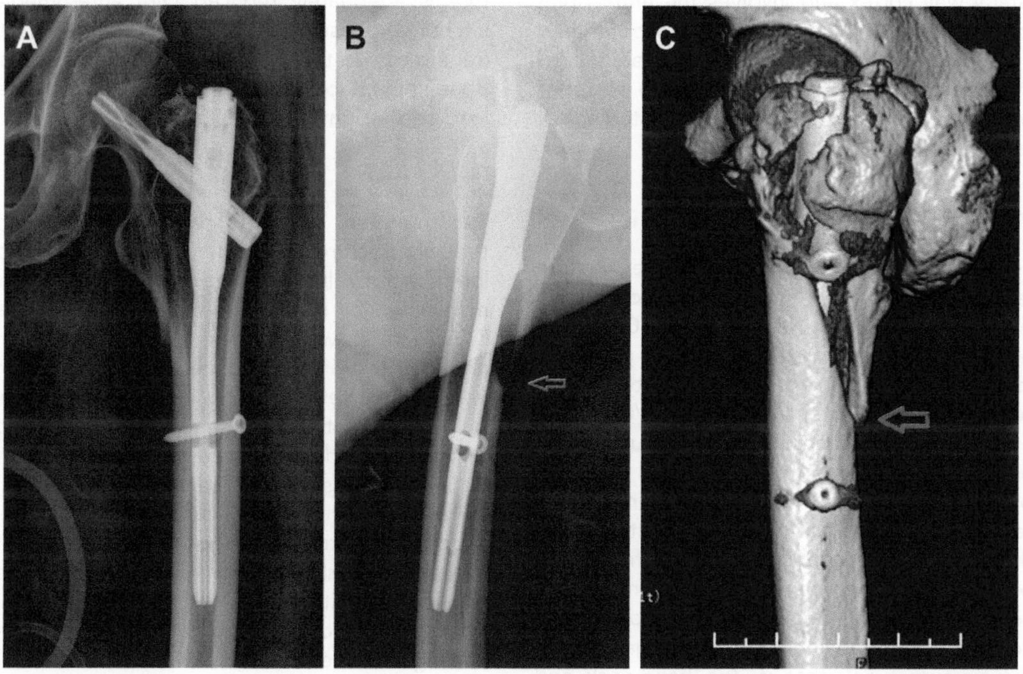

Fig. 9. Pertrochanteric A2.3 fracture with a large posterior coronal banana-like fragment involving greater trochanter, posterior crest, and lesser trochanter extending to the subtrochanteric region. The fracture was fixed with a normal-sized short nail (BEST FITN with 19.5 cm in length and 10 mm in diameter). (*A*, *B*) Postoperative AP and lateral radiographs. The distal nail-tip shifted anteriorly and abutted with the cortex. (*C*) Postoperative 3-D–CT demonstrated that the helical blade passed through the coronal fracture line on the lateral wall cortex. There was a coronal instability. ([*A*, *B*] *Courtesy of* Beijing BEST Bio-Technical Co. Ltd, Beijing, China; with permission.)

Table 4
Postoperative stability score

		Description		Score
Fracture reduction quality	Garden alignment	AP view	Normal or slight valgus[a]	1
		Lateral view	180°, angulation <20°	1
	Anteromedial cortex apposition	AP view	Positive or neutral medial cortex support	1
		Lateral view	Anterior cortex smooth continuity	1
Surgical technique	Implant seating position	AP view	Central or lower third, accept TAD or Cal-TAD	1
		Lateral view	Central or minor posterior, Parker ratio 40%–50%	1
Using intramedullary nail		Central occupation of medullary canal, metallic lateral wall		1
Postoperative lateral wall intact		Counterweight balance		1
Good: 8 points; acceptable: 6–7 points; poor: ≤5 points				

[a] Slight valgus means the valgus angle of no more than 10°.

is especially prominent for extrashort nails with very shorter nail-tip length distal to the interlocking screw (Fig. 8).

If the lesser trochanter fragment extends proximally to the greater trochanter and distally to the subtrochanteric region, it forms a large coronal fragment that runs over the midline on lateral wall cortex and involves the entry point for head-neck implant. There is also potentially a pendulum-like movement if short nail is used in a pertrochanteric fracture with large posterior banana-like fragment, leading to instability at least in the coronal plane (Fig. 9).

POSTOPERATIVE STABILITY SCORE

For the stability of reconstructions after fracture reduction and fixation, 5 influencing factors have been summarized by Kaufer[66] in 1980, that is, bone quality (osteoporosis), fragment geometry (comminution), fracture reduction quality, implant selection, and implant placement (TAD/Cal-TAD).

As the preconditioning factor, fracture reduction is the first step in treatment and always is paramount compared with other factors.[67] After reduction and internal fixation, the stability of the pertrochanteric/intertrochanteric fracture is primarily dependent on the attainment of firm contact between the anterior and/or medial cortices of the 2 major fragments (regardless of the fracture type), that is, the head-neck and femoral shaft. In addition, the placement of the internal fixation device also is important in relation to its seating position in reference to the femoral head. Furthermore, the use of an intramedullary nail also plays a major role, because its position in the central canal can prevent head-neck fragment from over-sliding and provide a rigid metal buttress. Otherwise, when a side plate is used, the head-neck fragment needs to slide more distance to reach the lateral wall (natural cortex or metallic plate) to get a mechanical buttress. In the authors' opinion, if the fracture is adequately reduced with anteromedial inferior cortex support and sustained by implants (regardless of the type used), then the overall bone-implant construct is stable and can bear load and weight bearing (Table 4).[3,68]

SUMMARY

The treatment of pertrochanteric/intertrochanteric hip fractures has undergone favorable evolution and revolution during the past 20 years, as manifested by new technical concepts, such as TAD, lateral wall, cortex support reduction, and the instrument success of intramedullary nailing. This review article identifies what may be crucial in determining the stability reconstruction and provides guidance regarding technical details that assist in decreasing postoperative complications. Anteromedial cortex-to-cortex support reduction is a key element, because it allows limited sliding to provide both good mechanical stability to share the loads from the implant and biological environment for fracture healing to achieve better clinical outcomes.

ACKNOWLEDGMENT

The authors would like to thank Dr. Ying-Qi Zhang, Dr. Shuang Li and Dr. Wen-Feng Xiong for their contributions in this topic during their doctoral degree program.

DISCLOSURE

The authors do not have any conflicts of interest, financial or otherwise, relevant to the material presented in this article.

REFERENCES

1. Waddell JP. Fractures of the proximal femur: improving outcomes. Philadelphia: Elsevier Saunders; 2011.
2. Egol KA, Leucht P. Proximal femur fractures: an evidence-based approach to evaluation and management. Switzerland: Springer; 2018.
3. Chang SM. Geriatric intertrochanteric hip fractures. Beijing (China): Science Publisher; 2019 [In Chinese].
4. Kanis IA, Oden A, McCloskey EV, et al. A systematic review of hip fracture incidence and probability of fracture worldwide. Osteoporos Int 2012;23:2239–56.
5. Hagino H, Furukawa K, Fujiwara S, et al. Recent trends in the incidence and lifetime risk of hip fracture in Tottori, Japan. Osteoporos Int 2009;20:543–8.
6. Orwig DL, Chan J, Magaziner J. Hip fracture and its consequences: differences between men and women. Orthop Clin North Am 2006;37:611–22.
7. Della Rocca GJ, Crist BD. Hip fracture protocols: what have we changed? Orthop Clin North Am 2013;44:163–82.
8. Mäkinen TJ, Gunton M, Fichman SG, et al. Arthroplasty for Pertrochanteric Hip Fractures. Orthop Clin North Am 2015;46:433–44.
9. Niu E, Yang A, Harris AH, et al. Which fixation device is preferred for surgical treatment of intertrochanteric hip fractures in the United States? A survey of orthopaedic surgeons. Clin Orthop Relat Res 2015;473:3647–55.
10. Zhang YQ, Chang SM, Xiong WF, et al. Fracture mapping of proximal femoral lateral wall. Chin J Clin Anat 2017;35:121–5 [in Chinese].
11. Li J, Tang S, Zhang H, et al. Clustering of morphological fracture lines for identifying intertrochanteric fracture classification with Hausdorff distance-based K-means approach. Injury 2019;50:939–49.
12. Gotfried Y. The lateral trochanteric wall: a key element in the reconstruction of unstable pertrochanteric hip fractures. Clin Orthop Relat Res 2004;425:82–6.
13. Palm H, Jacobsen S, Sonne-Holm S, et al. Integrity of the lateral femoral wall in pertrochanteric hip fractures: an important predictor of a reoperation. J Bone Joint Surg Am 2007;89A:470–5.
14. Haq RU, Manhas V, Pankaj A, et al. Proximal femoral nails compared with reverse distal femoral locking plates in intertrochanteric fractures with a compromised lateral wall, a randomised controlled trial. Int Orthop 2014;38:1443–9.
15. Ma Z, Chang SM. Where is the lateral femoral wall? Int Orthop 2014;38:2645–6.
16. Sun LL, Li Q, Chang SM. The thickness of proximal lateral femoral wall. Injury 2016;47:784–5.
17. Hsu CE, Chiu YC, Tsai SH, et al. Trochanter stabilising plate improves treatment outcomes in AO/OTA 31-A2 intertrochanteric fractures with critical thin femoral lateral walls. Injury 2015;46:1047–53.
18. Kellam JF, Meinberg EG, Agel J, et al. Fracture and Dislocation Classification Compendium-2018: International Comprehensive Classification of Fractures and Dislocations Committee. J Orthop Trauma 2018;32:S1–170.
19. Cho JW, Kent WT, Yoon YC, et al. Fracture morphology of AO/OTA 31-A trochanteric fractures: a 3D CT study with an emphasis on coronal fragments. Injury 2017;48:277–84.
20. Chang SM, Ma Z, Du SC, et al. Anatomic study on the proximal femoral lateral wall and its clinical implications for geriatric intertrochanteric fractures. Chin J Clin Anat 2016;34:39–44 [in Chinese].
21. Ma Z, Yao XZ, Chang SM. The classification of intertrochanteric fractures based on the integrity of lateral femoral wall: Letter to the editor, Fracture morphology of AO/OTA 31-A trochanteric fractures: A 3D CT study with an emphasis on coronal fragments. Injury 2017;48:2367–8.
22. Futamura K, Baba T, Homma Y, et al. New classification focusing on the relationship between the attachment of the iliofemoral ligament and the course of the fracture line for intertrochanteric fractures. Injury 2016;47:1685–91.
23. Gao Z, Lv Y, Zhou F, et al. Risk factors for implant failure after fixation of proximal femoral fractures with fracture of the lateral femoral wall. Injury 2018;49:315–22.
24. Kim Y, Bahk WJ, Yoon YC, et al. Radiologic healing of lateral femoral wall fragments after intramedullary nail fixation for A3.3 intertrochanteric fractures. Arch Orthop Trauma Surg 2015;135:1349–56.
25. Do JH, Kim YS, Lee SJ, et al. Influence of fragment volume on stability of 3-part intertrochanteric fracture of the femur: a biomechanical study. Eur J Orthop Surg Traumatol 2013;23:371–7.
26. Marmor M, Liddle K, Pekmezci M, et al. The effect of fracture pattern stability on implant loading in OTA type 31-A2 proximal femur fractures. J Orthop Trauma 2013;27:683–9.
27. Xiong WF, Zhang YQ, Chang SM, et al. Lesser trochanteric fragments in unstable pertrochanteric hip fractures: a morphological study using three-dimensional computed tomography (3-D CT) reconstruction. Med Sci Monitor 2019;25:2049–57.

28. Sharma G, Gn KK, Khatri K, et al. Morphology of the posteromedial fragment in pertrochanteric fractures: A three-dimensional computed tomography analysis. Injury 2017;48:419–31.
29. Ehrnthaller C, Olivier AC, Gebhard F, et al. The role of lesser trochanter fragment in unstable pertrochanteric A2 proximal femur fractures - is refixation of the lesser trochanter worth the effort? Clin Biomech (Bristol, Avon) 2016;42:31–7.
30. Kim GM, Nam KW, Seo KB, et al. Wiring technique for lesser trochanter fixation in proximal IM nailing of unstable intertrochanteric fractures: A modified candy-package wiring technique. Injury 2017;48: 406–13.
31. Baumgaertner MR, Curtin SL, Lindskog DM, et al. The value of the tip-apex distance in predicting failure of fixation of peritrochanteric fracture fixation. J Bone Joint Surg Am 1995;77:1058–64.
32. Chang SM, Zhang YQ, Ma Z, et al. Fracture reduction with positive medial cortical support: a key element in stability reconstruction for the unstable pertrochanteric hip fractures. Arch Orthop Trauma Surg 2015;135:811–8.
33. Li S, Sun GX, Chang SM, et al. Simulated postoperative weight-bearing after fixation of a severe osteoporotic intertrochanteric fracture. Int J Clin Exp Med 2017;10:8544–54.
34. Li S, Chang SM, Zhang LZ, et al. Effects of reduction with different anterior and medial cortical supports on stability after intramedullary nailing for unstable intertrochanteric fractures: a biomechanical comparison. Chin J Orthop Trauma 2019;21:57–64 [in Chinese].
35. Cho MR, Lee JH, Kwon JB, et al. The Effect of Positive Medial Cortical Support in Reduction of Pertrochanteric Fractures with Posteromedial Wall Defect Using a Dynamic Hip Screw. Clin Orthop Surg 2018;10:292–8.
36. Ramachandran K, Manoj KKA, Sankar AV. Critical analysis of factors determining mechanical failures in proximal femoral nailing. Int J Res Orthop 2019;5:275–82.
37. Li J, Zhang L, Zhang H, et al. Effect of reduction quality on post-operative outcomes in 31-A2 intertrochanteric fractures following intramedullary fixation: a retrospective study based on computerised tomography findings. Int Orthop 2018;43:1951–9.
38. Chang SM, Zhang YQ, Du SC, et al. Anteromedial cortical support reduction in unstable pertrochanteric fractures: a comparison of intra-operative fluoroscopy and post-operative three dimensional computerised tomography reconstruction. Int Orthop 2018;42:183–9.
39. Tsukada S, Okumura G, Matsueda M. Postoperative stability on lateral radiographs in the surgical treatment of pertrochanteric hip fractures. Arch Orthop Trauma Surg 2012;132:839–46.
40. Kozono N, Ikemura S, Yamashita A, et al. Direct reduction may need to be considered to avoid postoperative subtype-P in patients with an unstable trochanteric fracture: a retrospective study using a multivariate analysis. Arch Orthop Trauma Surg 2014;134:1649–54.
41. Kim Y, Dheep K, Lee J, et al. Hook leverage technique for reduction of intertrochanteric fracture. Injury 2014;45:1006–10.
42. O'Malley MJ, Kang KK, Azer E, et al. Wedge effect following intramedullary hip screw fixation of intertrochanteric proximal femur fracture. Arch Orthop Trauma Surg 2015;135:1343–7.
43. Tao YL, Ma Z, Chang SM. Does PFNA II avoid lateral cortex impingement for unstable peritrochanteric fractures? Clin Orthop Relat Res 2013;471:1393–4.
44. Prasarn ML, Cattaneo MD, Achor T, et al. The effect of entry point on malalignment and iatrogenic fracture with the Synthes lateral entry femoral nail. J Orthop Trauma 2010;24:224–9.
45. Xu Z, Zhang M, Yin J, et al. Redisplacement after reduction with intramedullary nails in surgery of intertrochanteric fracture: cause analysis and preventive measures. Arch Orthop Trauma Surg 2015;135:751–8.
46. Hak DJ, Bilat C. Avoiding varusmalreduction during cephalomedullary nailing of intertrochanteric hip fractures. Arch Orthop Trauma Surg 2011;131:709–10.
47. Butler BA, Selley RS, Summers HD, et al. Preventing wedge deformities when treating intertrochanteric femur fractures with intramedullary devices: A technical tip. J Orthop Trauma 2018;32:e112–6.
48. Maupin JJ, Steinmetz RG, Hickerson LE. A percutaneous threaded wire as a clamp technique for avoiding wedge deformity while nailing intertrochanteric femur fractures. J Orthop Trauma 2019;33:e276–9.
49. Chon CS, Kang B, Kim HS, et al. Implications of three-dimensional modeling of the proximal femur for cephalomedullary nailing: An Asian cadaver study. Injury 2017;48:2060–7.
50. Kuzyk PR, Zdero R, Shah S, et al. Femoral head lag screw position for cephalomedullary nails: a biomechanical analysis. J Orthop Trauma 2012;26:414–21.
51. Li S, Chang SM, Jin YM, et al. A mathematical simulation of the tip-apex distance and the calcar-referenced tip-apex distance for intertrochanteric fractures reduced with lag screws. Injury 2016;47: 1302–8.
52. Sawaguchi T, Sakagoshi D, Shima Y, et al. Do design adaptations of a trochanteric nail make sense for Asian patients? Results of a multicenter study of the PFNA-II in Japan. Injury 2014;45:1624–31.
53. Chang SM, Song DL, Ma Z, et al. Mismatch of short straight cephalomedullary nail (PFNA-II) with the anterior bow of the femur in Asian population. J Orthop Trauma 2014;28:17–22.

54. Peña OR, Gómez Gélvez A, Espinosa KA, et al. Cephalomedullary nails: factors associated with impingement of the anterior cortex of the femur in a hispanic population. Arch Orthop Trauma Surg 2015;135:1533–40.
55. Hu SJ, Chang SM, Ma Z, et al. PFNA-II proximal end protrusion over the greater trochanter in the Asian population: a postoperative radiographic study. Indian J Orthop 2016;50:641–6.
56. Zhang S, Zhang K, Wang Y, et al. Using three-dimensional computational modeling to compare the geometrical fitness of two kinds of proximal femoral intramedullary nail for Chinese femur. Scientific World J 2013;2013:978485.
57. Su XY, Zhao Z, Zhao JX, et al. Three-dimensional analysis of the curvature of the femoral canal in 426 Chinese femurs. Biomed Res Int 2015;2015: 318391.
58. Abdelaal AH, Yamamoto N, Hayashi K, et al. Radiological assessment of the femoral bowing in Japanese population. SICOT J 2016;2:2.
59. Chapman T, Sholukha V, Semal P, et al. Femoral curvature variability in modern humans using three-dimensional quadric surface fitting. Surg Radiol Anat 2015;37:1169–77.
60. Zhang S, Zhang Y, Hu S, et al. Imaging study on design and geometric match of a new type of short femoral intertrochanteric nail with anterior curvature. Chin J Repair Reconstr Surg 2016;30:1200–4 [in Chinese].
61. Chang SM, Hu SJ, Ma Z, et al. Femoral intertrochanteric nail (fitn): a new short version design with an anterior curvature and a geometric match study using postoperative radiographs. Injury 2018;49:328–33.
62. Baldwin PC 3rd, Lavender RC, Sanders R, et al. Controversies in intramedullary fixation for intertrochanteric hip fractures. J Orthop Trauma 2016;30: 635–41.
63. Hou Z, Bowen TR, Irgit KS, et al. Treatment of pertrochanteric fractures (OTA 31-A1 and A2): long versus short cephalomedullary nailing. J Orthop Trauma 2013;27:318–24.
64. Horwitz DS, Tawari A, Suk M. Nail Length in the Management of Intertrochanteric Fracture of the Femur. J Am Acad Orthop Surg 2016;24:e50–8.
65. Zhang Y, Zhang S, Wang S, et al. Long and short intramedullary nails for fixation of intertrochanteric femur fractures (OTA 31-A1, A2 and A3): A systematic review and meta-analysis. Orthop Traumatol Surg Res 2017;103:685–90.
66. Kaufer H. Mechanics of the treatment of hip injuries. Clin Orthop Relat Res 1980;146:53–61.
67. Haidukewych GJ. Intertrochanteric fractures: ten tips to improve results. J Bone Joint Surg Am 2009;91:712–9.
68. Zhang S, Hu S, Du S, et al. Concept evolution and research progress of stability reconstruction for intertrochanteric fracture. Chin J Repair Reconstr Surg 2019;33:1203–9 [in Chinese].

Pediatrics

The Burden of Pediatric Musculoskeletal Diseases Worldwide

Richard M. Schwend, MD

KEYWORDS

• Global burden of disease • Disability-adjusted life year • Years of life lived with a disability • Cost effective analysis • Surgery • Pediatric orthopedics • Musculoskeletal impairment

KEY POINTS

- Global burden of disease has a variety of definitions and meanings, but in general it refers to the economic and human costs resulting from poor health.
- The disability-adjusted life year is a measure of life lost from premature death and life not lived at 100% health and is the preferred metric to compare the health burden of various dissimilar diseases in populations.
- Because children will have many years lived with a disability, and surgical treatment early has been proven to be cost effective, resources should be provided for their early treatment.
- Recommendations from the Global Initiative for Children's Surgery have been made for optimizing children's surgical care.

INTRODUCTION

One-half of the world's population lack access to primary or surgical care.[1] Two-thirds lack access to orthopedic care. Only 10% of global health resources are provided for conditions that represent 90% of the global burden of disease (GBD). Surgery has long been neglected in the distribution of resources for global health. Approximately 30% of the global burden of disease (GBD) is from surgical treatable conditions. More than one-third of the world's population live in low-income countries (LIC), but they receive only 3.5% of the world's surgical care.[2] The Lancet Commission on Global Surgery reported that 5 billion people do not have access to safe and affordable surgical and anesthesia care, most of whom live in low-resource settings, with up to 50% being children.[3] The surgical burden of trauma and infections worldwide is related to falls, motor vehicle collisions (MVCs), war-related causes, iatrogenic causes, and nutrition.[1] With greater life expectancy globally, modernization through road traffic, and mechanization of the work environment, high-energy trauma is creating surgical challenges in children and working adults that can affect families through many generations.

GLOBAL BURDEN OF DISEASE

Burden of disease has a variety of definitions and meanings, but in general it refers to the economic and human costs resulting from poor health. The World Health Organization (WHO) measures global burden of disease (GBD) using standard methodology including the disability-adjusted life year (DALY), years lived with a disability (YLD), years of life lost (YLL), and life expectancy. The DALY metric was first developed in 1990 to better describe the burden of disease in a consistent manner across diseases, risk factors, and regions.[4] The DALY is a metric that quantifies the (financial) burden of disease, injuries, and health risk factors into a single measurement.[5] It is a measure of life lost from premature death and life lived not at 100% health. The formula is:

Department of Orthopaedic Surgery and Musculoskeletal Sciences, Children's Mercy Hospital, 2401 Gillham Road, Kansas City, MO 64112, USA
E-mail address: rmschwend@cmh.edu

Orthop Clin N Am 51 (2020) 207–217
https://doi.org/10.1016/j.ocl.2019.11.005

DALYx = YLLx + YLDx
DALYx = DALY for a particular condition x
YLLx = YLL due to premature death caused by that condition
YLDx = years of life lived with disability

This method may be used by countries in their health situation assessment and financial allocation for a variety of health-related conditions. For example, in the 1990 to 2016 review of the GBD study, although global childhood death rates have declined, YLD has been stagnant because of aging population, with resulting increases in obesity and diabetes.[6] A complementary concept is the HALE, which quantifies the number of years of life that expected to be lived in good health.[7]

WHY IS GLOBAL BURDEN OF DISEASE SO IMPORTANT?

Estimation techniques allow one to identify the diseases with the most burden in 171 countries globally.[8] GBD uses standardized and validated methods to all available databases, adjusting for major sources of bias. The higher the quality of the data, the more likely that the estimation techniques will represent real reported data. It is important to distinguish the diseases that result in death versus those that cause poor health, as there is a major difference in the appropriate response with resource allocation. Governments use GBD for priority-setting, policy making, and comparing disease effects within and between populations, changes over time, and financial costs. For example, neither clubfoot nor DDH typically results in death, but which of these conditions leads to a greater burden of disease as an adult can only be answered with good quality data. With good GBD data, decisions about priority allocation of scarce surgical resources can be decided better.[3,9]

GDB estimates depend on careful analysis from many data sources. The Global Burden of Disease study has been in continual development since 1990, from the Institute for Health Metrics and Evaluation (IHME) at University of Washington.[4] Recent GDB estimates (1990–2016) published in 2017 used 90,000 data sources, each of which had hundreds to billions of data points. The actual details of the process are most important. Before a data point can be used, it must be vetted and confirmed, which can take up to 50% to 80% of staff research time. Miscoded data must be reassigned, and data need to be transformed by estimation of the true data points. The actual details of the process can be found elsewhere.[10]

WHAT IS DISABILITY-ADJUSTED LIFE YEAR USED FOR?

DALY is a measure of life lost from premature death and life not lived at 100% health. From the WHO GBD study the DALY became the preferred metric to compare the health burden of various dissimilar diseases. It is applied to populations rather than to individuals. It is a composite of both mortality and morbidity, which is something to be avoided. As opposed to the QALY (quality-adjusted life year) it is a negative measure, a measure of disease within a population. Bickler and colleagues[11] have recommended a methodology for estimating the burden of surgical conditions and unmet need for surgical care. They recommend that the burden of surgical conditions should be expressed as DALYs, that unmet surgical need be expressed as potential DALYs avertable, and that DALYs averted be used as a measure of the impact of surgical care. Murray has stressed that the DALY is based on economic and ethical fairness principles to account for nonfatal health outcomes that can guide policy makers to deliver more cost-effective and equitable health care.[12]

COST-EFFECTIVE ANALYSIS

Murrey utilized the DALY to develop cost-effective analysis (CEA) as an analytical tool that correlates the effectiveness of a health intervention to its costs, in terms of dollar per DALY averted.[13] Recent data for CEA show that surgical care is cost-effective in low- and middle-income countries (LMICs) compared with the much higher surgical care costs in the United States and other high-income countries (HICs). Common relative costs/DALY averted include $48,000/DALY averted for a 60-year-old man in the United States receiving a hip arthroplasty, $3800/DALY for a tibia nailing in a young adult in the United States, $400/DLY for antiretroviral therapy for human immunodeficiency virus (HIV) in Africa, and $35 to 90/DALY averted in LMICs for surgical interventions in a district hospital.[14] As a response to these data and much persistence from surgical leadership, the WHO has recently promoted essential surgical services through their Emergency and Essential Surgical Care Project (EESC) and Global Initiative.[15]

WHAT IS THE GLOBAL BURDEN OF DISEASE FOR MUSCULOSKELETAL CONDITIONS?

Much research has come out of the 2010 GBD study to estimate the GBD of disease for musculoskeletal conditions.[9] 2004 estimates showed a burden of nontraumatic musculoskeletal conditions of 2.5% of the entire global burden.[16] By 2010, this had increased to 4.4%, and by 2016 the GDB for nontraumatic musculoskeletal conditions was 5.9% of GDB. However, there are no good data for the common pediatric conditions, especially globally, and estimating GDB for the pediatric musculoskeletal conditions is elusive. In an effort to describe burden of disease, incidence data are one estimate of population burden. Maps of GBD are elusive because of changes in disease prevalence over time and health inequalities within and among populations. Musculoskeletal conditions may be under-reported. For example, many children have missed infections that never get counted. If a child dies from sepsis and pneumonia, the infected humerus may not be counted. Likewise, the untreated child with a septic hip that results in a destroyed hip as an adult may never get counted as an infection. Undernutrition is the leading factor for health loss in children and can put many at risk for musculoskeletal infections, but this is not counted as a musculoskeletal condition.[17]

WHAT ARE THE MOST COMMON PEDIATRIC ORTHOPEDIC CONDITIONS IN DEVELOPING COUNTRIES?

A quality well-funded Rwanda study of musculoskeletal impairments (MSIs) with validated methodology involved a prospective door to door survey of 6757 individuals of all ages.[18,19] MSIs were identified for all ages, with a total of 352 cases (5.2% overall prevalence). MSI was highest in those over 60 years of age (24%), with most cases 43.7% considered moderate, and most of these (96%) requiring further treatment.[19] For the 3526 children under 16 years of age who were screened, MSI was present in 2.6%. Approximately 23% of cases were caused by congenital deformity; 14% were neurologic. Twelve percent were trauma; 3% were infection, and 46% were other pathology.[18] However, the researchers were not able to calculate the DALYs for most of the conditions that begin in childhood. They estimated that for this country of 8.4 million people, half of whom are children, 1.2% of those under 16 years (50,000) required orthopedic surgery. For example, the prevalence of clubfoot was 0.7 cases per 1000 population, which is similar to known prevalence of 1 case per 1000 population in other studies, and would require treatment of almost 60,000 people in their entire population. The study showed that in Rwanda, there is a large burden of MSI that is mostly untreated. The survey methodology should be used in other LMICs, but can be expensive at a cost of $100,000.

A survey by Qudsi and colleagues[20] in Haiti showed that the most common pediatric musculoskeletal conditions were infection, trauma, clubfoot, limb deformity, DDH, and neuromuscular conditions (**Fig. 1**).[20] However, the comfort level of the orthopedic clinicians was different. They were most comfortable with treating infection and trauma because of the frequency of

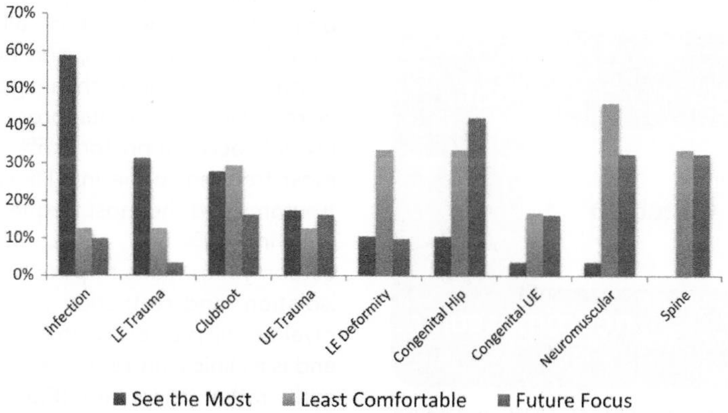

Fig. 1. Patterns of need and desire. Survey of providers in Haiti asking them what conditions they see the most, are least comfortable with, and would like future training. Percentages are percentage of individuals who included each diagnosis as 1 of their top 3 choices for each question. Missing rates for each question category ranged from 39% to 53% (considered missing if 0 diagnoses provided). Infection, osteomyelitis and septic arthritis. LE, lower extremity; UE, upper extremity. (*From* Qudsi RA, Roberts HJ, Bhashyam AR. et al. A self-reported needs assessment survey of pediatric orthopaedic education in Haiti. J Surg Educ 2018;75(1):144; with permission.)

these conditions and their practical urgency. They were least comfortable with DDH, limb deformity, and spine. These conditions are typically not so urgent, not so obvious early on, and when neglected, require more technically demanding resources. Clubfoot was in between in terms of their comfort level.

GLOBAL MUSCULOSKELETAL CONDITIONS IN CHILDREN THAT HAVE IMPLICATIONS INTO ADULT LIFE

Five pediatric orthopedic conditions that contribute to GBD and have implications for MSI later in life are infections, trauma, clubfoot, DDH, and cerebral palsy (**Fig. 2**). They also have a long period of time of YLD for the individual and DALYs for the population that are important for policymakers to estimate so that relative economic value and policy decisions can be made. These 5 conditions have in common that they can be treated with a combination of early detection, conservative management such as rehabilitation and devices, and surgery, which is more effective when provided early rather than later in the disease natural history. Musculoskeletal infections are of particular importance, because they are associated with so many of the other pediatric conditions (see **Fig. 2**).

INFECTIONS

Musculoskeletal infections can be acquired from trauma, hematogenous, or as a result of elective surgical procedures such as arthroplasty. As countries become more developed, post-traumatic and hematogenous infection risk may decline,

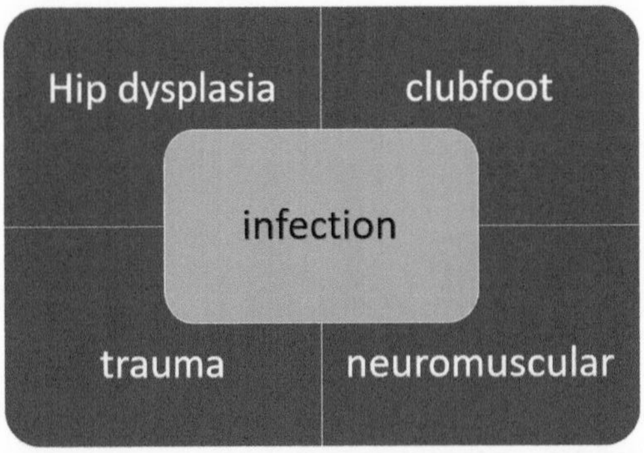

Fig. 2. Infections, trauma, clubfoot, DDH, and neuromuscular conditions are 5 important conditions seen globally that have significant implications for future YLD for the individual and DALYs for the population. Infections are central to these conditions as infection can complicate the surgical treatment but also be the result of neglected treatment, such as trauma.

but the prevalence of iatrogenic infections may increase, so the burden will not go away. Group A streptococcal diseases is 1 example, with a worldwide burden of over 500,000 deaths per year, a total of 111 million cases of pyoderma, although its greatest global burden is still rheumatic heart disease.[21] Essentially no DALY data exist for musculoskeletal infections in children. Nevertheless, Malizos has advocated that a targeted action plan should be in place so that the burden of MSK infections is included in the agenda for global health care priorities.[22]

Osteomyelitis and Septic Arthritis

There are 12 million children with osteomyelitis in the least developed countries. Osteomyelitis continues to be a worldwide problem because of the lack of surgical care and because of the reality that antibiotics have not been as successful against bone infections as for other infectious conditions.[23] Untreated acute osteomyelitis and septic arthritis remain a common cause of chronic osteomyelitis and late sequelae leading to a destroyed hip or other joint. Street[24] reported a prevalence of osteomyelitis in New Zealand of 1 case per 4000 population with, an over-representation of Maori and Pacific islanders. The burden of osteomyelitis was also studied in Fiji over a 5-year period.[25] The most common associated factors preceding the infection were trauma in 55% of cases, skin sepsis in 32% of cases and with 54% of the infections becoming chronic.[25] Malcius and colleagues[26] evaluated the prevalence of pediatric acute osteomyelitis in Lithuania and found that although the prevalence had increased, the clinical course was less complicated. Five hospitals in Uganda were sampled during a 1-year period.[27] Ten percent of all outpatient visits were for osteomyelitis, and 80% of cases were in patients younger than age 20 years. There were 9354 surgical total procedures, with osteomyelitis accounting for 3.5%. The tibia was the most frequent bone in 31% cases, and sequestrectomy was the most frequent surgical procedure in 60% of cases. Untreated chronic osteomyelitis leads to poor overall health, social isolation, and restriction from school.[28] Osteomyelitis disproportionately affects the young and is a clinical and surgical burden, best treated early rather than late (**Fig. 3**). Unfortunately, there are no published DALY or YLD data for pediatric osteomyelitis or septic arthritis.

Tuberculosis

Tuberculosis (TB) is a major global public health problem, with latent TB affecting 1.91 billion

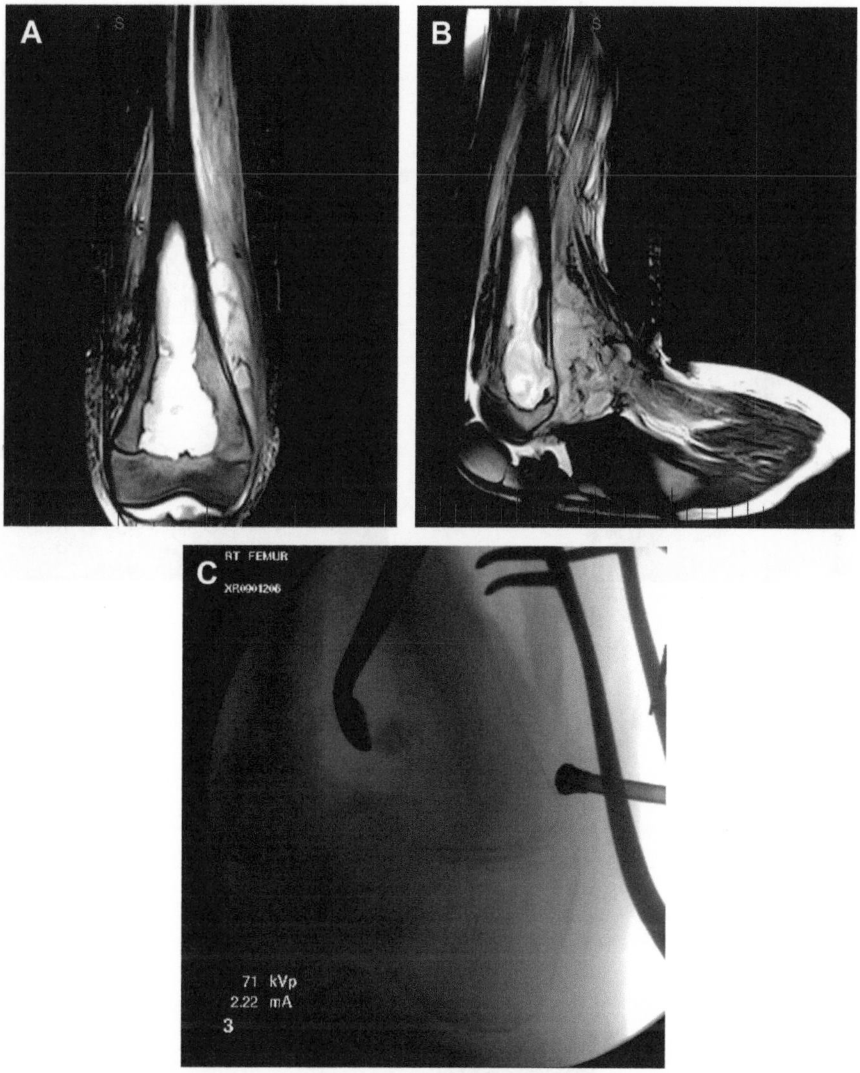

Fig. 3. Case of 10-year-old boy with hematogenous osteomyelitis of the distal femur. When diagnosed early, confirmed on these (*A, B*) MRI images, (*C*) effective surgical drainage and short course antibiotic therapy can be effective. If left untreated, growth arrest, arthritis, and chronic osteomyelitis can result, leading to a lifetime of YLD.

people (95% confidence interval [CI] 1.79 billion to 2.03 billion). Those with latent TB are at risk for developing active disease, with age, human immunodeficiency virus (HIV), malnutrition, diabetes, and alcohol being risk factors. Globally there were 10.4 million incident cases of TB in 2016, 331,00 multidrug-resistant cases, and 19,800 extensively drug-resistant cases. Overall, musculoskeletal involvement is seen in less than 10% of all cases of TB, and half of these have involvement of the spine. This is a much smaller proportion of the population with musculoskeletal TB and an even smaller proportion of TB in children. However, TB of the spine remains a serious cause of paralysis worldwide (Fig. 4). Incident cases of TB and musculoskeletal TB contribute to DALYs for the population. Maps of TB incidence do not always show the actual burden in a population. For example, although there are relatively few reported cases in sub-Saharan Africa, the incident cases are high because of the frequency of infections. A systematic analysis for the Global Burden of Disease study 2010 showed that tuberculosis was an important cause of YLD in sub-Saharan Africa.[29]

TRAUMA

Trauma-related conditions are the leading cause of childhood death after 1 year of age in the United States. GBD from trauma is increasing overall.[30] Injury mortality is even higher in

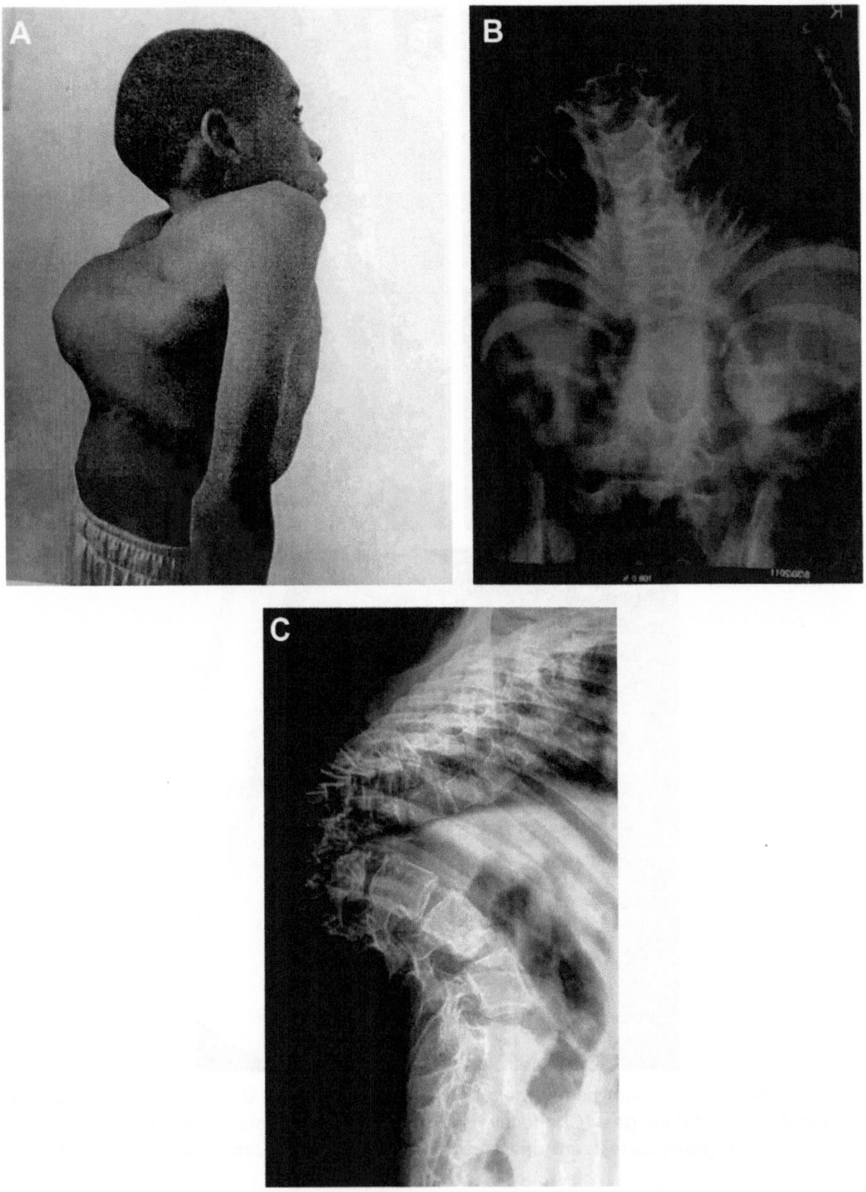

Fig. 4. (*A–C*) Tuberculosis of the spine when untreated medically can result in collapse, deformity, and myelopathy. Once it is at this stage, greater resources are needed to care for the child, resulting in unacceptable risk to the child and diversion of health resources from prevention of other conditions. Unskilled attempts to correct a major spine deformity with inadequate training and resources can result in paralysis, which is a death sentence in many poor countries.

LMIC, estimated to be double that of HIC. For every reported death, there are many more nonfatal injuries that may result in temporary or permanent disability (Fig. 5). As is true with mortality, disability disproportionately affects LIMC. A survey from Ghana showed a high rate of disability beyond 30 days, much higher than in the United States.[31,32] Because most of these, (68%) were extremity related, they should be treatable with basic orthopedic care and rehabilitation, unlike the greater resources needed in for the more frequent intracranial injuries seen in HMIC countries. In LMIC, road traffic injuries have become a great source of disability. The GBD study has shown the leading cause of nonfatal injuries from road traffic are intracranial injuries, open wounds, eg fractures, femur fractures, and internal injury.[33] Similar to the Ghana study, the 2106 GBD study data showed a higher prevalence of limb injuries from MVC, further proving the need for basic orthopedic management globally.[33]

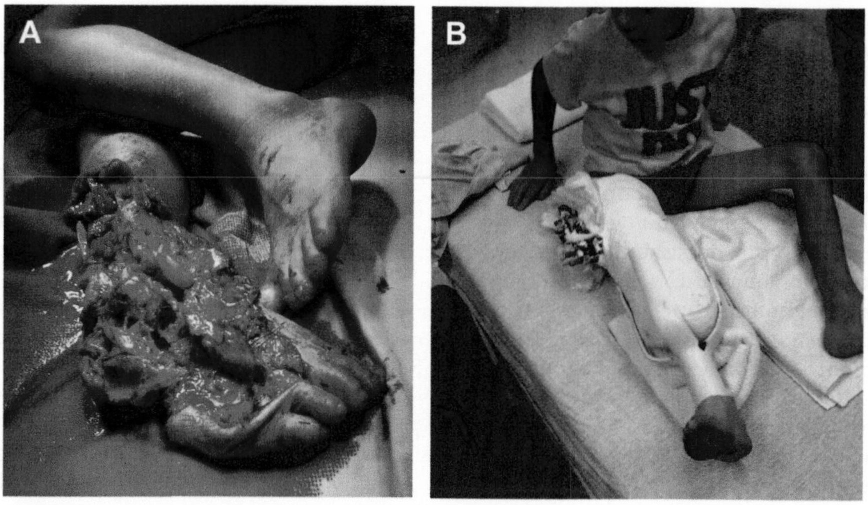

Fig. 5. As the LMIC become more developed, high-energy trauma becomes more frequent. (*A*) This includes injuries from MVC, mechanized farm equipment, and blast injuries from unexploded land mines in war zones. (*B*) Despite the severity of these injuries, amputation and simple prosthetic fitting can be done with available local technology.

CLUBFOOT

Globally, congenital idiopathic clubfoot is the most common serious musculoskeletal birth defect (Fig. 6). Worldwide prevalence is 1 case to 2 cases per 1000 population, resulting in 150,000 to 200,000 infants born with clubfoot. Eighty percent of children with clubfoot are born in countries with limited resources.[34] Thousands of children and adults in LMIC have neglected and untreated clubfoot, leading to later problems with shoe wear, pain, difficulty walking, and social and cultural issues. Cultural bias and prejudice can result in a life of poverty, lack of educational opportunities, and challenges to find a marital partner. The Ponseti treatment method has become a standard of care in over 100 countries of all levels of income. It is particularly well suited for use in LMICs, as the casting and supervised bracing program can be done by well-trained community health workers, rather than by physicians. In LMICs, braces can be made with local resources. Ponseti programs have been developed with the goal to provide treatment for every child born with a clubfoot. Sustainable funding, clinical programs, access to care, long distances from treatment centers, training, safe tenotomy, affordable braces, and quality control with program data analysis are ongoing challenges. A cost-effectiveness analysis has not been done comparing the cost/DALY of clubfoot treatment with that of other conditions such as DDH prevention with early treatment. A published care delivery value chain (CDVC) has recommended 6 steps to assure optimal program success[35]:

- Early diagnosis
- Development of high-volume Ponseti centers
- Trained nonphysician health workers
- Engaging families in care
- Addressing barriers to access
- Providing follow-up in the patient's own community

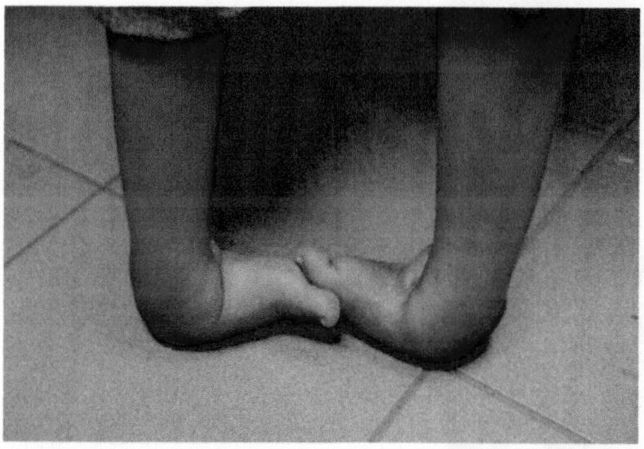

Fig. 6. Clubfoot is the most common serious musculoskeletal birth defect. Because it is obvious at birth and is a social stigma, parents are usually willing to go through the stress and expense of Ponseti method cast treatment before it becomes a functional disability. For similar reasons, parents are also accepting of surgical treatment of other obvious limb deformities.

DEVELOPMENTAL HIP DYSPLASIA

Developmental hip dysplasia (DDH) is a wide spectrum of conditions from mild instability to frank dislocation at birth, and from asymptomatic dysplasia to frank arthritis in the adult (Fig. 7A). The prevalence is 1.5 cases to 25 cases per 1000 live births. The burden of disease in terms of DALYs and YLD is an important concept for DDH, because this is often a lifelong condition with implications for function and disability during the working and later years. However, there has been little published on this, nor is there information how DALYs and YLD compare with other common pediatric conditions such as clubfoot, infection, or trauma. DDH is different than clubfoot, since early on it is a hidden condition, so late recognition and treatment or no treatment may occur. DDH is one of the more common reasons for an adult to have end-stage arthritis.

Primary prevention may be the most cost-effective step that can be done to influence the later prevalence of DDH. The risk for DDH is greater in cultures that practice tight swaddling with the hips maintained in an extended position. In many African and some Asian countries, infants are routinely carried with their hips abducted around the mother's back, and DDH is uncommon (Fig. 7B). Other cultures that practice tight swaddling have high rates of DDH (Fig. 7C). Tight swaddling with poor access to early primary care and hip examination in the newborn and infant can lead to late or unrecognized hip dysplasia. Tight swaddling should be discouraged. The following statement has been issued by the International Hip Dysplasia Institute with a statement of support from the

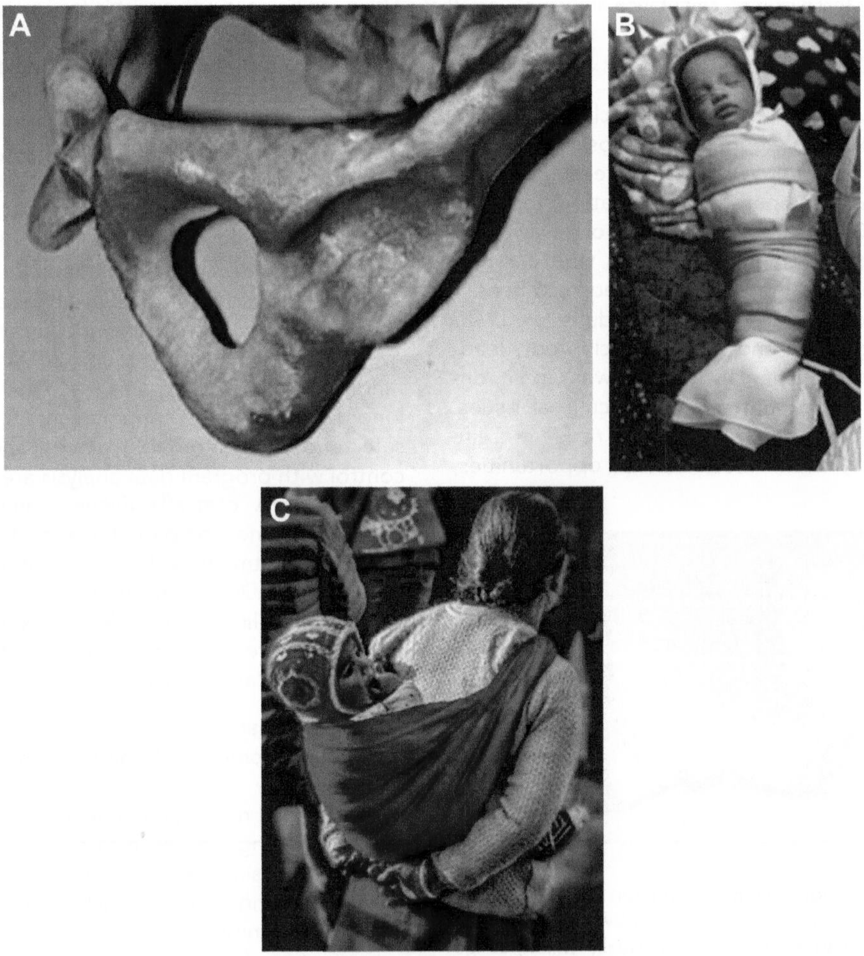

Fig. 7. (*A*) DDH commonly shares the feature of a deficient egg-shaped acetabulum. BecauseDDH is frequently not noticed at birth and early on has minimal symptoms, parents may not seek early treatment. Late treatment then requires more specialized surgical management, which may not be safely available. (*B*) Tight swaddling can lead to hip dysplasia and should be discouraged. (*C*) Baby wearing with the hips abducted promotes healthy hip development.

Pediatric Orthopedic Society of North America: "It is the recommendation of the International Hip Dysplasia Institute that infant hips should be positioned in slight flexion and abduction during swaddling. The knees should also be maintained in slight flexion. Additional free movement in the direction of hip flexion and abduction may have some benefit. Avoidance of forced or sustained passive hip extension and adduction in the first few months of life is essential for proper hip development."

CEREBRAL PALSY AND NEUROMUSCULAR CONDITIONS

The prevalence of cerebral palsy (CP) is as high as 2 to 3 cases per 1000 births worldwide, with many cases undiagnosed or misdiagnosed. On the other hand, approximately 10% of children seen in a CP clinic may have another diagnosis than CP (Fig. 8). In resource-poor environments, total rates of overall disability have been found to be 82 to 160 cases per 1000 population, and neurologic impairment to be 19 to 61 cases per 1000 population for children age 2 to 9 years.[36] In high-income countries CP is associated with prematurity and low birth weight. In LMIC it is associated with inadequate prenatal care, home deliveries, poor access to emergency obstetric interventions, and postnatal infections.[36] DALYs have not been calculated for CP, nor have they been compared with other common childhood musculoskeletal conditions.

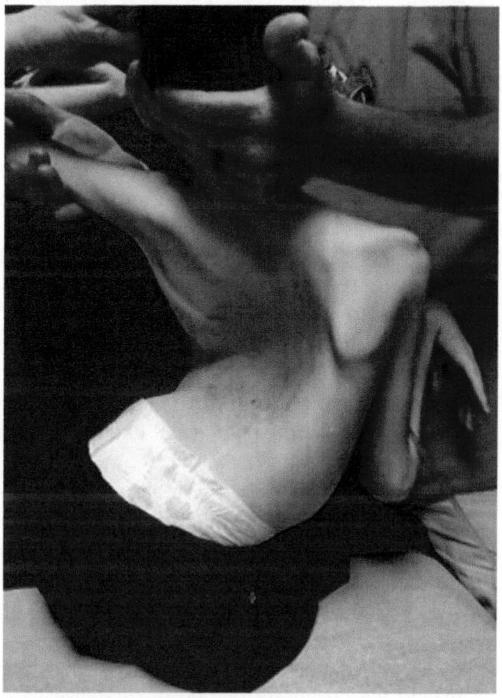

Fig. 8. CP is the most common neurologic condition seen in pediatric orthopedics. Globally, many patients with GMFCS 5 CP do not survive childhood. If they do, scoliosis can become severe if untreated. With time, it can not only cause discomfort with sitting, but can also affect respiration and nutrition. Basic surgical treatment of the limbs for ambulatory children is more cost-effective and safer when resources are limited.

The Gross Motor Functional classification system (with classes 1–5) is used for classifying the severity of involvement and function. In LMIC, nonambulatory children with GMFCS 5 may not survive and rarely receive more specialized surgical services such as spinal deformity or major hip reconstruction. Nepal is an example of an LMIC in which children with less motor impairment such as spastic hemiplegia may nevertheless have greater functional disability than children from HIC.[37] This may be because of neglect, lack of educational opportunities, and rehabilitation services. In LMIC, simple surgical treatment such as tendon transfer and tenotomy to maintain or improve function in conjunction with rehabilitation and orthotic devices is preferred for ambulatory children with GMFCS 1 to 3 functional level who could benefit by greater ease of walking or upper extremity function.[37]

SUMMARY

Because of YLD and the large proportion of children in a population, these pediatric musculoskeletal conditions can contribute greatly to the GBD, now and later. The 5 common pediatric conditions (infection, trauma, DDH clubfoot and CP/NM, and others) should be part of future GBD studies. DALYs should be determined so that policy makers can allocate appropriate resources for these conditions that may affect children and families for generations. However, one cannot and should not wait for a GBD study to be completed before action is taken. Prevention and treatment of these conditions should become WHO essential surgical services. Recommendations from the Global Initiative for Children's Surgery (GICS) for optimizing children's surgical care include: establishing standards and integrating them into national surgical plans for each level of care, a children's hospital for each country, establishment and support of regional training hubs for all children's surgical specialties, and establishing regional research support centers.[3]

DISCLOSURE

The author has no commercial or financial conflicts of interest related to this article. There was no funding for this article.

REFERENCES

1. Joshipura M, Mock C, Gosselin RA. Global burden of musculoskeletal conditions. In: Gosselin RA, Spiegel DA, Foltz M, editors. Global Orthopedics. 2nd edition. Chum (Switzerland): Springer; 2020. p. 9–11.
2. Weiser TG, Regenbogen SE, Thompson KD, et al. An estimation of the global volume of surgery: a modelling strategy based on available data. Lancet 2008;372(9633):139–48.
3. Goodman LF, St-Louis E, Yousef Y, et al. The global initiative for children's surgery: optimal resources for improving care. Eur J Pediatr Surg 2018;28(1): 51–9.
4. Available at: http://www.healthdata.org/gbd. Accessed September 22, 2019.
5. Murray CJ. Quantifying the burden of disease: the technical basis for disability-adjusted life years. Bull World Health Organ 1994;72(3): 429–45.
6. GBD 2016 Disease and Injury Incidence and Prevalence Collaborators. Global, regional and national incidence, prevalence, and years lived with disability for 328 diseases and injuries for 195 countries, 1990-2016: a systemic analysis for the Global Burden of Disease Study 2016. Lancet 2017;390: 1211–59.
7. GBD 2017 DALYs and HALE Collaborators. Global, regional, and national disability-adjusted life-years (DALYs) for 359 diseases and injuries and healthy life expectancy (HALE) for 195 countries and territories, 1990-2017: a systematic analysis for the Global Burden of Disease Study 2017. Lancet 2018;392(10159):1859–922.
8. GBD 2016 SDG Collaborators. Measuring progress and projecting attainment on the basis of past trends of the health-related sustainable development goals in 188 countries: an analysis from the Global Burden of Disease Study 2016. Lancet 2017;390:1423–59.
9. Hoy DG, Smith E, Cross M, et al. The global burden of musculoskeletal conditions for 2010: an overview of methods. Ann Rheum Dis 2014;73(6):982–9.
10. Available at: https://medium.com/acting-on-data/what-data-sources-go-into-the-gbd-c1857b9ba7f5. Accessed September 22, 2019
11. Bickler S, Ozgediz D, Gosselin R, et al. Key concepts for estimating the burden of surgical conditions and the unmet need for surgical care. World J Surg 2010;34(3):374–80.
12. Murray CJ, Acharya AK. Understanding DALYs (disability-adjusted life years). J Health Econ 1997; 16(6):703–30.
13. Murray CJL, Lopez AD, editors. The global burden of disease. Boston: Harvard University Press; 1996.
14. Debas H, Gosselin RA, McCord TA. Surgery. In: Jamison D, editor. Disease control priorities in developing countries. Washington, DC: Oxford University Press; 2006. p. 1245–60.
15. Spiegel DA, Abdullah F, Price RR, et al. World Health Organization global initiative for emergency and essential surgical care: 2011 and beyond. World J Surg 2013;37:1462–9 (open access).
16. Lopez AD, Mathers CD. Global burden of disease and risk factors. New York: Oxford University Press; 2016.
17. Lopez AD, Mathers CD, Ezzati M, et al. Global and regional burden of disease and risk factors, 2001: systematic analysis of population health data. Lancet 2006;367(9524):1747–57.
18. Atijosan O, Simms V, Kuper H, et al. The orthopaedic needs of children in Rwanda: results from a national survey and orthopaedic service implications. J Pediatr Orthop 2009;29(8):948–51.
19. Matheson JI, Atijosan O, Kuper H, et al. Musculoskeletal impairment of traumatic etiology in Rwanda: prevalence, causes and service implications. World J Surg 2011;35(12):2635–42.
20. Qudsi RA, Roberts HJ, Bhashyam AR. A self-reported needs assessment survey of pediatric orthopaedic education in Haiti. J Surg Educ 2018;75(1):140–6.
21. Carapetis JR, Steer AC, Mulholland EK, et al. The global burden of group a streptococcal diseases. Lancet Infect Dis 2005;5(11):685–94.
22. Malizos KN. Global forum: the burden of bone and joint infections: a growing demand for more resources. J Bone Joint Surg Am 2017;995:e20.
23. Lew DP, Waldvogel FA. Osteomyelitis. Lancet 2004; 364(9431):369–79.
24. Street M, Puna R, Huang M, et al. Pediatric acute hematogenous osteomyelitis. J Pediatr Orthop 2015;35(6):634–9.
25. Munshi B, MacFater W, Hill AG, et al. Paediatric osteomyelitis in Fiji. World J Surg 2018;42(12):4118–22.
26. Malcius D, Trumpulyte G, Barauskas V, et al. Two decades of acute hematogenous osteomyelitis in children: are there any changes? Pediatr Surg Int 2005;21(5):356–9.
27. Stanley CM, Rutherford GW, Morshed S, et al. Estimating the healthcare burden of osteomyelitis in Uganda. Trans R Soc Trop Med Hyg 2010;104(2): 139–42.
28. Jones DS, Podolsky SH, Greene JA. The burden of disease and the changing task of medicine. N Engl J Med 2012;366:2333–8.
29. Vos T, Flaxman AD, Naghavi M, et al. Years lived with a disability (YLD) for 1160 sequelae of 289

diseases and injuries 1990-2010: a systematic analysis for the Global Burden of Disease Study 2010. Lancet 2012;380(9859):628.
30. Mokdad AH, Jaber S, Aziz MI, et al. The state of health in the Arab world, 1990-2010: an analysis of the burden of diseases injuries and risk factors. Lancet 2014;383(9914):309–20.
31. Mock CN, Abantanga F, Cummings P, et al. Incidence and outcome of injury in Ghana: results of community-based survey. Bull World Health Organ 1999;77:955–64.
32. The lancet, global burden of diseases, injuries, and risk factors study 2013. Available at: http://www.thelancet.com/global-burden-of-disease. Accessed December 21, 2019.
33. GBD 2017 Disease and Injury Incidence and Prevalence Collaborators. Global, regional and national incidence, prevalence, and years lived with a disability for 354 diseases and injuries for 105 countries and territories, 1990-2017: a systematic analysis for the Global Burden of Disease Study 2017. Lancet 2018;392(10159):1789–858.
34. Owen RM, Penny JN, Mayo A, et al. A collaborative public health approach to clubfoot intervention in 10 low-income and middle-income countries: 2-year outcomes and lessons learnt. J Pediatr Orthop B 2012;21:361–5.
35. Harmer L, Rhatigan J. Clubfoot care in low-income and middle-income countries. From clinical innovation to a public health program. World J Surg 2014;38:839–48.
36. Gladstone M. A review of the incidence and prevalence, types and aetiology of childhood cerebral palsy in resource-poor settings. Ann Trop Paediatr 2010;30(3):181–96.
37. LeBrun DG, Banskota B, Banskota AK, et al. Socioeconomic status influences functional severity of untreated cerebral palsy in Nepal: A prospective analysis and systematic review. Clin Orthop Relat Res 2019;477(1):10–21.

Development of a Global Pediatric Orthopedic Outreach Program in Ecuador Through Project Perfect World

Past, Present, and Future Directions

Eric Fornari, MD[a,*], Richard M. Schwend, MD[b], Jacob Schulz, MD[a], Christopher Bray, MD[c], Matthew R. Schmitz, MD[d]

KEYWORDS

• Global health • Education • Training • Ethics • Pediatric orthopedics

KEY POINTS

- Global health should focus on not only the delivery of care, but also the promotion of local capacity and infrastructure building.
- Developing global health delivery vehicles requires dedicated team members and long-term relationships with host nations.
- Education and prevention strategies should be a part of all global health initiatives to help host nations.

INTRODUCTION

Over the last half century, knowledge and understanding of the effective delivery of global health has undergone significant growth and development.[1–9] As the world has become more interconnected, we have witnessed first-hand the rapid evolution of this field. What started with well-meaning but relatively unstructured medical mission trips has evolved into an independent discipline of medicine with a growing body of literature helping to shape how this work will be best carried out in the future.[4,6,7,10–15]

As an orthopedic surgeon, there are a number of different ways one can be involved with global outreach.[4] Dr Kaye Wilkens, a renowned pediatric orthopedic surgeon at the forefront of this work, described 3 different mechanisms for support.[16] The first is direct surgical help: teams that come for discreet periods to perform surgery in low- and middle-income countries (LMIC). Direct surgical help is often criticized for not providing education to local health workers; however, we have found that this can be one of the most powerful ways to learn, by local and visiting teams working together, side by side.

The second is training, which can be direct training of local surgeons during a medical mission or bringing selected surgeons from LMICs to institutions that can provide appropriate subspecialty training in formal fellowships

[a] Albert Einstein College of Medicine, The Children's Hospital at Montefiore, 3400 Bainbridge Avenue, 6th Floor, Bronx, NY 10467, USA; [b] Department of Orthopaedics and Musculoskeletal Medicine, Children's Mercy Hospital, 2401 Gillham Road, Kansas City, MO 64108, USA; [c] Department of Orthopedic Surgery, Prisma Health Upstate, Steadman Hawkins Clinic of the Carolinas, 701 Grove Road, Greenville, SC 29605, USA; [d] Department of Orthopaedics, San Antonio Military Medical Center, 3851 Roger Brooke Drive Fort, Sam Houston, TX 78234, USA
* Corresponding author.
E-mail address: efornari@montefiore.org

Orthop Clin N Am 51 (2020) 219–225
https://doi.org/10.1016/j.ocl.2019.12.002

or observerships. The third is local education: creating and supporting continuing medical education courses in the LMIC.[16] In practice, any successful and meaningful program incorporates all 3 mechanisms for engagement.[1,12,16] Furthermore, sustaining the outreach effort ultimately requires ongoing assessment to ensure quality and ethical standards are met through data-driven analysis.[12,17]

At its core, any global outreach program should be founded on the promotion of local capacity building while using the delivery of culturally sensitive care.[5,7,8,12,14] Regardless of the mechanism or vehicle, the primary focus of any global program should include an emphasis on local infrastructural support, surgical education, and the empowerment of local health care providers.[5,12,13] As physicians, and especially surgeons, it most important to go about this work in a thoughtful, systematic manner that ensures our goals and expectations are aligned with those we are setting out to engage and assist.[5,11–13,17–19]

In this article, the authors present our experience working at the Roberto Gilbert Hospital in Guayaquil, Ecuador, through Project Perfect World (PPW), a 501(c)3 charitable foundation dedicated to the delivery of health care to the children of the world who would not otherwise have access. The development of this pediatric orthopedic program over the last 20 years has been heavily shaped by expanded knowledge and understanding of how this work is best carried out to have a truly long-term, sustainable impact. This evolution is the result of the vision, commitment, and hard work of a diverse team of individuals, both from the United States, but importantly from Ecuador, dedicated to achieving a common goal. What started as short-term trips providing surgical care has transformed into a multilayered program that fosters engagement, education, and learning. It is through these mechanisms that the program works to achieve its overall mission of improving the health of the world's children through quality medical intervention, mentoring with local medical colleagues, and infrastructure development.

SURGICAL OUTREACH LOGISTICS

Identifying a Vehicle

One of the major steps in participating in a global outreach program is identifying and working with an entity that will help to facilitate the trip. There are a variety of potential vehicles to help promote global outreach and provide medical care in LMICs. These range from formal agreements between training institutions in the United State and abroad, religious organizations that help to sponsor outreach trips, and nonprofit organizations with a goal of helping deliver and sustain such outreach projects. The PPW Foundation is a secular charitable foundation that was started as a memorial by Bob Simpson and has organized at least 2 trips annually for more than 20 years to provide orthopedic care for the children of Ecuador. The vision of PPW is to develop close and long-term professional relationships with the local hospital staff to help them provide quality medical care and orthopedic services now and in the future. PPW accomplishes the goal of cultural competence, bidirectional education, and capacity building through their biannual surgical outreach trips. Einstein stated, "Example is not another way to teach, it is the only way." We base our educational program on this principle of closely working together with our hosts to provide, through a trusting relationship, a 2-way exchange of ideas and methods.

The surgical outreach trips occur each spring and fall and are located at the Roberto Gilbert Hospital in Guayaquil, Ecuador, where the foundation has a long-standing relationship with the local children's hospital and staff as well as important community leaders.

Developing a Team

Once a location and vehicle are identified, one must set up the traveling team. This process involves identifying motivated personnel with multiple job types and skill sets. The trips to Guayaquil involve 3 to 4 pediatric orthopedic surgeons, along with 3 to 4 anesthesiologists, including someone skilled in regional anesthetic blocks. Understanding the potential need of the target population and likely case mix helps to determine the personnel required. We have used RedCap as our database, with more than 800 patients entered. This resource provides patients needing surgical care to be identified well in advance, allowing medical optimization and surgical planning to occur. One of the nonprofit foundations we use is the First Hand Foundation. This foundation has provided funding if they are provided specific details of the proposed surgical care for a child in advance, another advantage of having a reliable database.

The PPW Ecuadorian trips generally plan to be self-sustained and take nursing support (for both the operating room and recovery room), operating room technician support, along with sterile processing technicians so as not to be a burden on the local children's hospital manpower resources. In 2008, we began bringing a sterile processing person on each trip, which has provided education and quality assurance in infection prevention. This infrastructure assistance has greatly improved the sterile processing standard work for the hospital's entire surgical suite. We are unaware of any major infections since this program started.

The team typically brings 20 to 30 personnel, including nonmedical participants who serve as translators and help with transporting patients between the operating theaters and the wards. In addition, we have added 1 to 2 orthotists and a prosthetist who serve a vital role as an adjunct to surgical management providing nonoperative treatment. The overall team structure can vary and depends on the location and patient population being served. Establishing a long-term relationship with continuity helps to better prepare the team leaders to successfully construct a highly effective team.

There are several principles that we have adopted over the years and followed:

- Safety always.
- Focus on long-term, sustainable relationships.
- We are guests in their country. We follow their rules and are respectful and compassionate always.
- If someone sees something that is not right, it is his or her responsibility to speak up. Keeping quiet is no excuse.
- If any team member feels that a surgery cannot be done safely, it will not be done until issues are resolved.
- Culturally sensitive informed patient consent must be provided in their language. This issue is extremely important, because families are desperate for care and so the consenting aspect may be in question. This is one reason surgeries are often scheduled a year in advance, to give the families time.
- Resolve interpersonal conflicts early and professionally.
- We are all replaceable, so always be training those who will come after you.
- Enjoy the children and families we care for. Enjoy each other and the work we do.

Fundraising

Participation in global outreach programs comes with a monetary cost. From travel and housing to the cost of supplies, this can be one of the larger obstacles to overcome in the development of a successful program. The PPW Ecuadorian trips use a year-round fundraising strategy to help minimize individual costs for the biannual trips. Private donations, monetary and equipment donations from medical supply companies, and donations from individual participants help to fund the trips. In addition, bringing and storing your own implants and supplies help to decrease the host burden in LMIC. Each trip and locale is unique, depending on housing availability and resources available. Each trip to Guayaquil costs approximately $75,000, with a majority of those costs being airfare and hotel for 25 people for the 8 days. We have partnered with the Damian House, a local faith-based entity that helps to care for adult patients with Hansen's disease (leprosy) and their staff help with translation services, food preparation, and local transportation for our group to help defray costs for the trip. Our trip participants reciprocate by helping with a variety of tasks at the local facility (painting, maintenance) and by bringing much-needed medical and clothing supplies to donate to the facility.

Local Support

As discussed, local support is paramount to a successful trip. Assistance from the hospital is critical with clinical space, operating room time, and the ability to purchase certain medications and anesthetics that cannot be transported. In addition, we use storage at the local children's hospital where we can safely pack away our supplies for the next trip in 6 months. The hospital serves as a receiving entity when we ship supplies for upcoming trips and helps to support the program during the weeks that we are there. Inventory control of surgical supplies is critical when deciding on surgeries; before each procedure, we meticulously determine what we have available so as to avoid intraoperative issues. Open communication is critical between the groups. We typically coordinate our trips to happen during a national holiday, when the hospital's clinics and operating rooms would normally be closed to elective business, so as to lessen the burden on our hosts. In addition, holding clinic or patient evaluations on otherwise slow days (such as a Sunday) helps to decrease the footprint of a visiting medical team. It is important to be cognizant of the impact that a global outreach program can have in a potentially negative way by occupying clinic and operating room space that the hospital needs to use for paying patients for financial success of the host institution.

Weekly Overview

Schedules can vary and depend greatly on the resources and clinical space that are available to the traveling team. The 1-week trips to Guayaquil involve traveling on Saturday and seeing a large clinic of new patients and follow-up patients on Sunday. For the past 18 years, our host orthopedic colleagues have attended these clinics with us to jointly evaluate the children. This has been an excellent example of sharing the mutual interest of our specialty and working collaboratively to arrive at the best treatment plan for a child. Sunday evening, after the clinical evaluations are complete, we set the surgical schedule for the week. This schedule depends on the number of operating rooms available during the upcoming week (and available resources). Some children who would benefit from surgery in the United States may not have the opportunity to undergo a similar procedure in the host nation because of equipment available or follow-up, and so on. This is one of the more difficult portions of the trip—setting the surgical schedule and effectively triaging patients who would benefit most. We travel with enough personnel to run 2 operating rooms full time and in the evenings, and we sometimes split out into a third room depending on case volume, complexity, and local resource availability. We perform operations Monday through Friday. Local residents and nurses care for the postoperative patients overnight. Regional anesthesia is used often because postoperative pain control is limited to acetaminophen and ibuprofen in most cases, with a small amount of narcotics distributed to the family to use for the patient overnight. On Saturday we then clean, pack up, and store our equipment on before traveling back to the United States on Sunday.

Follow-up

Follow-up care is also extremely important for the patients and host physicians. We have developed close relationships with the local orthopedic surgeons and, after we depart, each patient has a follow-up plan specific to their surgical procedure (ie, cast off at 6 weeks, radiographs taken). We keep in communication with the local surgeons via email if they have any questions or concerns and plan on patient follow-up with the second PPW team at their trip 6 months later. This is a rudimentary form of telemedicine or virtual health with email communication. There is obvious potential to expand the role of telemedicine in the future with regular virtual follow-up appointments and consultations that should be considered. We maintain a registry of surgical patients using a password protected cloud-based database (RedCap) and continue to follow them annually during our trips. The local medical community communicates with the families about the timing of our trips, allowing for appropriate follow-up for the patients. Establishing a long-term relationship with local teams is best for the care of the patients undergoing surgery, but also helps to improve the capacity of the local surgeons to assume care for the current and future patients through continual process improvement and education.

Collateral Benefits

As a result of a strong commitment from all stakeholders involved with the project, we have recognized many additional benefits and started numerous other programs. These include a new orthotics building and training program; Ponseti treatment program that is run by the Ecuadorian staff; 10 years of a successful spinal deformity program[20]; safe, sterile processing for the entire hospital; the hiring of 2 spine surgeons at the hospital; collaboration with the intensive care unit, rehabilitation, and physical therapy programs; an exchange program with neurosurgery; and the mentoring and training of a generation of medical students and residents.

Challenges

Despite many wins, there remain serious challenges. Although surgical care has been shown to be cost effective in terms of disability-adjusted life-years, the funding still must be raised to have these programs succeed. Political unrest can delay or end a program at any time. Local surgeons need to earn a living, so they may not be able to take time away from their practices to spend the entire week working with the team. Issues of liability, malpractice coverage, and how to care for or compensate a child who has a major complication or is permanently harmed are ethical issues that have not been discussed enough and certainly have not been resolved.[12] Outcomes research is just in infancy, with challenges of funding, institutional review board process, informed patient consent, and on-site resources to run prospective registries.

NEXT STEPS

Now that we have established a commitment to the local population based on trust and capacity building, the groundwork has been laid to further develop our program, again with the unified goal of improving the pediatric orthopedic care for the children of Ecuador. We plan to use 3 main avenues to accomplish this goal: education, research, and prevention strategies.

Education

A successful global outreach program must use bidirectional education. During our time in country, we seek to provide as many educational opportunities as possible for the local medical community. During the biannual trips, these efforts include didactic sessions for local medical students and residents, combined teaching rounds on the wards, and live interactive surgical demonstrations with the local staff. We encourage the local physicians to serve as cosurgeons for the surgical procedures with step-by-step instructions. During the Sunday clinic, the local surgeons are present to show difficult cases and help to develop individualized treatment plans for each of the patients. They educate us on some of the cultural differences and obstacles for care, helping us to better understand the impact of disease and programs. Medical students and orthopedic residents work with us in the clinic and operating rooms as translators, but more important they are there to learn about the musculoskeletal care of children. We in turn learn from them, about health care in Ecuador, and continuously work to improve our Spanish language skills.

We understand that engagement of the local pediatric orthopedic community is paramount to the programs' success. We have used the POSNA Children's Orthopedics in Underserved Regions (COUR) scholarship to foster this engagement.[21] The COUR scholarship program pairs a local pediatric orthopedist with a POSNA member. The scholar travels to North America to attend the POSNA annual meeting or IPOS and then participates in an observership at their sponsor's institution. The goal is to build and foster relationships that lead to ongoing collaboration and learning. There has been 1 past POSNA COUR scholar from Ecuador. This individual and his sponsor have maintained a close, collaborative working relationship. Together they have coordinated 2 POSNA-sponsored local CME events as precourses to the annual Sociedad Ecuadorian de Orthopedia y Traumatologia meeting. The very first course was held in 2010 and was a Ponseti clubfoot course. The second was in 2017 and focused on early detection of developmental dysplasia of the hip (DDH). A national course with a focus on pediatric orthopedic trauma will be held in 2020.

Also in 2020 will be a half-day DDH course for primary care providers and pediatricians. This program represents efforts to reach the primary care community with DDH primary prevention and early detection, and is the result of collaboration between POSNA, International Hip Dysplasia Institute, International Hip Dysplasia Registry, and I'm a HIPpy Foundation. We look forward to continuing to be involved with these local educational initiatives, which are key to building strong local relationships and support. They demonstrate our ongoing dedication to the overall advancement of pediatric orthopedic care in the country and region.

Outcomes Assessment/Analysis and Research

The next phase of the program's growth and development is bringing data-driven analysis to the surgical care and outcomes. The availability of RedCap and other online databases provide for real time record keeping to track the patients. Furthermore, about two-thirds of incoming medical students and resident trainees are interested in doing international work.[22,23] Studies show us that if we engage them early, then they are more likely to continue this work as they start their careers.[24] As a result, there are many stakeholders with a strong interest and incentive to make these programs successful.[21–24] Population health, epidemiology of disease, and surgical outcomes research are great mechanisms for engagement and involvement for those trainees interested in doing global outreach work.

In Ecuador, we are proceeding on a few different fronts. We have compiled a comprehensive database of more than 130 postoperative patients with DDH in the program that we have treated surgically during the course of our biannual trips, over the past 18 years. The goal is to complete a retrospective study of outcomes and to then prospectively measure results with validated patient-reported outcome measures. Medical students and orthopedic residents have joined on these trips to assist with this initiative. Their structured involvement provides them pivotal early career experiences participating in the delivery of global outreach work while at the same time establishing a proper foundation on how this work should be approached and carried out.

Prevention Strategies

Year after year, we continue to encounter untreated DDH. Although this condition is not always preventable, with the exception of avoiding tight swaddling, early diagnosis and relatively simple treatment strategies can be used to decrease the life-long burden of hip dysplasia. One of the CME courses we developed for 2020 will be a half-day course on DDH for pediatricians and primary care providers. With the support of POSNA, the International Hip Dysplasia Institute, International Hip Dysplasia Registry, and I'm a HIPpy Foundation plans are in place to provide this educational program aimed at early diagnosis and basic management strategies. The International Hip Dysplasia Registry has been working on developing global care pathways in India, China, and Ecuador, led by Dr Kevin Shea from Stanford University and Dr Kishore Mulpuri from BC Children's Hospital. We have collaborated to conduct surveys of all the attendees on current treatment trends to help us better understand some of the local obstacles to delivery of care so that we can best devise how to implement an effective and comprehensive DDH care pathway tailored to local needs and resources available. In doing so, this provides the best chance to truly have an impact in addressing how DDH is approached and treated.

SUMMARY

The field of global health has gone through substantial growth and development over the last few decades. At its core, the rationale behind this work and impetus for involvement are clear: to improve the quality of life and function of those who would otherwise not have access. What started as medical missions have transformed into short-term experiences in global health and multifaceted programs aimed at limiting the burden of musculoskeletal disease in the LMIC.[9,13,20] To be truly impactful and successful, these programs require a strong commitment to cultural competence, bidirectional education, and capacity building.[1,12] Technology has made the world small in many ways. It is incumbent on us to take advantage of the resources we are now afforded and put them to use as vehicles of positive change.

DISCLOSURE

The authors all report no commercial or financial conflicts of interest or any funding sources pertinent or related to this work.

REFERENCES

1. Watts HG. Children's orthopaedics in underdeveloped regions: making it better. J Pediatr Orthop 2001;21:563–4.
2. Cobey JC. Physicians and surgeons volunteering in developing countries: a personal perspective. Clin Orthop Relat Res 2002;396:65–72.
3. Rankin EA. Volunteer experience overseas. Clin Orthop Relat Res 2002;396:80–3.
4. Pezzella AT. Volunteerism and humanitarian efforts in surgery. Curr Probl Surg 2006;43:848–929.
5. Kim JY, Farmer P, Porter ME. Redefining global health-care delivery. Lancet 2013;382:1060–9.
6. Dormans JP, Fisher RC, Pill SG. Orthopaedics in the developing world: present and future concerns. J Am Acad Orthop Surg 2001;9:289–96.
7. Shah S, Lin HC, Loh LC. A comprehensive framework to optimize short-term experiences in Global Health (STEGH). Global Health 2019;15(1):27.
8. Sykes KJ. Short-term medical service trips: a systematic review of the evidence. Am J Public Health 2014;104:e38–48.
9. Crump JA, Sugarman J, Working Group on Ethics Guidelines for Global Health Training (WEIGHT). Ethics and best practice guidelines for training experiences in global health. Am J Trop Med Hyg 2010;83:1178–82.
10. Lozano R, Naghavi M, Foreman K, et al. Global and regional mortality from 235 causes of death for 20 age groups in 1990 and 2010: a systematic analysis for the Global Burden of Disease Study 2010. Lancet 2012;380(9859):2095–128.
11. Farmer PE, Kim JY. Surgery and global health: a view from beyond the OR. World J Surg 2008; 32(4):533–6.
12. Pean CA, Premkumar A, Pean MA, et al. Global orthopaedic surgery: an ethical framework to prioritize surgical capacity building in low and middle-income countries. J Bone Joint Surg Am 2019; 101(13):e64.
13. Melby MK, Loh LC, Evert J, et al. Beyond medical "Missions" to impact-driven Short-Term Experiences in Global Health (STEGHs): ethical principles to optimize community benefit and learner experience. Acad Med 2016;91(5):633–8.
14. Crump JA, Sugarman J. Ethical considerations for short-term experiences by trainees in global health. JAMA 2008;300:1456–8.
15. Snyder J, Dharamsi S, Crooks VA. Fly-by medical care: conceptualizing the global and local social responsibilities of medical tourists and physician voluntourists. Global Health 2011;7:6.
16. Wilkins KE. Providing outreach continuing education in countries with limited resources. Clin Orthop Relat Res 2008;466:2413–7.
17. Wendler D, Emanuel EJ, Lie RK. The standard of care debate: can research in developing countries be both ethical and responsive to those countries' health needs? Am J Public Health 2004;94(6):923–8.
18. DeWane M, Grant-Kels JM. The ethics of volunteerism: whose cultural and ethical norms take precedence? J Am Acad Dermatol 2018;78(2):426–8.
19. Wall AE. Ethics in global surgery. World J Surg 2014;38(7):1574–80.

20. Fletcher AN, Schwend RM. The Ecuador pediatric spine deformity surgery program. An SRS-GOP site 2008-20916. Spine Deform 2019;7(2):220–7.
21. Fornari ED, Sabharwal S, Schwend RM. The POSNA-COUR international scholar program. results of the first 7 years. J Pediatr Orthop 2017;37:570–4.
22. Association of American Medical Colleges. Matriculating student questionnaire: 2012 all schools summary report. Washington, DC: Association of American Medical Colleges; 2012.
23. Khan OA, Guerrant R, Sanders J, et al. Global health education in U.S. medical schools. BMC Med Educ 2013;13:3.
24. Drain PK, Primack A, Hunt DD, et al. Global health in medical education: a call for more training and opportunities. Acad Med 2007;82:226–30.

Hand and Wrist

Ulnar Abutment Syndrome in the Athlete

Thomas R. Acott, MD[a], Jeffrey A. Greenberg, MD, MS[b,*]

KEYWORDS

• Ulnar abutment syndrome • Ulnocarpal impaction • Ulnar-wrist pain • Athlete
• Ulnar metaphyseal closing wedge osteotomy

KEY POINTS

- Ulnar abutment syndrome most commonly occurs in those with positive ulnar variance, but may occur in neutral or negative ulnar variance.
- Patients usually present with insidious onset ulnar wrist pain with a positive ulnocarpal stress test.
- Nonoperative treatment may be attempted based on the athlete's sport, season (in season or off season), and functional demands.
- Multiple procedures are available to offload the ulnocarpal joint; treatment ideally should be tailored to the individual athlete.

INTRODUCTION

It has been estimated that 3% to 9% of all athletic injuries involve the hand and wrist, and up to one-half of injuries are the result of overuse.[1,2] Overuse injuries are common in racket sports, rowing, volleyball, baseball, and gymnastics.[2,3] Although the majority of daily activities may be accomplished with 40° of wrist extension, 40° of wrist flexion, and 40° of radial-ulnar deviation,[4] the demands for athletic performance are often greater and largely sport dependent. Basketball requires 50° of extension and 70° of wrist flexion in the shooting hand, baseball pitchers require 32° of extension and 94° of wrist flexion, and golfers require 45° of radial-ulnar motion.[1] Gymnastics, unlike other sports, requires weight bearing on the upper extremity combined with hyperextension and radial and ulnar deviation of the wrist. As a result, wrist injuries are common in both female and male gymnasts, with up to 88% of participants experiencing wrist pain.[3,5] Increased demands on the wrist owing to athletics may predispose to specific injury patterns, and influence treatment decisions as athletes may not be willing to undergo motion-limiting immobilization, and may make treatment decisions based on their sporting season.

Ulnar abutment syndrome or ulnocarpal impaction is a degenerative condition resulting from excessive load transfer across the ulnocarpal joint associated with abutment of the ulnar pole against the ulnar carpus. It most commonly occurs in the ulnar positive variant wrist, but may occur in neutral or ulnar negative variance.[6] Prolonged impaction leads to degenerative changes in the triangular fibrocartilage complex (TFCC), chondromalacia of the lunate, triquetrum, and distal ulnar head, instability of the lunotriquetral joint, and finally, degenerative arthrosis of the ulnocarpal and distal radioulnar joints (DRUJ).

BIOMECHANICS

Approximately 18% of the axial load across the wrist is borne by the TFCC and ulnar head in an ulnar neutral wrist in neutral alignment.[7] Increased load transfer across the TFCC and ulnar head occurs with positive ulnar variance, ulnar deviation, and during relative ulnar lengthening that occurs in pronation and power grip. The axial load borne by the ulnocarpal

[a] The Core Institute, 9321 W Thomas Road, Suite 205, Phoenix, AZ 85037; [b] Indiana Hand to Shoulder Center, 8501 Harcourt Road, Indianapolis, IN 46260, USA
* Corresponding author.
E-mail address: handdr@mac.com

Orthop Clin N Am 51 (2020) 227–233
https://doi.org/10.1016/j.ocl.2019.11.007

articulation increases to 42% when ulnar variance increases 2.5 mm, and decreases to 4% when ulnar variance decreases by 2.5 mm.[7] Athletes that participate in frequent pronation and power grip activities, such as seen in baseball and other racquet sports (tennis), may be affected. Ulnar positive variance can be congenital or acquired.[8] Acquired ulnar positive variance may be seen in gymnasts or football lineman with distal radial physeal growth arrest as a result of repetitive loading of the distal radial physis that occurs before skeletal maturity.[3,5,9]

PRESENTATION

Patients often present with an insidious onset of ulnar wrist pain, usually without any single traumatic event.[8,10] Patients often complain that ulnar-sided wrist pain is exacerbated by activities that cause a relative increase in ulnar variance, such as power grip, pronation, and ulnar deviation. This pain is often relieved by rest.

PHYSICAL EXAMINATION

Patients often exhibit tenderness to palpation at the fovea or proximal pole of the lunate.[10,11] Symptoms may be reproduced in a position of extension and ulnar deviation. Pronation also may reproduce symptoms owing to the relative ulnar lengthening that occurs.[12] An ulnocarpal stress test may elicit symptoms; this test is performed by placing the patient's wrist in maximal ulnar deviation while applying an axial load while the wrist is taken passively through a range of pronosupination.[11,12] The test is considered positive if it elicits pain. Patients with ulnocarpal abutment often do not exhibit any DRUJ instability, but a comprehensive physical examination should evaluate for other etiologies of ulnar wrist pain.

IMAGING

Plain radiographs are often helpful in the diagnosis of ulnocarpal abutment and are useful to exclude other etiologies of ulnar wrist pain (eg, carpal malalignment, fractures of the carpus, metacarpal base, distal ulna, hook of the hamate, Kienböck's disease, and arthrosis). Ulnar variance should be assessed on a zero rotation posteroanterior radiograph. A pronated grip view is also helpful to assess dynamic positive ulnar variance, which has been shown to increase in pronation and power grip an average of 2.5 mm[13,14] (**Fig. 1**). Changes on radiographs are often subtle.[13] Subchondral sclerosis and cystic change may be present in the proximal ulnar lunate, the proximal radial triquetrum, or the ulnar head.[10,13] Degenerative arthrosis is uncommon. MRI may establish a diagnosis in patients with normal appearing radiographs and can be useful in establishing a diagnosis during the early stages before plain radiographic changes are present. Findings on MRI include cartilage fibrillation of the ulnar head and ulnar carpus, edema and hyperintensity on T2-weighted images, and low-intensity T1-weighted images, as well as degenerative changes of the TFCC including central disc perforations and lunotriquetral ligament injury[10,13] (**Fig. 2**). Findings localized to the ulnar aspect of the lunate help confirm the diagnosis of ulnocarpal

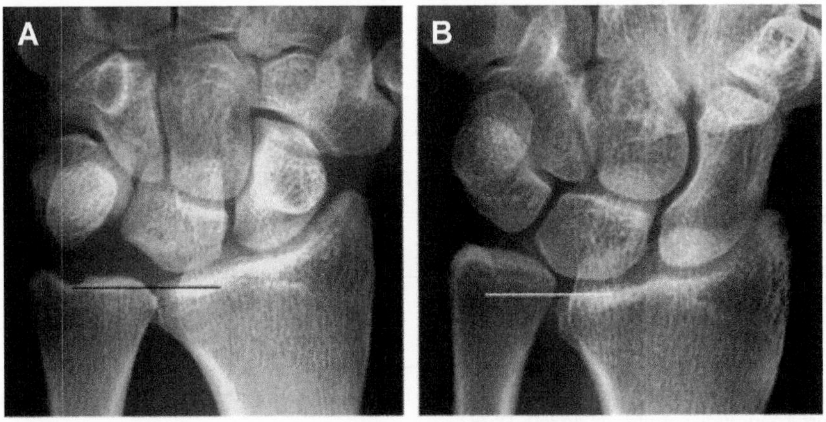

Fig. 1. Effect of gripping on ulnar variance. (*A*) Conventional posteroanterior radiograph of the wrist in neutral deviation shows slightly positive ulnar variance (*line*). (*B*) Radiograph obtained during forearm pronation combined with a firm grip shows a significant increase in ulnar variance (*line*). (*From* Cerezal L, del Piñal F, Abascal F, et al. Imaging findings in ulnar-sided wrist impaction syndromes. RadioGraphics 2002;22(1):107; with permission.)

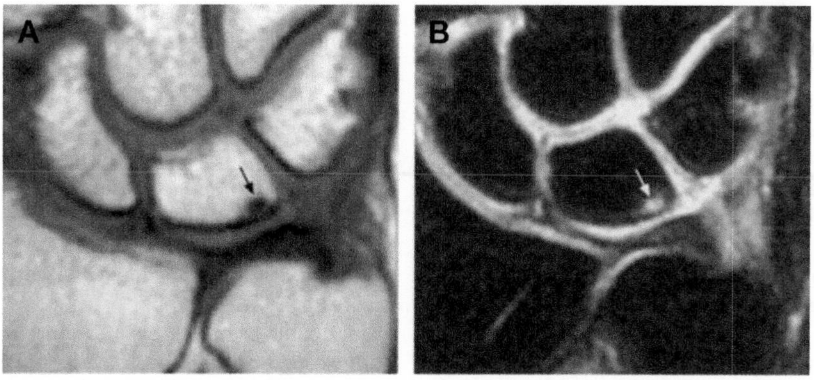

Fig. 2. Ulnar impaction syndrome in a 24-year-old man with neutral variance and ulnar-sided wrist pain. (*A*) Coronal T1-weighted (500/15) MRI demonstrates a small focus of low signal intensity in the subchondral ulnar corner of the lunate bone (*arrow*). (*B*) Corresponding coronal fat-suppressed T2-weighted (3000/50) MRI shows focal loss of lunate articular cartilage and high signal intensity marrow edema within the corresponding area of the lunate bone (*arrow*). The TFCC is intact. An arthroscopic wafer procedure was performed, resulting in complete resolution of symptoms. (*From* Cerezal L, del Piñal F, Abascal F, et al. Imaging findings in ulnar-sided wrist impaction syndromes. RadioGraphics 2002;22(1):110; with permission.)

abutment as compared with the diffuse findings seen in Kienbock's disease. MRI findings often return to normal after surgical intervention.[15]

NONOPERATIVE TREATMENT

Initial nonoperative treatment is usually recommended despite the athletes' activity. Depending on the patient's sport, specialized braces may be worn that accommodate sport-specific demands on wrist motion; such braces, for example, may be worn by gymnasts. These braces often limit terminal ulnar deviation and wrist extension and reduce ulnocarpal joint pressure[3] (**Fig. 3**). Medications such as nonsteroidal anti-inflammatories as well as taping and training modification may also be attempted to help control symptoms. Alterations in grip size, type of grip, string composition and string tension can be made for racquet players. Alterations in swing mechanics and changes in practice duration and intensity can be instituted. Corticosteroid injections may be useful for acute exacerbation of symptoms, and may have diagnostic benefit. A short (4–6 weeks) period of immobilization may be attempted as another nonoperative option, particularly during the off season.[5] Nonoperative treatment may allow for a symptomatic athlete to complete their current sporting season before pursuing surgical treatment. Athletes should be counseled on whether there is any long-term harm in delaying surgical treatment to the off season.

There is little scientific data regarding conservative treatment of ulnocarpal impaction in athletes; Roh and colleagues[16] found that, in nonathletes, 60% showed improvement with conservative treatment, however 25% went on to require ulnar shortening osteotomy (USO). Female sex, prolonged duration of symptoms, and findings on MRI were predictive of failure of conservative treatment. Despite these findings, nonoperative treatment is unlikely to be a definitive treatment in the athlete, and symptoms are likely to recur at some point after return to sport.[9,17]

OPERATIVE TREATMENT

Surgical treatment focuses on mechanically decreasing ulnocarpal joint load, with the goal of returning athletes to competitive play in a safe and timely manner.[12] Options include arthroscopic or open wafer resection procedure, diaphyseal USO, and ulnar metaphyseal

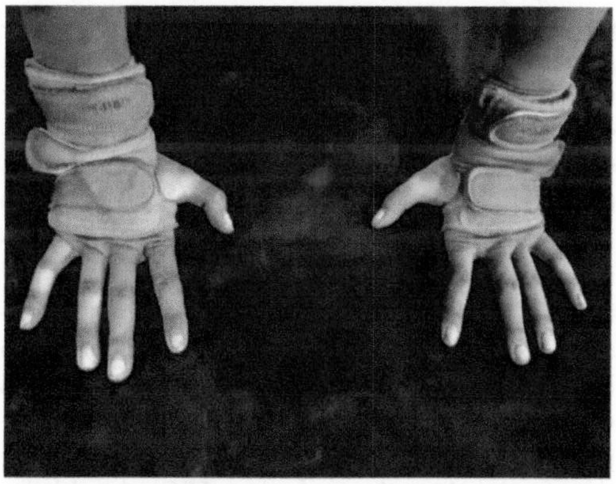

Fig. 3. A brace that can be used to limit wrist dorsiflexion. (*From* Benjamin HJ, Engel SC, Chudzik D. Wrist Pain in Gymnasts: A Review of Common Overuse Wrist Pathology in the Gymnastics Athlete. Curr Sports Med Rep 2017;16(5):324; with permission.)

closing wedge osteotomy. Concomitant arthroscopy is performed to address associated pathology that often includes TFC and osteochondral lesions. Arthroscopy also allows treatment of any concurrent carpal pathology.[17] Arthroscopic debridement of central TFCC tears alone in ulnar positive wrists has been shown to have high failure rates (13%–60%) and some form of ulnar variance correction should be performed.[12,18] Arthroscopic debridement alone may be considered in those with ulnar neutral or ulnar negative variance, although patients may require secondary ulnar shortening if they fail debridement alone.[18] The goal of ulnar shortening is to surgically create ulnar neutral or ulnar negative variance up to 2 mm.[9,19]

During a wafer resection procedure, the distal 2 to 3 mm of the distal ulna are removed. This procedure may be performed arthroscopically or open. Regardless of the technique, the radioulnar ligaments, their foveal insertion, and the distal radioulnar articular surfaces are preserved.[17,20] If performed arthroscopically, it is important to fully pronate and supinate the forearm to confirm acceptable ulnar head removal and to confirm adequate resection using fluoroscopy.[11,20] Griska and Feldon[20] recommended arthroscopic wafer resection only in patients with a central TFCC defect that allows arthroscopic access to the ulnar head. The benefit of the wafer procedure is that it avoids the risks of nonunion and symptomatic hardware that may require secondary removal.[12,20] An ulnar positive variance of greater than 4 mm is a contraindication to a wafer resection.[16] Persistent hemarthrosis from the exposed cancellous bone surface may lead to a prolonged recovery time.[19]

Diaphyseal USO is a common procedure with predictably good results. This procedure preserves the ulnar head articular surface while removing 2 mm or more of the ulnar diaphysis; stabilization is achieved with contemporary internal fixation techniques. In addition to offloading the distal ulna, the diaphyseal USO increases DRUJ stability by tightening the radioulnar ligaments. Nishiwaki and colleagues[21] found that diaphyseal ulnar shortening may tension and restabilize the DRUJ in patients with intact or partially torn radioulnar ligaments; this effect does not hold true in the case of a complete radioulnar ligament injury, in which case the foveal insertion of the TFC should be reestablished.

Ulnar shortening may also be performed via an ulnar metaphyseal closing wedge osteotomy, originally described by Slade and Gillon.[22] The benefits of the metaphyseal closing wedge osteotomy are that it avoids the risks of nonunion and symptomatic, prominent hardware. Placing the osteotomy in the metaphysis just proximal to the articular surface allows for rapid bony healing. This method is the senior author's preferred surgical technique.

Ulnar Metaphyseal Closing Wedge Osteotomy

Diagnostic arthroscopy is generally performed before osteotomy, but may be performed after osteotomy. The ulnocarpal, radiocarpal, and midcarpal joints are inspected and concurrent pathology is treated. Special attention is given to the TFCC; central tears amenable to debridement are common and debridement of the central disc back to a stable rim is performed. Peripheral TFCC tears should be addressed at the time of surgery. The ulnocarpal joint and lunate are inspected arthroscopically and any loose cartilage or osteochondral lesions are debrided. Arthroscopy may be difficult in patients with significant ulnar positive variance; delaying arthroscopy until completion of the ulnar shortening may facilitate arthroscopy in these patients.

A dorsal approach to the wrist is made through the floor of the fifth dorsal compartment. The extensor digiti minimi is retracted ulnarly, and the DRUJ is entered via an L-shaped capsulotomy proximal to the TFCC. The TFCC is protected to prevent injury during the procedure, as is the dorsal sensory branch of the ulnar nerve. Pronation, dorsal-directed force on the ulnar head, and volar-directed force on the radius may assist in visualization of the distal and dorsal ulnar head.[19]

A radially based closing wedge osteotomy of the distal ulna is then performed. The distal limb is placed parallel to the distal ulnar articular cartilage just proximal to the articulation with the sigmoid notch, and a second diagonal limb is placed as to intersect the transverse limb at the ulnar border of the ulna. This diagonal limb is placed 2 to 5 mm proximal to the transverse limb, and a wedge of distal ulna metaphysis is removed (**Fig. 4**). A headless compression screw is placed across the osteotomy from the dorsal radial corner of the ulnar head to the ulna border of the ulnar diaphysis, engaging the ulnar cortex (**Fig. 5**). Care is made to avoid violation of the ulnar seat, which articulates with the lesser sigmoid notch of the radius.

The DRUJ capsule and extensor retinaculum are then repaired, and the skin is closed.

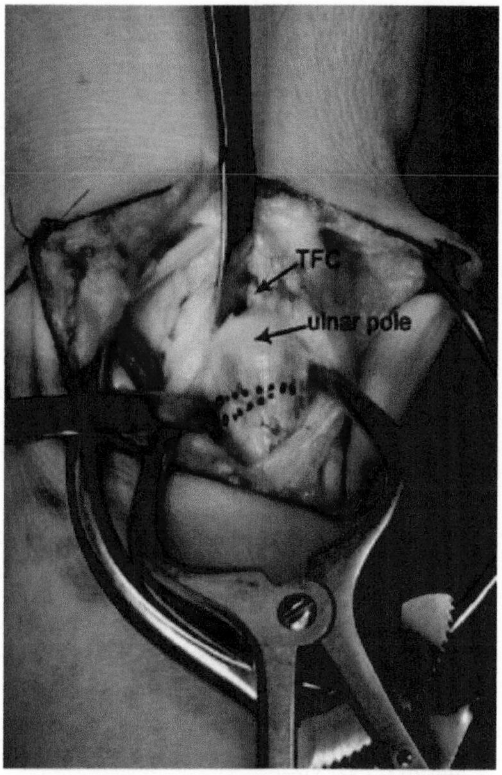

Fig. 4. Anatomic specimen showing osteotomy cuts for distal ulnar metaphyseal closing wedge osteotomy.TFC, triangular fibrocartilage. (*From* Crosby NE, Greenberg JA. Ulnar-sided wrist pain in the athlete. Clin Sports Med 2015;34(1):139; with permission.)

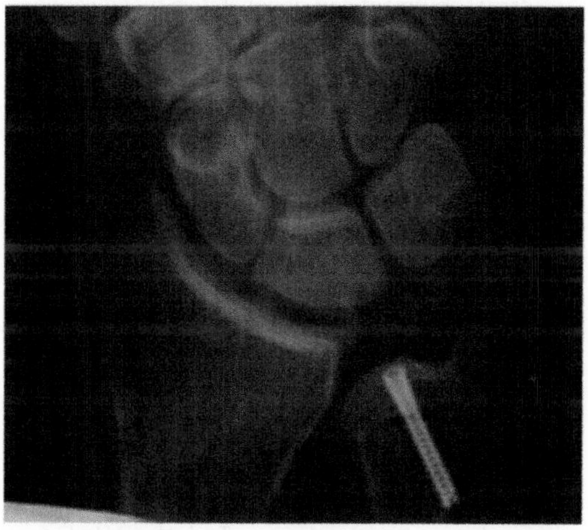

Fig. 5. Posteroanterior radiograph demonstrating headless compression screw fixation of closing wedge osteotomy of distal ulnar metaphysis. (*From* Crosby NE, Greenberg JA. Ulnar-sided wrist pain in the athlete. Clin Sports Med 2015;34(1):140; with permission.)

Patients are immobilized in a short arm splint for 4 to 6 weeks, during which time radiographs are obtained to assess bony healing. Gentle range of motion is begun when bony union is appreciated, followed by increased activity and sport-specific rehabilitation.

A separate but less common entity is ulnar styloid impaction syndrome. This impaction occurs between a long ulnar styloid and the triquetrum and can cause similar ulnar-sided wrist pain; however, it involves the triquetrum and lunotriquetral ligament rather than the lunate. Surgical treatment consists of ulnar styloid resection with care made to preserve the proximal ulnar styloid to preserve the deep radioulnar ligament insertion.[12,13]

COMPLICATIONS AND OUTCOMES

Complications after diaphyseal USO include nonunion, delayed union, symptomatic hardware, and malalignment of the DRUJ that affects forearm rotation.[10] Union rates exceed 90% and are decreased in smokers.[9] Nonunion is also a complication after metaphyseal closing wedge osteotomy, along with injury to dorsal sensory branches of the ulnar nerve, stiffness secondary to arthrotomy, and intraoperative ulnar head fracture.[10,19] Nonunion after either technique generally requires reoperation and nonunion repair with revision internal fixation. Both ulnar shortening techniques alter the tracking line and mechanics of the DRUJ and potentially predispose the DRUJ to delayed degenerative changes. Care should be made to avoid overshortening, which may increase forces across the DRUJ and potentially lead to degenerative arthritis.[23] Complications after wafer resection include intraoperative ulnar styloid fracture, injury to the deep radioulnar ligaments or their insertion, damage to the DRUJ articular surface, and inadequate or excessive resection.[20]

To date, no study has investigated ulnar shortening procedures in athletes. McAdams and associates[15] found that high-level athletes (varsity high school and higher) returned to play 3 months after procedures for TFCC tears. Concurrent ulnar wrist pathology including ulnar abutment may delay return to play.

Studies comparing the wafer resection procedure and USO demonstrate similar results. Constantine and colleagues[24] compared open wafer resection and diaphyseal USO and found no significant difference in regards to grip strength (85%–98% of unaffected extremity), pain relief, range of motion, or return to work. There were increased secondary procedures in the USO group, the most common being hardware removal. Similarly, Bernstein and colleagues[25] found that diaphyseal USO and arthroscopic wafer resections provide similar pain relief, improved grip strength (84%–86% unaffected extremity), and restoration of function, however, USO was associated with an increased incidence of secondary procedures (HWR) and tendonitis. Similar findings were demonstrated by Smet and colleagues[26] with similar postoperative Disabilities of the Arm, Shoulder, and Hand and visual analog scale scores seen in patients undergoing arthroscopic wafer resections and diaphyseal ulnar shortening osteotomies. Patients undergoing wafer resection returned to work earlier than those with diaphyseal USO (6.1 months vs 7.0 months). Given the recovery time, missed competition, and small risk in delaying surgical treatment, many athletes can be successfully surgically managed in their off season.

Multiple surgical procedures exist for ulnar shortening in the athlete with similar outcomes, each with their distinct complications. Treatment (nonoperative and operative) should be tailored to the athlete; their individual sport, in-season versus off-season timing, and their unique functional demands, with the goal of returning the athlete to competitive play in a safe and timely manner.

DISCLOSURE

The authors have nothing to disclose.

REFERENCES

1. Rettig AC. Athletic injuries of the wrist and hand. Part I: traumatic injuries of the wrist. Am J Sports Med 2003;31(6):1038–48.
2. Rettig AC. Athletic injuries of the wrist and hand: part II: overuse injuries of the wrist and traumatic injuries to the hand. Am J Sports Med 2004;32(1): 262–73.
3. DiFiori JP, Caine DJ, Malina RM. Wrist pain, distal radial physeal injury, and ulnar variance in the young gymnast. Am J Sports Med 2006;34(5): 840–9.
4. Ryu JY, Cooney WP, Askew LJ, et al. Functional ranges of motion of the wrist joint. J Hand Surg Am 1991;16(3):409–19.
5. Webb BG, Rettig LA. Gymnastic wrist injuries. Curr Sports Med Rep 2008;7(5):289–95.
6. Tatebe M, Nakamura R, Horii E, et al. Results of ulnar shortening osteotomy for ulnocarpal impaction syndrome in wrists with neutral or negative ulnar variance. J Hand Surg Br 2005;30(2):129–32.
7. Palmer AK, Werner FW. Biomechanics of the distal radioulnar joint. Clin Orthop Relat Res 1984; 187(187):26–35. Available at: http://www.ncbi.nlm.nih.gov/pubmed/6744728.
8. Benjamin HJ, Engel SC, Chudzik D. Wrist pain in gymnasts: a review of common overuse wrist pathology in the gymnastics athlete. Curr Sports Med Rep 2017;16(5):322–9.
9. Osterman AL. Central TFC tear/ulnar impaction injuries in professional football players. Hand Clin 2012;28(3):343–4.
10. Crosby NE, Greenberg JA. Ulnar-sided wrist pain in the athlete. Clin Sports Med 2015;34(1):127–41.
11. Sachar K. Ulnar-sided wrist pain: evaluation and treatment of triangular fibrocartilage complex tears, ulnocarpal impaction syndrome, and lunotriquetral ligament tears. J Hand Surg Am 2012;37(7): 1489–500.
12. Henderson CJ, Kobayashi KM. Ulnar-sided wrist pain in the athlete. Orthop Clin North Am 2016; 47(4):789–98.
13. Cerezal L, del Piñal F, Abascal F, et al. Imaging findings in ulnar-sided wrist impaction syndromes. Radiographics 2002;22(1):105–21.
14. Tomaino MM. The importance of the pronated grip x-ray view in evaluating ulnar variance. J Hand Surg Am 2000;25(2):352–7.
15. McAdams TR, Swan J, Yao J. Arthroscopic treatment of triangular fibrocartilage wrist injuries in the athlete. Am J Sports Med 2009;37(2):291–7.
16. Roh YH, Kim S, Gong HS, et al. Prognostic value of clinical and radiological findings for conservative treatment of idiopathic ulnar impaction syndrome. Sci Rep 2018;8(1):9891.
17. Jarrett CD, Baratz ME. The management of ulnocarpal abutment and degenerative triangular fibrocartilage complex tears in the competitive athlete. Hand Clin 2012;28(3):329–37, ix.
18. Nagle DJ. Triangular fibrocartilage complex tears in the athlete. Clin Sports Med 2001;20(1):155–66.
19. Khouri JS, Hammert WC. Distal metaphyseal ulnar shortening osteotomy: technique, pearls, and outcomes. J Wrist Surg 2014;3(3):175–80.
20. Griska A, Feldon P. Wafer resection of the distal ulna. J Hand Surg Am 2015;40(11):2283–8.
21. Nishiwaki M, Nakamura T, Nakao Y, et al. Ulnar shortening effect on distal radioulnar joint stability: a biomechanical study. J Hand Surg Am 2005;30(4): 719–26.
22. Slade JF, Gillon TJ. Osteochondral shortening osteotomy for the treatment of ulnar impaction syndrome: a new technique. Tech Hand Up Extrem Surg 2007;11(1):74–82.
23. Nishiwaki M, Nakamura T, Nagura T, et al. Ulnar-shortening effect on distal radioulnar joint pressure: a biomechanical study. J Hand Surg Am 2008;33(2):198–205.

24. Constantine KJ, Tomaino MM, Herndon JH, et al. Comparison of ulnar shortening osteotomy and the wafer resection procedure as treatment for ulnar impaction syndrome. J Hand Surg Am 2000; 25(1):55–60.
25. Bernstein MA, Nagle DJ, Martinez A, et al. A comparison of combined arthroscopic triangular fibrocartilage complex debridement and arthroscopic wafer distal ulna resection versus arthroscopic triangular fibrocartilage complex debridement and ulnar shortening osteotomy for ulnocarpal abutment syndrome. Arthroscopy 2004;20(4):392–401.
26. Smet LD, Vandenberghe L, Degreef I. Ulnar impaction syndrome: ulnar shortening vs. arthroscopic wafer procedure. J Wrist Surg 2014;3(2):98–100.

Operative Distal Radial Fractures

A Comparison of Time to Surgery After Evaluation by Surgical and Nonsurgical Providers in a Walk-in Clinic

Matthew N. Fournier, MD*, Joseph T. Cline, MD,
Adam Seal, BS, Richard A. Smith, PhD,
Thomas W. Throckmorton, MD,
Benjamin M. Mauck, MD[1]

KEYWORDS

• Distal radial fracture • Evaluation • Nonsurgical providers • Walk-in clinic

KEY POINTS

- Initial evaluation by a nonsurgical provider in a walk-in orthopedic clinic setting was associated with a slightly longer delay between initial evaluation and surgical treatment than in a conventional hand surgeon's clinic, but this difference may not be clinically significant.
- Patients initially seen in a hand surgeon's office had fewer office visits than those seen in a walk-in clinic.
- Evaluation by a nonsurgical provider was not associated with a significantly increased duration to definitive treatment compared with evaluation by a surgical provider.

INTRODUCTION

Most orthopedic care historically has been delivered by orthopedic surgeons, but, as the needs of orthopedic clinical practice change under dynamic regulatory conditions, nonsurgeon providers are playing an increasingly important role.[1] Although the surgeon continues to direct the health care team, providers, such as family medicine and physical medicine physicians, physician assistants (PAs), and nurse practitioners (NPs), commonly are used to fill various roles in care delivery to patients.[2–5] These providers may be used in a variety of capacities, from assisting in surgery to running an independent clinic, but the goal of providing efficient, cost-effective, quality care to patients remains constant. Overuse injuries, simple fractures, and conservative care for degenerative conditions represent a significant portion of the outpatient clinical care provided by orthopedic hand surgeons, but many of these issues can be managed safely and effectively by care providers without a surgical background.[5] Practices may choose to supplement the care team with nonsurgical providers to meet increasing clerical or clinical duties that cannot feasibly be undertaken by surgical providers. Practices also may offer walk-in or after-hours triage clinics that are available for patients outside of normal business hours. Nonsurgical providers can bolster the number of staff available to see patients in this setting, thereby avoiding an undue demand

University of Tennessee-Campbell Clinic Department of Orthopaedic Surgery and Biomedical Engineering, 1211 Union Avenue, Suite 510, Memphis, TN 38104, USA
[1] Senior Author.
* Corresponding author.
E-mail address: mfournie@uthsc.edu

Orthop Clin N Am 51 (2020) 235–239
https://doi.org/10.1016/j.ocl.2019.11.006

on busy orthopedic surgeons.[6] In both cases, musculoskeletal care is made available to patients in a way that maximizes a practice's ability to see patients and minimizes financial barriers associated with employing more surgical providers. By referring patients in whom conservative management has failed, these providers also increase the percentage of patients requiring operative care in a surgeon's clinic.

Although nonsurgical providers are well integrated into clinical orthopedic practice in many centers, objective data analyzing the care they provide compared with orthopedic surgeons are lacking.[2,3,5,7] When a nonsurgical provider evaluates a patient with a surgical problem, a transfer of care becomes necessary. This transition of care can take many forms, ranging from a real-time phone call to the surgeon to discuss the patient and potentially schedule surgical treatment to scheduling a 1-week follow-up for reevaluation. Transfers of care can result in delays that are not present when a patient is evaluated and treated by a single surgical provider. The purpose of this study was to evaluate whether initial evaluation by a nonsurgical provider in an orthopedic walk-in setting delayed the care of operative distal radial fractures. The authors hypothesized that evaluation by nonsurgical providers would not significantly delay the surgical care of these patients.

MATERIALS AND METHODS

After Institutional Review Board approval, a retrospective chart review identified skeletally mature patients who were initially seen in an orthopedic walk-in clinic for evaluation of an acute distal radial fracture between January 2010 and December 2017, and who subsequently had surgical fixation of their injury. Only acute injuries, defined as fractures less than 2 weeks old, were included. The cohort was divided based on whether the initial evaluation was conducted by a surgical or nonsurgical provider. Surgical providers included orthopedic surgeons and fellows trained in a variety of subspecialties, and nonsurgical providers included family medicine physicians, physiatrists, NPs, and PAs. All providers were employed by the same single-specialty orthopedic group, and only patients who presented on a walk-in basis, without a previously scheduled appointment, were included. Nonsurgical providers see patients without the direct oversight of an orthopedic surgeon in this setting, although surgeons are available for consultation should the provider deem it necessary. Patients who underwent a trial of nonoperative management of any duration at the direction of any provider were excluded from analysis.

A control group of patients who were evaluated and managed solely in a fellowship-trained hand surgeon's clinic also were identified. These patients were seen at a regularly scheduled appointment and subsequently had closed or open reduction and fixation of a distal radial fracture by the same surgeon. Demographic information was collected for both groups, including age, gender, race, payor status, and injury characteristics. Days until surgical treatment, days until evaluation by surgical provider, number of clinic visits, and number of providers seen in the episode of care prior to surgery were considered primary endpoints. Statistical analysis of the results was completed using descriptive statistics, Student *t* tests, analysis of variance (ANOVA), and chi-square testing for association. *P* values less than .05 were considered statistically significant.

Table 1
Cohort demographics

	Patients Seen by Surgical Provider	Patients Seen by Nonsurgical Provider	Control Group	*P* Value
Patients (n)	72	63	61	
Gender (n)				.786
Male	16	11	12	
Female	56	52	49	
Mean age (y)	55.8	54.8	54.5	.899
Race (n)				.757
White	61	53	52	
African American	10	9	6	
Other	1	1	3	

Table 2
Comparison of days to treating surgeon

	N	Mean	SD	*P* Value
Surgical providers	72	5.33	3.84	.17[a]
Nonsurgical providers	63	4.52	2.96	—

[a] *P* value comparing means for operative and nonoperative groups' days to treating surgeon.

RESULTS

Of 135 patients who were initially seen in a walk-in clinic and had surgical fixation of a distal radial fracture, 80% were female, and the average age was 55.3 (15–83) years; 72 patients initially were seen by an orthopedic surgeon and 63 by a nonsurgical provider. There were no significant differences between groups regarding gender, age, race, or payor status (Table 1).

Operative Versus Nonoperative Providers

There were no significant differences between the surgical and nonsurgical groups with regard to the number of days elapsed between initial walk-in evaluation and first visit with the surgical provider (Table 2). Patients initially evaluated by a surgical provider were seen by their treating surgeon an average of 5.3 days later, whereas patients in the nonsurgical group were seen after an average of 4.5 days ($P = .17$). Likewise, no significant delay was found when comparing the time to surgery between the surgical and nonsurgical groups (Table 3). The patients seen by a surgical provider had fixation at an average of 9 days after their initial visit compared with 8.5 days for the nonsurgical cohort ($P = .53$). Approximately 89% of patients from both groups had their procedure after 2 clinic visits, with no significant differences noted between the mean number of total providers or clinic visits between the groups (Table 4).

Single-surgeon Control Group

The control group of patients who were evaluated and treated solely by a fellowship-trained hand surgeon were found to have significantly fewer days between evaluation and surgery as well as fewer total clinic visits. These patients had surgery an average of 5.2 days after their initial office visit compared with 9 days and 8.5 days for the surgical and nonsurgical cohorts, respectively ($P = .001$). Of the control patients, 96% attended only 1 office visit before surgery compared with 2 visits by 88% of both the surgical and nonsurgical cohorts ($P = .001$).

DISCUSSION

Societal demands on the musculoskeletal workforce continue to grow, due in large part to a growing and aging population. Some estimates call for a 40% increase in the number of Americans over the age of 65 by 2030.[3] During the same time frame, the supply of physicians is predicted to remain stagnant, with a modest increase of 0.5% per year.[8] Advanced practice providers (APPs), including PAs and NPs, are expected to help offset this disparity, with recent surveys suggesting increasing enrollment in APP programs.[1,9] In the future, APPs and nonsurgical physicians likely will play an increasingly important role in the delivery of musculoskeletal care, and orthopedic surgeons will be responsible for the safe and efficient integration of these providers into the clinical setting.

Despite the increasing prevalence of APPs and nonsurgical physicians in the orthopedic setting, there is little objective evidence to compare the care they provide. A recent study evaluated the clinical and financial impact of integrating PAs into the orthopedic trauma service at a level 2 community hospital. A decrease in time elapsed between registration and initial evaluation was shown, as well as time until surgery, in addition to a decrease in overall length of stay.[10] The investigators concluded that the use of PAs improved efficiency without compromising patient care. Other studies have investigated APPs in a variety of nonorthopedic clinical settings and found them to provide safe and efficient care.[11,12] Finally, research suggests

Table 3
Comparison of days to surgery

	N	Mean	SD	95% CI	*P* Value
Surgical providers	72	9.03	4.92	7.87–10.18	.530[a]
Nonsurgical providers	63	8.5	4.3	7.44–9.61	—
Control group	61	5.2	4.63	4.31–6.15	.001[b]

[a] *P* value for Student *t* test comparing means for operative and nonoperative days to surgery.
[b] *P* value for ANOVA comparing mean days to surgery for all 3 groups.

Table 4
Comparison of total clinic visits

	Number of Clinic Visits			$P = .001$[a]
	1	2	3	4
Surgical providers (n [%])	3 (4.2)	64 (88.9)	4 (5.6)	1 (1.4)
Nonsurgical providers (n [%])	0 (0)	56 (88.9%)	7 (11.1)	0 (0)
Control group (n [%])	59 (96.7)	2 (3.3)	0 (0)	0 (0)

[a] *P* value for chi-square test for independence.

that patients generally receive a comparably satisfying health care experience when cared for by an APP or a surgeon, although there are some scenarios when patients may prefer a visit with an orthopedic surgeon.[4,7]

The purpose of this study was to evaluate whether evaluation by a nonsurgical provider in a walk-in orthopedic clinic delayed the eventual surgical care of operative distal radial fractures compared with initial evaluation by a surgeon. This study found no significant differences when comparing days to evaluation by the treating surgeon or total days to surgery between the surgical and nonsurgical groups. This is consistent with studies that have found comparable care between physicians and APPs,[2,4,7,10–12] suggesting that nonsurgical providers are able to efficiently transfer the care of operative injuries to surgeons without introducing a significant delay.

This study also showed that patients seen and evaluated in a fellowship-trained hand surgeon's clinic are likely to undergo their definitive procedure slightly sooner than patients seen by either provider type in a walk-in setting. The authors attribute this difference of approximately 3 days to the ability of the hand surgeon to assess the injury and commence surgical planning in the same clinic visit without any transfer of care. This likely also explains the ability of the hand surgeon to arrange the procedure after a single clinic visit compared with an average of 2 clinic visits in the walk-in groups. Although this difference in surgical timing was statistically significant, a delay of 3 days is unlikely to have a clinically significant effect on the injuries included in this study. Work by Weil and colleagues[13] suggested similar outcomes in patients with distal radial fractures treated after a delay of more than 21 days compared with acute fixation. A delay of 3 days is unlikely to significantly increase the difficulty of the operation or mandate the use of alternative fixation techniques.

The results of this study suggest that for patients with an acute distal radial fracture who prefer to be evaluated in a walk-in clinic setting, evaluation by a nonsurgical provider does not introduce significant delay compared with evaluation by a surgeon in the same setting. They also can expect care that is clinically comparable that provided in a hand surgeon's clinic.

There are limitations of this study in addition to those associated with its retrospective design. The patients in this study were all evaluated in a walk-in clinic staffed by providers from a single orthopedic group. Nonsurgical providers in this group have direct access to surgeons in both the walk-in setting and in the regular clinic setting. This scenario may not be applicable to nonsurgical providers in smaller practices where exposure to surgical providers is more limited, and it certainly is not generalizable to APPs who evaluate orthopedic injuries in nonorthopedic settings, such as community urgent care clinics. The results of this study likely are best applied to nonsurgical providers who are integrated into larger, well-established orthopedic groups with broad, fellowship-trained surgeon representation. The authors also acknowledge the potential for selection bias with the exclusion of patients who underwent a trial of nonoperative management by any provider, because these patients may have more uncertainty and possible variation in their course of treatment. The authors found no other studies that directly compare the care of operative distal radial injuries by orthopedic surgeons with care by nonsurgical providers. Further research is necessary to evaluate the care provided by APPs and nonsurgical physicians as their role in musculoskeletal care delivery becomes increasingly prominent.

REFERENCES

1. Salsberg E. The nurse practitioner, physician assistant, and pharmacist pipelines: continued growth. 2015. Available at: http://healthaffairs.org/blog/2015/05/26/the-nurse-practitioner-physician-assistant-and-pharmacist-pipelines-continued-growth/. Accessed June 12, 2019.

2. Althausen PL, Shannon S, Owens B, et al. Impact of hospital-employed physician assistants on a Level II community-based orthopaedic trauma system. J Orthop Trauma 2016;30(Suppl 5):S40–4.
3. Day CS, Boden SD, Knott PT, et al. Musculoskeletal workforce needs: are physician assistants and nurse practitioners the solution? AOA critical issues. J Bone Joint Surg Am 2016;98(11):e46.
4. Manning BT, Bohl DD, Luchetti TJ, et al. Physician extenders in hand surgery: the patient's perspective. Hand (N Y) 2019;14(1):127–32.
5. Ward WT, Eberson CP, Otis SA, et al. Pediatric orthopaedic practice management: the role of midlevel providers. J Pediatr Orthop 2008;28(8): 795–8.
6. Anderson TJ, Althausen PL. The role of dedicated musculoskeletal urgent care centers in reducing cost and improving access to orthopaedic care. J Orthop Trauma 2016;30(Suppl 5):S3–6.
7. Manning BT, Bohl DD, Hannon CP, et al. Patient perspectives of midlevel providers in orthopaedic sports medicine. Orthop J Sports Med 2018;6(4). 2325967118766873.
8. Auerbach DI, Staiger DO, Buerhaus PI. Growing ranks of advanced practice clinicians - implications for the physician sorkforce. N Engl J Med 2018; 378(25):2358–60.
9. Hooker RS, Muchow AN. Supply of physician assistants: 2013-2026. JAAPA 2014;27(3):39–45.
10. Christmas AB, Reynolds J, Hodges S, et al. Physician extenders impact trauma systems. J Trauma 2005;58(5):917–20.
11. Costa DK, Wallace DJ, Barnato AE, et al. Nurse practitioner/physician assistant staffing and critical care mortality. Chest 2014;146(6):1566–73.
12. Kleinpell RM, Ely EW, Grabenkort R. Nurse practitioners and physician assistants in the intensive care unit: an evidence-based review. Crit Care Med 2008;36(10):2888–97.
13. Weil YA, Mosheiff R, Firman S, et al. Outcome of delayed primary internal fixation of distal radius fractures: a comparative study. Injury 2014;45(6):960–4.

Shoulder and Elbow

Global Perspectives on Management of Shoulder Instability

Decision Making and Treatment

Lisa G.M. Friedman, MD, MA[a,*], Laurent Lafosse, MD[b],
Grant E. Garrigues, MD[a]

KEYWORDS

• Shoulder • Instability • Dislocation • Subluxation • Bankart • Latarjet • Arthroscopy

KEY POINTS

- The shoulder depends on dynamic and static stabilizers because it has little inherent stability, making it prone to instability.
- There are several classification systems; none perfectly take into account the complexity of diagnosis, treatment, and prognosis for all the different types of instability.
- Patients with unidirectional traumatic instability, particularly young patients engaging in high-risk activities, have a high risk of recurrent instability when treated nonoperatively.
- Patients with unidirectional traumatic instability with bone loss or recurrence after surgery can be treated effectively with a variety of bone block procedures.
- Patients with multidirectional instability should be treated with a long course of physical therapy before surgery. Young age, laxity, and high-risk sports are negative prognostic factors.

FUNCTIONAL ANATOMY OF THE GLENOHUMERAL JOINT

The glenohumeral joint has the largest range of motion of any joint in the human body. This feat is due to the unique anatomy, with very little intrinsic osseous stability.[1]

Dynamic stabilization is offered by the muscles of the rotator cuff and the periscapular musculature, as well as the long-head of the biceps brachii. The rotator cuff, as well as middle deltoid, function to dynamically compress the humeral head against the glenoid, a phenomenon known as concavity compression. Dynamic stability is also afforded to the shoulder through neuromuscular control. This combines an individual's sense of joint proprioception and ability to perform reactive muscle contractions to stabilize the humeral head during motion.[1] Like a seal balancing a ball on its nose, scapulohumeral balance is achieved by varying the scapular position in space to provide a mobile but stable platform to balance the humerus within the glenoid.[2]

Additional stability is afforded to the glenohumeral joint through its static stabilizers. The glenoid labrum functions to deepen the glenoid fossa by 50%.[3,4] It is also the attachment site for many of the glenohumeral ligaments. Together, the coracohumeral ligament, superior glenohumeral ligament, middle glenohumeral ligament, and inferior glenohumeral ligament complex are individual thickenings of the capsule that prevent instability in various positions of rotation.[1,5] In addition, the overall watertight seal of the capsule provides stability globally by maintaining

[a] Midwest Orthopaedics at Rush, Rush University Medical Center, 1611 West Harrison Street, Chicago, IL 60612, USA; [b] Clinique Générale, Alps Surgery Institute, 4 Chemin de la Tour la Reine, 74000 Annecy, France
* Corresponding author.
E-mail address: Lisa.Friedman@rushortho.com
twitter: @Shoulder2LeanOn (L.G.M.F.); @Grant_Garrigues (G.E.G.)

Orthop Clin N Am 51 (2020) 241–258
https://doi.org/10.1016/j.ocl.2019.11.008

a negative intra-articular pressure.[1,6] This negative intra-articular pressure creates a relative vacuum seal between the glenohumeral joint that also contributes to articular stability through viscous and intermolecular forces.[1,7]

Instability of the shoulder is a common orthopedic problem worldwide and orthopedic surgery clinicians and researchers from around the globe continue to search for optimal solutions for patients; individual patient activity and anatomy present specific challenges.

DIAGNOSIS

Patients with unidirectional instability typically describe that their symptoms began with a traumatic event resulting in dislocation or subluxation. These instability events can become ongoing and recurrent. In unidirectional traumatic instability, there is structural damage such as labral tears or fractures to the glenoid rim or humeral head. In most cases, surgery is indicated to repair those structural injuries to prevent recurrent instability.[8,9] For posterior instability, injuries typically occur with dynamic posterior loading activities, with the arm flexed, adducted, and internally rotated.[10] Anterior instability typically results from trauma in external rotation and a hyperabducted position when an anterior directed forces displaces the humeral head from the glenoid.[4]

For patients with multidirectional instability (MDI), instability must be distinguished from laxity, with laxity being an objective term used to describe translation of the humeral head upon the glenoid and instability referring to an abnormal amount of laxity that results in symptoms.[11,12] Patients with MDI may or may not be able to recall an inciting traumatic event. In MDI, the primary structural problem is excessive redundancy of the capsule. MDI can exist in the presence of a structural lesion such as a labral tear or an osseous defect, indicating a traumatic etiology. In other cases, MDI can exist in the setting of excessive ligamentous laxity, which can be either congenital or owing to numerous microtrauma such as in competitive athletes or manual laborers.[11]

There are anatomic lesions that are often seen as a result of instability. These common pathologies, as well as their incidence, are summarized in **Table 1**.

PHYSICAL EXAMINATION

For patients with instability, the physical examination involves inspection for atrophy and scapular winging, as well as palpation to discern areas of tenderness. Range of motion and strength deficits should also be noted. Patients older than 40 years of age often have acute rotator cuff tears associated with dislocation, making strength testing especially essential in this population.[13] Examination maneuvers to discern labral pathology are indicated as well. The glenohumeral capsular structures tighten and relax with both translation and rotation. Although there are many special tests described elsewhere in this article that emphasize the translation side of this equation, a careful range of motion examination is critical. The range of motion examination should be slow and controlled, not proceeding past any point of apprehension, with special caution in the patient with a recent traumatic dislocation, to avoid an iatrogenic dislocation.

There are multiple specific tests designed to assess for shoulder instability that are summarized in **Table 2**.

Imaging

Plain radiographs should be obtained for the patient with the complaint of instability. These should include a Grashey anteroposterior view in neutral rotation, a scapular Y, and axillary lateral. These views are important to assess whether the shoulder is currently reduced, and, if not, the direction of the instability as well as any concomitant fractures.[14] In addition, there are other views that are helpful, especially in the setting of glenohumeral instability. The Stryker-Notch view shows the articulation of the glenoid and the humeral head and is used for assessing for Hills-Sachs lesions. The West Point axillary view, named for the US Military Academy where it was developed, is a tangential view of the anteroinferior glenoid rim and is the best view for visualizing glenoid rim pathology such as bony Bankart lesions.[15] The Bernageau view, named for Jacques Bernageau of Paris, France, is obtained with a 30° craniocaudal tilt directed toward the spine of the scapula while the patient stands or sits in an anterior oblique position with the arm abducted to 135°. The purpose of this view is to visualize the anteroinferior segment of the glenoid rim without the superimposition of the superior glenoid.[16]

Advanced imaging is often helpful. Three-dimensional computed tomography imaging is often the preferred measure for evaluating for bone loss, because 2-dimenaional computed tomography scans can overestimate or underestimate the amount of bone loss based on patient positioning within the computed

Table 1
Anatomic lesions and their incidence commonly seen in the shoulder as a result of instability

Anatomic Lesion	Description	Incidence
Bankart lesion	Avulsion off the anterior inferior aspect of the glenoid labrum and capsule from the glenoid rim	96%–97%[4]
Bony Bankart	Bankart with a fracture of the anteroinferior glenoid	—
Reverse Bankart	Avulsion off the posterior inferior aspect of the glenoid labrum and capsule from the glenoid rim from posterior dislocation	—
Perthes lesion	Nondisplaced tear of the anteroinferior labrum with intact medial scapular periosteum.	—
Anterior labroligamentous periosteal sleeve avulsion	Complete detachment of the anteroinferior labrum that becomes medially displaced and inferiorly rotated on the glenoid rim and scapular neck.	12.5% (acute instability) 31% (chronic instability)[109]
Glenoid articular disruption	Damage to chondrolabral junction, which occurs at anteroinferior portion of the glenoid fossa	—
Humeral avulsion of the glenohumeral ligament	Rupture of the humeral attachment of the IGHL with or without bony avulsion	7.5%–9.3%[110]
Posterior humeral avulsion of the glenohumeral ligament	Humeral attachment of the posterior band of IGHL and capsule tears from the posterior humeral neck	—
Glenoid avulsion of the glenohumeral ligament	Avulsion of the IGHL from the glenoid with seperation from the labrum	—
Hill-Sachs	Contre-coup impaction fracture of the posterior humeral head from its contact on the anterior glenoid rim.	93%[111]
Reverse Hill-Sachs	Impaction fracture to the anterior humeral head as a result of a posterior dislocation	—
Kim Lesion	An avulsion of the deep portion of the posteroinferior labrum and glenoid cartilage	—
Patulous inferior capsule	Pathognomonic finding of MDI	—

Abbreviations: IGHL, inferior glenohumeral ligament complex.

tomography gantry and does not allow for humeral subtraction.[17] In contrast, historically, MRI has been used to evaluate for soft tissue injuries typically seen in instability.[18] There is some debate over the usefulness of arthrography to enhance MRI to increase the diagnostic yield. A study by Magee[19] demonstrated increased sensitivity in the diagnosis of partial thickness articular surface supraspinatus tears, anterior labral tears, and superior labrum anterior to posterior tears compared with conventional MRI studies. Studies have demonstrated that MRI can measure glenoid bone loss accurately.[20–22]

CLASSIFICATION

There are multiple classification systems that attempt to define and guide treatment for

Table 2
Physical examination maneuvers and their specificities and sensitivities used to assess for shoulder instability

Test	Description	Specificity	Sensitivity
Anterior apprehension test	Affected arm is brought into 90° of external rotation and 90° of abduction. Apprehension of impending instability is a positive test.	95.4%	65.6%[112]
Relocation test	Apprehension is relieved when the shoulder is manually stabilized by applying a posteriorly directed force to the humeral head.	90.2%	64.6%[112]
Combined apprehension test and relocation test		98%	81%[113]
Load and shift	The humeral head is first "loaded" into the glenoid fossa and then shifted anteriorly and then graded between 0 (minimal displacement) and 3 (dislocated without spontaneous reduction).	89.9%–100%	8.0–71.7[114]
Anterior/posterior drawer test	The humeral head is shifted anteriorly or posteriorly in the glenoid fossa.	85.0%–92.7%	53.0%–58.3%.[114]
Jerk test	Patient positioned in 90° of abduction and 90° of internal rotation while stabilizing the scapula. The humerus is axially loaded and adducted. Painful or audible subluxation of the humeral head off the glenoid is a positive test for posterior or posteroinferior labral pathology.	98%	73%[115]
Kim test	Patient is positioned in 90° of abduction and 90° of internal rotation. The proximal forearm is held and adducted and elevated to 45°, while a posterior and axial load is applied through the shoulder. The presence of pain is indicative of posteroinferior labral pathology.	94%	80%[115]

(continued on next page)

Test	Description	Specificity	Sensitivity
Sulcus sign	Inferiorly directed force applied with the arm at the side. Inferior displacement of the humeral head that does not improve with external rotation is positive for superior glenohumeral ligament and coracohumeral ligament deficiency.	97% with a 2-cm cutoff	28% with a 2-cm cutoff[116]
Gagey hyperabduction test	Shoulder girdle is stabilized and the shoulder is passively abducted. Patients who can passively abduct over 105° suggests excessive laxity, particularly through the IGHL.	89.0%	66.7%[114]
Hyperextension internal rotation test[117] (Fig. 1)	The affected shoulder is placed in hyperextension and internal rotation, placing the IGHL and inferior capsule under tension without risk of dislocation in clinic. Patients with instability owing to incompetence of the IGHL and inferior capsule will have increased extension angles compared with the contralateral, unaffected side.		
Beighton score	Scale for quantifying the global level of joint hypermobility in patients. It takes into account passive dorsiflexion of the fifth metacarpophalangeal joints, passive hyperextension of the elbows, passive hyperextension of the knees, passive apposition of the thumbs to the forearm, and forward flexion of the trunk such that the palms contact the ground with a maximum score of 9.	—	As a screening examination for shoulder laxity specifically: 0.40–0.48.[118]

Abbreviation: IGHL, inferior glenohumeral ligament complex.

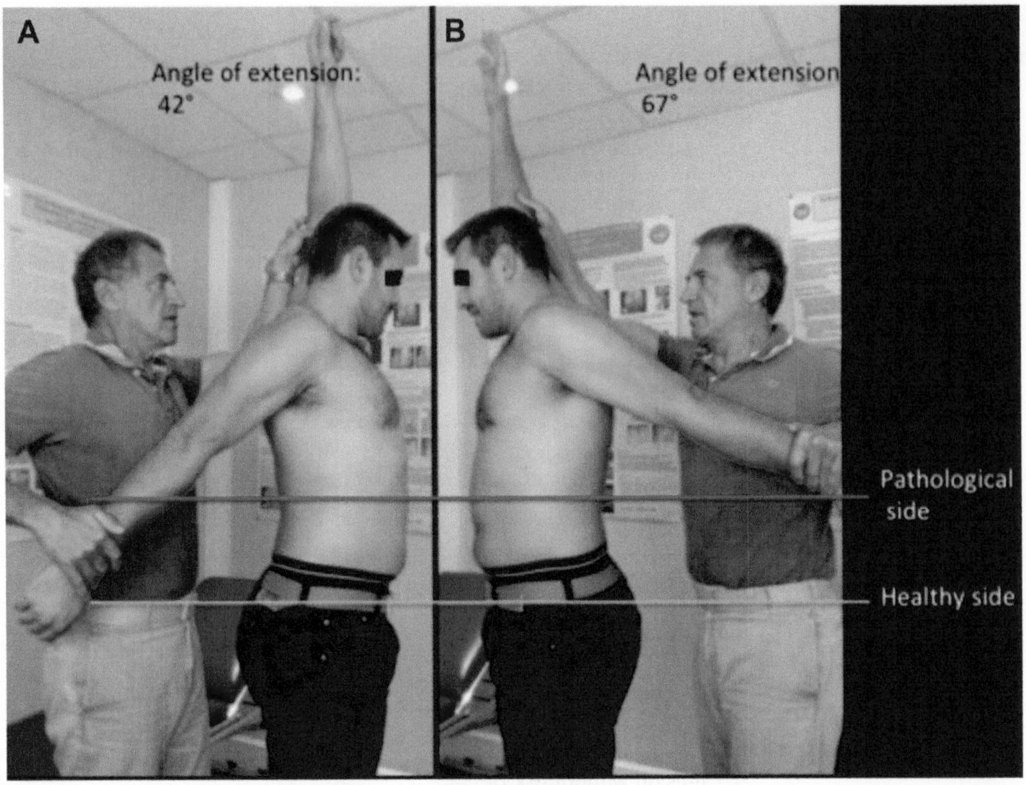

Fig. 1. Hyperextension and internal rotation test, demonstrating differences in extension angle between A) healthy and B) pathological shoulders. (*Reproduced* from Lafosse T, Fogerty S, Idoine J, et al. Hyper extension-internal rotation (HERI): A new test for anterior gleno-humeral instability. Orthop Traumatol Surg Res 2016;102(1):8. Copyright © 2016 published by Elsevier Masson SAS. All rights reserved.)

various causes of instability. It has been difficult to develop a single comprehensive system.

One method to classify shoulder instability is by pathology. Thomas and Matsen[23] sought to divide instability into 2 distinct groups using the acronyms TUBS and AMBRI. TUBS (for traumatic, unidirectional, Bankart, and surgery) is defined by unidirectional instability—either anterior or posterior that is associated with a traumatic origin. AMBRI (for atraumatic, multidirectional, bilateral, rehabilitation, and inferior capsular shift) describes the group first defined by Neer and Foster[24] in their 1980 case series in which they discussed the clinical entity of MDI as anterior and/or posterior as well as inferior instability and distinguished it from unilateral shoulder instability. The approach to MDI is typically a prolonged course of rehabilitation before considering surgical intervention—historically an inferior capsular shift or, more commonly today, arthroscopic capsular plication.

The Stanmore triangle, which was developed by Bayley and colleagues[25] at the Royal National Orthopedic Hospital in Stanmore, England, also characterizes shoulder instability according to pathology, but with less distinction between 3 different groups (Fig. 2). One pillar of the triangle is polar type I, traumatic structural, which is similar to Thomas and Matsen's TUBS group. Another pillar is the polar type II, atraumatic structural, which correlates with Thomas and Matsen's AMBRI group. The polar type III group consists of those with habitual, nonstructural instability who have abnormal muscle patterning. Both polar type II and type III are historically lumped together as MDI. These 3 groups exist on a spectrum with overlapping characteristics existing between each of the groups. For example, a patient with MDI and a labral tear can develop some degree of scapular dyskinesia and abnormal muscle patterning, moving them along a spectrum from polar type II to polar type III. Polar type I and II share less abnormal muscle patterning compared with polar type III, whereas polar type II and polar type III share less trauma compared with polar type I. Thus, a patient likely fits somewhere on the continuum between polar groups and may shift between points over time.[25]

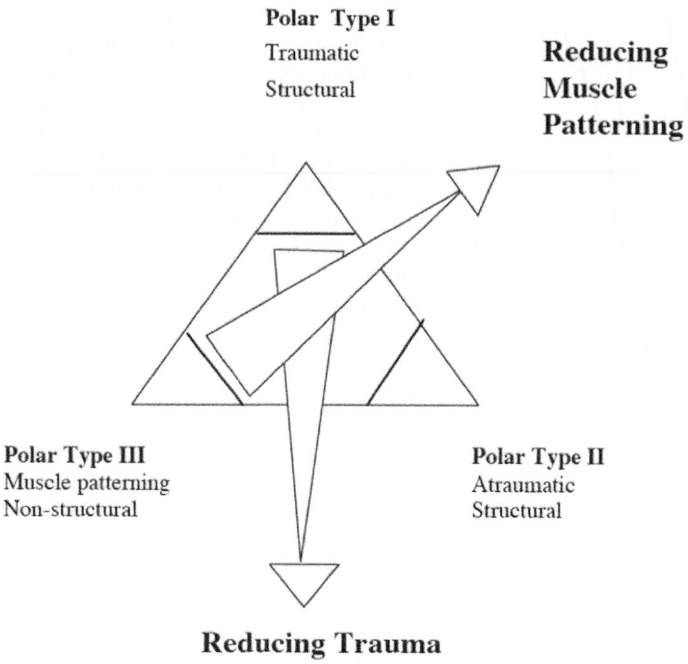

Fig. 2. Stanmore triangle shoulder classification, indicating the 3 pillars of instability. (*From* Lewis A, Kitamura T, Bayley J.I.L. Mini Symposium: Shoulder Instability (ii) The classification of shoulder instability: new light through old windows! Curr Orthop 2004;18(2):101; with permission.)

Another way to classify shoulder instability that has important implications for treatment is by the amount of bone loss. Quantifying the amount of bone loss and defining when bone loss on the glenoid and/or humeral side necessitates a change in surgical tactic has been an active area of research. The importance of defining substantial bone loss was found through a collaboration between Burkhart from Texas in the United States and De Beer of the Cape Shoulder Institute in Cape Town, South Africa, who followed 194 consecutive shoulders undergoing arthroscopic Bankart repairs. Although there was a 10.8% recurrence rate overall, patients without significant bone loss had a recurrence rate of 4%, and those with significant bone loss—as defined by an engaging Hill-Sachs lesion or an inverted pear-shaped glenoid—had a 67% recurrence rate.[26] Multiple studies have sought to quantify what constitutes critical glenoid bone loss, and this number has steadily been decreasing from initial concerns about the inverted pear glenoid with a glenoid width loss of greater than or equal to 25%.[27] More recently, a dose-dependent relationship between bone loss and a higher risk of recurrence and worse functional outcomes has been shown, even below the critical bone loss threshold, with a recent study by Shaha and colleagues[28] suggesting that the critical value of bone loss should be redefined at a lower threshold of 13.5%. On the humeral side, although it is less clear what the relationship is between recurrent instability and Hill-Sachs lesions, it seems that the risk increases with increasing lesion size.[29–31] Indeed, the amount of glenoid and humeral head bone loss is a major contributing factor to the success or failure of a stabilizing surgical procedure, especially those options that involve only soft tissue repair.[15,32]

Yamamoto and colleagues[33] from the Akita University School of Medicine in Akita, Japan, also classified bone loss by introducing the concept of whether lesions were considered on track or off track (Fig. 3). In this paradigm, the glenoid and the humeral head have a contact zone called the glenoid track. A significant amount of increasing bone loss in the glenoid or humeral head or a bipolar lesion increases the risk of engagement or dislocation and is considered an off-track lesion. An off-track lesion is, by definition, at high risk of being an engaging lesion, and would be a significant amount of bone loss that has a high rate of recurrence if not addressed.[34] Depending on the degree of bone loss, off-track lesions can be treated with Bankart repairs and remplissage or bone block procedures such as Bristow-Latarjet.[35] A helpful analogy is a car tire and a pothole; a sufficiently wide car tire can be thought of as the glenoid track and it will never fall into a small pothole, which represents the

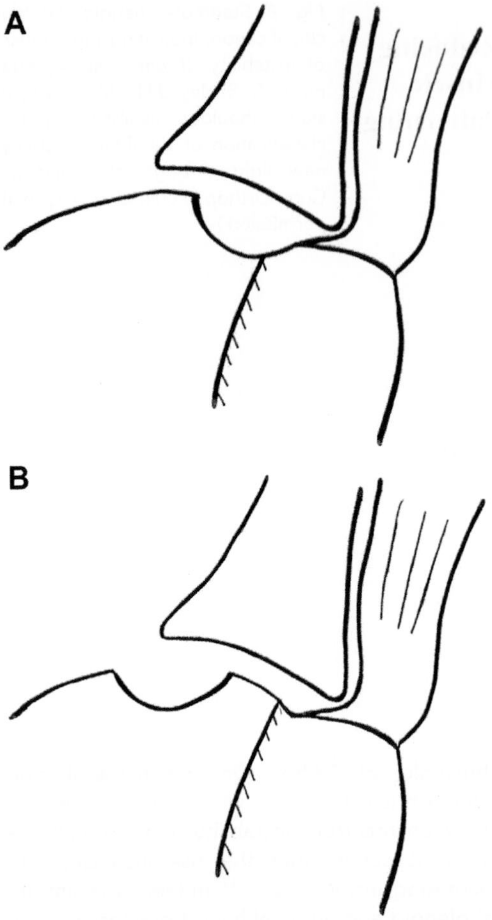

Fig. 3. Illustration of the concept of the glenoid track for a Hill-Sachs defect. (*A*) The Hill-Sachs defect remains within the glenoid track and thus is considered an "on-track" lesion that will not be engaging. (*B*) The Hill-Sachs defect is more medial and overrides the rim of the glenoid tract. Therefore, it is an "off-track" lesion with high probability of engaging, causing recurrent instability. (*From* Yamamoto N, Itoi E, Abe H, et al. Contact between the glenoid and the humeral head in abduction, external rotation, and horizontal extension: A new concept of glenoid track. J Shoulder Elbow Surg 2007;16(5):654; with permission.)

Hill-Sachs defect. However, if the pothole gets larger, or if the tire gets narrower, recurrent instability persists.

Some classification systems attempt to take into account various risk factors to create comprehensive treatment algorithms—moving beyond bone loss alone. The Instability Severity Index Score is one such scoring system developed by Balg and Boileau[36] from Nice, France, after their case-control study of 131 patients who developed anterior recurrent instability after arthroscopic Bankart repair. Among other factors (**Table 3**), the scoring system relies on patient age, sports involvement, and glenoid and humeral bone loss as assessed on standard radiographs. For patients who score higher than 6, the recurrence rate was a dismal 70% with an arthroscopic Bankart repair. The Instability Severity Index Score was validated by Loppini and colleagues[37] from Humanitas University in Milan, Italy, who found that, for patients who underwent anterior arthroscopic stabilization, the success rate with an Instability Severity Index Score of less than or equal to 3 was 93.7%, whereas the success rate was 54.6% if the Instability Severity Index Score was greater or equal to 6. For this reason, the recommendation is for a more substantial open stabilization procedure, such as a Bristow-Latarjet, for patients with high Instability Severity Index Score.[36] However, the appropriate cut-off value for the Instability Severity Index Score is an area of continued research and debate.[38]

MANAGEMENT

Shoulder instability is a common problem. Lennart Hovelius from the Gälve Hospital in Sweden found an incidence of shoulder dislocation of 1.7% in a Swedish population, with higher rate in males,[39] whereas Krøner and colleagues[40] from the Aarhus Municipal Hospital in Denmark found an incidence of 17 per 100,000 person-years in a Danish population, with the highest incidence in men between 21 and 30 years of age and women between 61 and 80 years of age. Zacchilli and Owens[41] studied the epidemiology of shoulder dislocations presenting to emergency departments in the United States and found an incidence rate of 23.9 in 100,000 person-years, which was also highest in young adult males.

The optimal treatment for the first time dislocator is a subject under debate. Patients who are treated with nonoperative treatment are often at high risk for redislocation, particularly younger patients and those who engage in high risk activity. Patients under 20 years of age are noted to have a recurrence rate as high as 94%.[42] In 1956, Rowe[43] found a redislocation rate of 38% of 313 patients at a mean follow-up of 4.8 years. Similarly, Hovelius[42] found a redislocation rate of 44% of 256 patients at the 5-year follow-up. Kirkley and her colleagues[44] from the Fowler Kennedy Sport Medicine Clinic at the University of Western Ontario in Canada randomized patients after a first dislocation to immobilization for 3 weeks followed by rehabilitation or early arthroscopic stabilization within 4 weeks of

Table 3
The Instability Severity Index Score, indicating points given to various factors to determine severity of instability

Prognostic Factor	Points
Age	
Age ≤20 y at the time of surgery	2
Age >20 y time of surgery	0
Sports participation	
Competitive sports participation preoperatively	2
Recreational or no sports participation preoperatively	0
Sports type	
Contact or forced overhead sport participation preoperatively	1
Other	0
Shoulder hyperlaxity	
Anterior or inferior shoulder hyperlaxity	1
Normal laxity	0
Bone Loss	
Hill Sachs visible in external rotation on an anteroposterior radiograph	2
Hall Sachs not visible in external rotation on an anteroposterior radiograph	0
Glenoid loss of contour on an anteroposterior radiograph	2
No loss of glenoid contour on an anteroposterior radiograph	0

Adapted from Balg F, Boileau P. The instability severity index score. A simple pre-operative score to select patients for arthroscopic or open shoulder stabilisation. J Bone Joint Surg Br 2007;89(11):1470-1477; with permission.

injury, followed by identical immobilization and rehabilitation. They found a significant decrease in redislocation rates, with the surgery group having a redislocation rate of 15.9% and the rehabilitation group having a redislocation rate of 47%. As measured by the Western Ontario Shoulder Instability Index, there was an improvement in disease-specific quality of life in the early arthroscopic stabilization group.[44] This group of patients was again followed to a 75-month follow-up and found that the difference in recurrence remained significant, as did the mean difference between the Western Ontario Shoulder Instability Index scores, although the shoulder function as measured by the American Shoulder and Elbow Surgeons and Disability of Arm Shoulder and Hand scores were not significant.[45] As a result, the case for early stabilization is strong, particularly in young patients and those who are contact and overhead athletes.

For those being treated nonoperatively, there is a lack of consensus about the usefulness of immobilization and in what position this should occur. Smith[46] from the Norfolk and Norwich University Hospital in England performed a review of the literature and found little consensus in the role of immobilization in preventing recurrence of instability, with some studies suggesting that immobilization plays a role in preventing recurrence and others indicating it does not. It seems age at dislocation, and not immobilization, is the biggest factor in predicting recurrence and failing to control for this factor prevented these studies from drawing definitive conclusions. Further, these studies failed to come to consensus about for how long patients should be immobilized.[46] Future study into this area is warranted. A developing area of study is the position of immobilization. Itoi and colleagues[47] from the Akita University Medical School in Japan performed a randomized control trial comparing immobilization in internal rotation to immobilization in 10° of external rotation after dislocation in 198 patients. The internal rotation group had a significantly higher recurrence rate of dislocation or subluxation at 42% than the external rotation group at 26%. In contrast, Liavaag and colleagues[48] from the Sørlandet Hospital in Arendal, Norway, performed a randomized controlled trial of 188 patients with primary anterior dislocations that were immobilized in either internal rotation or 15° of external rotation for 3 weeks. There were no significant differences in the recurrence rates of instability between the 2 groups. This lack of significance in the position of immobilization was also found by Finestone and colleagues[49] from the Assaf HaRofeh Medical Center in Be'er Ya'akov Israel in a population of military servicemen.

Because of the high risk of redislocation, many advocate for surgery for patients after the first traumatic, unidirectional instability event. A systematic review by Brophy and Marx[50] comparing nonoperative treatment to surgical treatment for first-time dislocators demonstrated that surgical repair was associated with a significantly lower rate of recurrence of 7% than nonoperative management of 46% at the 2-year follow-up. When extending this to longer term follow-up of 3 to 10 years, these differences become even more significant, with a recurrence rate of 10% for surgically treated patients and 58% for nonoperative treatment.[50] For many patients without significant bone loss, the procedure of choice for anterior unidirectional traumatic instability is typically a capsulolabral repair. This procedure, also known as a Bankart repair, involves repairing the torn antero-inferior labrum in an effort to reconstitute the labral bumper and retension the capsuloligamentous structures that insert on the labrum. Early studies and meta-analysis favored open repair over arthroscopic techniques.[51–53] However, these studies have a significant bias given that arthroscopic techniques have evolved rapidly in the last 30 years. A retrospective study by van Oostveen and colleagues[54] from the University Medical Center Utrecht in the Netherlands found modern suture anchors to have better outcomes after arthroscopic capsulolabral reconstruction, with fewer complications and lower recurrence rates, compared with transglenoid sutures. As technology, techniques, and material sciences have improved, capsulolabral reconstruction has increasingly become an arthroscopic technique. More recent studies have found recurrence rates with both open and arthroscopic techniques using suture anchors to be roughly equivalent.[55–57]

There are limitations to the indications of the use of arthroscopic soft tissue repair in the treatment of shoulder instability. Calvo and colleagues[58] from The Fundación Jiménez Diaz in Madrid, Spain, prospectively followed 61 patients treated with arthroscopic Bankart repair for anterior instability and found age of less than 28 years, ligamentous laxity, the presence of fracture of the glenoid rim involving more than 15% of the articular surface, and participation in contact or overhead sports to have a higher rate of recurrence after surgery, with bone loss being the most impactful factor. In addition, a recent study by Shaha and colleagues[28] demonstrated that bone loss as little as 13.5% has negative impact on functional outcome scores. A systematic review by Murphy and colleagues[59] from Dublin, Ireland, of long-term outcomes of arthroscopic Bankart repairs demonstrated a 31% recurrent instability rate, resulting in a 17% revision rate; 59.4% of patients had developed some incidence of instability arthropathy. These studies demonstrate that arthroscopic repair is not the panacea for all patients with instability and there is a need to pursue more substantial operations when indicated.

For those with glenoid bone loss or without significant bone loss, but failed primary arthroscopic repair, surgical treatment typically consists of a bone grafting procedure.[60] In a Latarjet procedure, first described by Michel Latarjet in 1954 of Lyon France, the entire horizontal pillar of the coracoid is fixated to the anterior glenoid rim to fill in the bone defect. A modification of this technique is the Bristow procedure, described by the South African born Arthur Helfet in 1958 and named after his mentor, British surgeon Rowley Bristow, in which the tip of the coracoid is fixated to the glenoid rim. An additional modification is the congruent arc, in which the medial aspect of the coracoid is transferred, and rotated 90° to create a more congruent surface with the glenoid.[61] A consequence of the procedure is that the conjoint tendon is shifted to a new position with the coracoid, producing a secondary stabilizing sling effect. There are a number of technical variations on how to perform this procedure in terms of how to approach the subscapularis, osteotomize the coracoid, orient the coracoid, fixate the graft, and repair the capsule.[60,62] Certainly, as an open procedure involving hardware and rearranged anatomy near the neurovascular structures, there are complications, but in general, the Latarjet procedure has proved to be very successful.[61,63,64] Indeed, a systematic review by Ialenti and colleagues[65] compared arthroscopic Bankart repair using modern suture anchors with open Bankart and Latarajet repairs and found that both arthroscopic Bankart and Larajet repairs had similar return to sport rates that were superior to open Bankart repairs.

However, the Latarjet repair had a significantly lower rate of dislocation than both arthroscopic and open Bankart repairs. The success of the Latarjet procedure was also demonstrated in a systematic review of 24 studies by Cowling and colleagues[62] from the James Cook University Hospital in Middlesbrough, England. They found an overall recurrent instability rate of 5.36% (range, 2.94%–43.00%). Although there was a wide range of surgical techniques described, the outcome was independent of technique. Patient selection was the biggest factor accounting for recurrence; when 1 report including epileptic patients with a high rate of recurrence was excluded, the recurrence rate decreased to 3.79% (range, 2.94%–10.00%).

In 2007, Lafosse and colleagues[66] from the Alps Surgery Institute in Annecy, France, described an arthroscopic technique for the Latarjet procedure. They prospectively collected outcomes on their first 100 arthroscopic Latarjet procedures. They found 91% had excellent results, 9% had a good result, and 80% of patients had excellent graft position. There was an average 18° loss of external rotation with complications including 2 hematomas, 1 graft fracture, 1 musculocutaneous nerve palsy, 4 nonunions, and 3 cases of graft lysis.[67] When 62 patients undergoing arthroscopic Latarjet procedures were followed for a minimum of 5 years, patients had high Western Ontario Shoulder Instability Index scores with only 1 patient reporting recurrent subluxations and no need for revision surgery, indicating it is a durable approach to the unstable shoulder.[68] Boileau and colleagues[69] from the Institut Universitaire Locomoteur & Sport in Nice, France, found that fixation with suture buttons in the place of screws for the arthroscopic Latarjet repair is also a safe and reliable technique. In 121 patients followed for this technique for at least 2 years, there was 3% recurrent instability rate, resulting in a 2.5% revision rate, and no neurologic or hardware failure. There were 4 nonunions that were associated with smoking. Graft position was flush to the glenoid rim in 95% of cases and subequatorial in 92%. Return to sport was 93%. In a French retrospective multicenter trial of 6 arthroscopic Latarjet specialists consisting of 1555 Latarjet cases, there were 4 severe neurologic complications (0.2%), 10 infections (0.6%), 7 hematomas (0.4%), 14 fractures of the graft (1.0%), and 30 cases of recurrent instability (2.0%), resulting in 58 revision surgeries (3.7%), demonstrating that arthroscopic Latarjet to be a safe and effective procedure.[70] In a French multicenter prospective comparative study comparing open and arthroscopic Latarjet repairs, the arthroscopic group had significantly less pain on postoperative days 3 and 7.[71] When compared with open Latarjet procedures, a systematic review by Hurley and colleagues[72] from Dublin, Ireland, found that arthroscopic Latarjet repairs had no significant differences in recurrent instability, total complications, or revision surgeries. Although arthroscopic Latarjet repair is a technically challenging procedure with a significant learning curve, it has the advantage of leaving the subscapularis intact, a critically important point, particularly in the unstable shoulder, as well as providing excellent visualization of graft position, the opportunity to recognize and address other intra-articular pathology concomitantly, and decreased pain in the immediate postoperative period.[67]

The distal tibia has a radius of curvature similar to the glenoid and has articular cartilage, and thus it is used as an allograft in the setting where the Latarjet procedure is not optimal—including cases of bone loss of more than 30% of the glenoid width, larger than can be reconstructed with the coracoid, and in cases where the coracoid is absent owing to prior surgery or trauma.[60] Early outcomes have been promising.[73] Similarly, tricortical iliac crest autograft (the Eben-Hybbinnette procedure) or allograft, although lacking articular cartilage, can be used for the same indications with good results with a low rate of recurrence.[60,74,75] Rahme and colleagues[76] from Uppsala University Hospital in Sweden reported less promising results with long-term follow-up of 77 shoulders. Although 74% of patients were satisfied, the recurrence rate was 20% and 47% of shoulders went on to develop arthrosis. The key difference between the Latarjet procedure and the other bone block procedures is the absence of the dynamic effect of the conjoint tendon sling and the repositioning of the subscapularis when the conjoint is not attached and threaded through a subscapularis split. The importance of these effects is difficult to test biomechanically and is a subject of intense debate. A systematic review by Longo and colleagues[77] from the Università Campus Bio-Medico di Roma in Italy, found the open Bristow-Latarjet and Eden-Hybinette procedures to have similar clinical outcomes, whereas the Eden-Hybinette repair had a higher rate of recurrence and development of osteoarthritis. Bone block procedures, in general and including the Latarjet repair, had a lower rate of recurrence compared with Bankart repairs. Just as the Latarjet repair is now being performed arthroscopically, skilled arthroscopists such as Markus Schiebel in Zurich, Switzerland, and Ettore Taverna in Milan, Italy, have developed arthroscopic approaches for iliac crest bone grafting.[78,79]

Off-track Hill-Sachs fractures are at risk for engaging with the glenoid and causing recurrent instability.[33] In cases of bipolar bone loss (bone loss on both the glenoid and humeral side), treating the glenoid side with a bony procedure as described elsewhere in this article may be preferred to lengthen the glenoid arc and create an on track Hill-Sachs lesion after reconstruction.[66,80] However, in the case of isolated humeral bone loss, there are a variety of procedures to treat Hill-Sachs defects, including humeral head osteotomy, anterior capsular plication, osteochondral allograft, humeroplasty, and resurfacing arthroplasty. These lesions are most frequently treated with a remplissage procedure, which is from the French for to fill-in, in which infraspinatus and posterior capsule is transferred into the defect. This infraspinatus tenodesis prevents the humeral head from translating anterior and subluxating and prevents the defect from engaging with the glenoid, effectively converting it from an intra-articular to an extra-articular defect.[81] A systematic review by Lazarides and colleagues[82] demonstrated arthroscopic remplissage to be a reliable procedure in conjunction with arthroscopic Bankart for unstable shoulders with subcritical bone loss, with good clinical outcomes, low rates of recurrence that averaged 5.8% across the 18 included clinical studies, with only a 0.4% complication rate, and, perhaps surprisingly, preserved external rotation, with losses that ranged between 9° and 14° among studies. A case control study by Cho and colleagues[83] from Kyung Hee University in Seoul, South Korea, compared arthroscopic Bankart repair with arthroscopic Bankart repair with remplissage for those with up to 25% bone loss. In this study, the recurrence rate in the Bankart group was 25.7% and 5.4% in the group with an added remplissage, which also had a higher postoperative Rowe score, all of which were significant findings.

The overall prevalence of posterior shoulder instability is 1.1 per 100,000 person-years.[84] Posterior unidirectional instability can be treated along much the same paradigm as anterior unidirectional instability. A posterior Bankart tear is often treated successfully with arthroscopic capsulolabral repair. A systematic review by DeLong and colleagues[85] of arthroscopic repair for unidirectional posterior instability demonstrated an overall recurrent instability rate of 8% to 10%. Results were worse in patients who had prior surgery—particularly thermal capsulorraphy, anchorless sutures, unappreciated MDI, who were overhead athletes, or who underwent open procedures. For associated reverse Hill-Sachs lesions, a McLaughlin procedure can be performed, in which the bone defect is filled in with the subscapularis tendon,[86] or a modified McLaughlin, in which the lesser tuberosity is transferred into the bone defect.[87] Case series of the modified McLaughlin procedure have demonstrated it to be a reliable procedure to treat posterior instability, with low rates of recurrence and good to excellent results.[88,89] The posterior glenoid rim can be reconstructed with a variety of bone blocks, including iliac crest bone block, distal tibia allograft, glenoid allograft, pedunculated acromial graft, and distal clavicular autograft.[10,90–93] Posterior instability can sometimes be the result of glenoid dysplasia. For patients with excessive glenoid retroversion, for which a maximum acceptable limit has not been established in the literature, a glenoid osteotomy can help to restore the glenoid to more neutral version.[10,94] However, although glenoid osteotomies can help to stabilize the shoulder in the short term, these procedures are challenging and fraught with complications, including the development of glenohumeral osteoarthritis, disordered scapulohumeral rhythm, and the development of anterior instability.[94,95] Posterior dislocations, in particular, are at risk for going undetected, resulting in chronic, locked dislocations. When the humeral head is dislocated for more than 6 months, it can lead to humeral head damage through avascular necrosis.[96] In these cases, hemiarthroplasty and total shoulder arthroplasty are effective salvage options.[97]

For patients with MDI, the recommendation is for a prolonged course of rehabilitation for at least 6 months that focuses on the dynamic stabilizers, given that surgical outcomes are less reliable than for patients with MDI than those with unilateral, traumatic instability.[12,98,99] Indeed, the difference in surgical outcomes was demonstrated by Burkhead and Rockwood,[98] who followed 115 patients undergoing rehabilitation for all types of instability. They found that 16% of patients with traumatic subluxation had good or excellent results with rehabilitation compared with 88% of patients who underwent rehabilitation for atraumatic subluxation, indicating the extent to which an accurate diagnosis is crucial and that traumatic instability and MDI represent distinct pathologies that ought to be treated with separate treatment algorithms. Rehabilitation programs typically focus on strengthening the rotator cuff, periscapular musculature, and proprioceptive retraining. Although there are many rehabilitation protocols, 2 popular rehabilitation programs are the Watson program, which focuses on scapular biomechanics before strengthening the deltoid and rotator cuff, before progressing into sport-specific ranges,[100] and the Rockwood program, which focuses on rotator cuff and deltoid strengthening, with the majority of exercises being done at 0° of elevation.[98] For MDI, studies have reported successful outcomes from a variety of rehabilitation protocols.[98,100–102] A systematic review by Warby and colleagues[103] on the effects of exercised based management by MDI concluded that there was great deal of variability owing to study heterogeneity and a great deal of bias across studies, indicating this an area in need of more research.

When dynamic stabilizers cannot effectively prevent instability in MDI, surgery is indicated to repair and augment the static stabilizers in the shoulder.[99,104] Although a systematic review by Warby and colleagues[105] comparing exercise based management versus surgery for MDI was hindered by low-quality evidence and bias, it found that surgery improved shoulder kinematics and increased the likelihood of return to sport. There was inconsistency over whether surgery or exercise improved functional scores more and there was insufficient evidence to make a recommendation for one intervention over the other. First pioneered by Neer in 1980, inferior capsular shift has been the mainstay of the treatment of the redundant capsule seen in MDI.[24] A systematic review by Longo and colleagues[106] demonstrated that open capsular shift and arthroscopic capsular plication are reliable treatment strategies with similar outcomes. They identified younger age, laxity, and demanding sports as negative prognostic factors. Thermal and laser assisted capsulorraphy was used briefly, but has been abandoned owing to the complication of rapid chondrolysis and attenuation of capsular tissue.[107,108]

SUMMARY

Shoulder instability is a common and challenging problem, often affecting some of our highest demand patients—the young and highly active. Worldwide, multiple strategies have been developed to address shoulder instability and, recently, significant progress has been made in attempting to match the right procedure to the right patient.

DISCLOSURE

The authors have nothing to disclose.

REFERENCES

1. Wilk KE, Arrigo CA, Andrews JR. Current concepts: the stabilizing structures of the glenohumeral joint. J Orthop Sports Phys Ther 1997. https://doi.org/10.2519/jospt.1997.25.6.364.
2. Lippitt S. The shoulder. 5th edition. Rockwood CA, Matsen F, Wirth MA, et al, editors. Developmental Anatomy of the Shoulder and Anatomy of the Glenohumeral Joint, Editor Commentary. Philadelphia: Elsevier; 2017. p. 32.
3. Lugo R, Kung P, Ma CB. Shoulder biomechanics. Eur J Radiol 2008. https://doi.org/10.1016/j.ejrad.2008.02.051.
4. Gil JA, DeFroda S, Owens BD. Current concepts in the diagnosis and management of traumatic, anterior glenohumeral subluxations. Orthop J Sports Med 2017. https://doi.org/10.1177/2325967117694338.
5. Burkart AC, Debski RE. Anatomy and function of the glenohumeral ligaments in anterior shoulder instability. Clin Orthop Relat Res 2002. https://doi.org/10.1097/00003086-200207000-00005.
6. Gohlke F, Essigkrug B, Schmitz F. The pattern of the collagen fiber bundles of the capsule of the glenohumeral joint. J Shoulder Elbow Surg 1994. https://doi.org/10.1016/S1058-2746(09)80090-6.
7. Habermeyer P, Schuller U, Wiedemann E. The intra-articular pressure of the shoulder: an experimental study on the role of the glenoid labrum in stabilizing the joint. Arthroscopy 1992. https://doi.org/10.1016/0749-8063(92)90031-6.
8. Hovelius L, Eriksson K, Fredin H, et al. Recurrences after initial dislocation of the shoulder. Results of a prospective study of treatment. J Bone Joint Surg Am 1983. https://doi.org/10.2106/00004623-198365030-00008.
9. Rowe CR. Acute and recurrent anterior dislocations of the shoulder. Orthop Clin North Am 1980;11(2):253–70.
10. Antosh IJ, Tokish JM, Owens BD. Posterior shoulder instability: current surgical management. Sports Health 2016. https://doi.org/10.1177/1941738116672446.
11. Gaskill T, Taylor D, Millett P. Management of multidirectional instability of the shoulder. J Am Acad Orthop Surg 2011;19:758–67.

12. Schenk TJ, Brems JJ. Multidirectional instability of the shoulder: pathophysiology, diagnosis, and management. J Am Acad Orthop Surg 1998;6(1):65–72.
13. Lizzio VA, Meta F, Fidai M, et al. Clinical evaluation and physical exam findings in patients with anterior shoulder instability. Curr Rev Musculoskelet Med 2017. https://doi.org/10.1007/s12178-017-9434-3.
14. Farrar NG, Malal JJG, Fischer J, et al. An overview of shoulder instability and its management. Open Orthop J 2013. https://doi.org/10.2174/1874325001307010338.
15. Provencher MT, Bhatia S, Ghodadra NS, et al. Recurrent shoulder instability: current concepts for evaluation and management of glenoid bone loss. J Bone Joint Surg Am 2010. https://doi.org/10.2106/JBJS.J.00906.
16. Bernageau J, Patte D, Debeyre J, et al. Value of the glenoid profile in recurrent luxations of the shoulder. Rev Chir Orthop Reparatrice Appar Mot 1976;62(2 suppl):142–7 [in French].
17. Gross DJ, Golijanin P, Dumont GD, et al. The effect of sagittal rotation of the glenoid on axial glenoid width and glenoid version in computed tomography scan imaging. J Shoulder Elbow Surg 2016. https://doi.org/10.1016/j.jse.2015.06.017.
18. Tirman PFJ, Steinbach LS, Belzer JP, et al. A practical approach to imaging of the shoulder with emphasis on MR imaging. Orthop Clin North Am 1997. https://doi.org/10.1016/S0030-5898(05)70306-0.
19. Magee T. 3-T MRI of the shoulder: is MR arthrography necessary? Am J Roentgenol 2009. https://doi.org/10.2214/AJR.08.1097.
20. Friedman LGM, Ulloa SA, Braun DT, et al. Glenoid bone loss measurement in recurrent shoulder dislocation: assessment of measurement agreement between CT and MRI. Orthop J Sports Med 2014. https://doi.org/10.1177/2325967114549541.
21. Gyftopoulos S, Beltran LS, Yemin A, et al. Use of 3D MR reconstructions in the evaluation of glenoid bone loss: a clinical study. Skeletal Radiol 2014. https://doi.org/10.1007/s00256-013-1774-5.
22. Stillwater L, Koenig J, Maycher B, et al. 3D-MR vs. 3D-CT of the shoulder in patients with glenohumeral instability. Skeletal Radiol 2017. https://doi.org/10.1007/s00256-016-2559-4.
23. Thomas SC, Matsen FA. An approach to the repair of avulsion of the glenohumeral ligaments in the management of traumatic anterior glenohumeral instability. J Bone Joint Surg Am 1989. https://doi.org/10.2106/00004623-198971040-00005.
24. Neer CS. JBJS classics inferior capsular shift for involuntary inferior and multidirectional instability of the shoulder. J Bone Joint Surg Am 1980;62(6):897–908.
25. Lewis A, Kitamura T, Bayley J. Mini symposium: shoulder instability (ii): the classification of shoulder instability: new light through old windows! Curr Orthop 2004;18(2):97–108.
26. Burkhart SS, De Beer JF. Traumatic glenohumeral bone defects and their relationship to failure of arthroscopic Bankart repairs: significance of the inverted-pear glenoid and the humeral engaging Hill-Sachs lesion. Arthroscopy 2000. https://doi.org/10.1053/jars.2000.17715.
27. Saliken DJ, Bornes TD, Bouliane MJ, et al. Imaging methods for quantifying glenoid and Hill-Sachs bone loss in traumatic instability of the shoulder: a scoping review. BMC Musculoskelet Disord 2015. https://doi.org/10.1186/s12891-015-0607-1.
28. Shaha JS, Cook JB, Song DJ, et al. Redefining "critical" bone loss in shoulder instability: functional outcomes worsen with "subcritical" bone loss. Am J Sports Med 2015. https://doi.org/10.1177/0363546515578250.
29. Randelli P, Ragone V, Carminati S, et al. Risk factors for recurrence after Bankart repair a systematic review. Knee Surg Sports Traumatol Arthrosc 2012. https://doi.org/10.1007/s00167-012-2140-1.
30. Cetik O, Uslu M, Ozsar BK. The relationship between Hill-Sachs lesion and recurrent anterior shoulder dislocation. Acta Orthop Belg 2007;73(2):175–8.
31. Boileau P, Villalba M, Héry JY, et al. Risk factors for recurrence of shoulder instability after arthroscopic Bankart repair. J Bone Joint Surg Am 2006. https://doi.org/10.2106/JBJS.E.00817.
32. Rowe CR, Zarins B, Ciullo JV. Recurrent anterior dislocation of the shoulder after surgical repair. Apparent causes of failure and treatment. J Bone Joint Surg Am 1984. https://doi.org/10.2106/00004623-198466020-00001.
33. Yamamoto N, Itoi E, Abe H, et al. Contact between the glenoid and the humeral head in abduction, external rotation, and horizontal extension: A new concept of glenoid track. J Shoulder Elb Surg 2007. https://doi.org/10.1016/j.jse.2006.12.012.
34. Shaha JS, Cook JB, Rowles DJ, et al. Clinical validation of the glenoid track concept in anterior glenohumeral instability. J Bone Joint Surg Am 2016. https://doi.org/10.2106/JBJS.15.01099.
35. Hatta T, Yamamoto N, Shinagawa K, et al. Surgical decision making based on the on-track/off-track concept for anterior shoulder instability: a case-control study. JSES Open Access 2019;3(1):25–8.
36. Balg F, Boileau P. The instability severity index score. A simple pre-operative score to select patients for arthroscopic or open shoulder stabilisation. J Bone Joint Surg Br 2007. https://doi.org/10.1302/0301-620X.89B11.18962.

37. Loppini M, Delle Rose G, Borroni M, et al. Is the instability severity index score a valid tool for predicting failure after primary arthroscopic stabilization for anterior glenohumeral instability? Arthroscopy 2019. https://doi.org/10.1016/j.arthro.2018.09.027.
38. Thomazeau H, Langlais T, Hardy A, et al. Long-term, prospective, multicenter study of isolated Bankart repair for a patient selection method based on the instability severity index score. Am J Sports Med 2019. https://doi.org/10.1177/0363546519833920.
39. Hovelius L. Incidence of shoulder dislocation in Sweden. Clin Orthop Relat Res 1982;(166):127–31.
40. Krøner K, Lind T, Jensen J. The epidemiology of shoulder dislocations. Arch Orthop Trauma Surg 1989. https://doi.org/10.1007/BF00932317.
41. Zacchilli MA, Owens BD. Epidemiology of shoulder dislocations presenting to emergency departments in the United States. J Bone Joint Surg Am 2010. https://doi.org/10.2106/JBJS.I.00450.
42. Hovelius L. Anterior dislocation of the shoulder in teen-agers and young adults. Five-year prognosis. J Bone Joint Surg Am 1987. https://doi.org/10.2106/00004623-198769030-00011.
43. Rowe CR. Prognosis in dislocations of the shoulder. J Bone Joint Surg Am 1956. https://doi.org/10.2106/00004623-195638050-00001.
44. Kirkley A, Griffin S, Richards C, et al. Prospective randomized clinical trial comparing the effectiveness of immediate arthroscopic stabilization versus immobilization and rehabilitation in first traumatic anterior dislocations of the shoulder. Arthroscopy 1999. https://doi.org/10.1053/ar.1999.v15.015050.
45. Kirkley A, Werstine R, Ratjek A, et al. Prospective randomized clinical trial comparing the effectiveness of immediate arthroscopic stabilization versus immobilization and rehabilitation in first traumatic anterior dislocations of the shoulder: long-term evaluation. Arthroscopy 2005. https://doi.org/10.1016/j.arthro.2004.09.018.
46. Smith TO. Immobilisation following traumatic anterior glenohumeral joint dislocation: a literature review. Injury 2006. https://doi.org/10.1016/j.injury.2005.06.005.
47. Itoi E, Hatakeyama Y, Sato T, et al. Immobilization in external rotation after shoulder dislocation reduces the risk of recurrence: a randomized controlled trial. J Bone Joint Surg Am 2007. https://doi.org/10.2106/JBJS.F.00654.
48. Liavaag S, Brox JI, Pripp AH, et al. Immobilization in external rotation after primary shoulder dislocation did not reduce the risk of recurrence: a randomized controlled trial. J Bone Joint Surg Am 2011. https://doi.org/10.2106/JBJS.J.00416.
49. Finestone A, Milgrom C, Radeva-Petrova DR, et al. Bracing in external rotation for traumatic anterior dislocation of the shoulder. J Bone Joint Surg Br 2009. https://doi.org/10.1302/0301-620X.91B7.22263.
50. Brophy RH, Marx RG. The treatment of traumatic anterior instability of the shoulder: nonoperative and surgical treatment. Arthroscopy 2009. https://doi.org/10.1016/j.arthro.2008.12.007.
51. Mohtadi NGH, Bitar IJ, Sasyniuk TM, et al. Arthroscopic versus open repair for traumatic anterior shoulder instability: a meta-analysis. Arthroscopy 2005. https://doi.org/10.1016/j.arthro.2005.02.021.
52. Yong GR, Jeong HH, Nam SC. Anterior shoulder stabilization in collision athletes: arthroscopic versus open Bankart repair. Am J Sports Med 2006. https://doi.org/10.1177/0363546505283267.
53. Freedman KB, Smith AP, Romeo AA, et al. Open Bankart repair versus arthroscopic repair with transglenoid sutures or bioabsorbable tacks for recurrent anterior instability of the shoulder: a meta-analysis. Am J Sports Med 2004. https://doi.org/10.1177/0363546504265188.
54. van Oostveen DPH, Schild FJA, van Haeff MJ, et al. Suture anchors are superior to transglenoid sutures in arthroscopic shoulder stabilization. Arthroscopy 2006. https://doi.org/10.1016/j.arthro.2006.07.006.
55. Petrera M, Patella V, Patella S, et al. A meta-analysis of open versus arthroscopic Bankart repair using suture anchors. Knee Surg Sports Traumatol Arthrosc 2010. https://doi.org/10.1007/s00167-010-1093-5.
56. Mahiroğullari M, Özkan H, Akyüz M, et al. Comparison between the results of open and arthroscopic repair of isolated traumatic anterior instability of the shoulder. Acta Orthop Traumatol Turc 2010. https://doi.org/10.3944/AOTT.2010.2289.
57. Godin J, Sekiya JK. Systematic review of arthroscopic versus open repair for recurrent anterior shoulder dislocations. Sports Health 2011. https://doi.org/10.1177/1941738111409175.
58. Calvo E, Granizo JJ, Fernández-Yruegas D. Criteria for arthroscopic treatment of anterior instability of the shoulder. A prospective study. J Bone Joint Surg Br 2005. https://doi.org/10.1302/0301-620X.87B5.15794.
59. Murphy AI, Hurley ET, Hurley DJ, et al. Long-term outcomes of the arthroscopic Bankart repair: a systematic review of studies at 10-year follow-up. J Shoulder Elbow Surg 2019. https://doi.org/10.1016/j.jse.2019.04.057.
60. Rabinowitz J, Friedman R, Eichinger JK. Management of Glenoid bone loss with anterior shoulder instability: indications and outcomes. Curr Rev Musculoskelet Med 2017. https://doi.org/10.1007/s12178-017-9439-y.

61. de Beer JF, Roberts C. Glenoid bone defects-open Latarjet with congruent arc modification. Orthop Clin North Am 2010. https://doi.org/10.1016/j.ocl.2010.02.008.
62. Cowling PD, Akhtar MA, Liow RYL. What is a Bristow-Latarjet procedure? A review of the described operative techniques and outcomes. Bone Joint J 2016. https://doi.org/10.1302/0301-620X.98B9.37948.
63. Burkhart SS, De Beer JF, Barth JRH, et al. Results of modified Latarjet reconstruction in patients with anteroinferior instability and significant bone loss. Arthroscopy 2007. https://doi.org/10.1016/j.arthro.2007.08.009.
64. Mook WR, Petri M, Greenspoon JA, et al. Clinical and anatomic predictors of outcomes after the Latarjet procedure for the treatment of anterior glenohumeral instability with combined glenoid and humeral bone defects. Am J Sports Med 2016. https://doi.org/10.1177/0363546516634089.
65. Ialenti MN, Mulvihill JD, Feinstein M, et al. Return to play following shoulder stabilization: a systematic review and meta-analysis. Orthop J Sports Med 2017. https://doi.org/10.1177/2325967117726055.
66. Lafosse L, Lejeune E, Bouchard A, et al. The arthroscopic Latarjet procedure for the treatment of anterior shoulder instability. Arthroscopy 2007. https://doi.org/10.1016/j.arthro.2007.06.008.
67. Lafosse L, Boyle S. Arthroscopic Latarjet procedure. J Shoulder Elbow Surg 2010;19(2):2–12.
68. Dumont GD, Fogerty S, Rosso C, et al. The arthroscopic Latarjet procedure for anterior shoulder instability: 5-year minimum follow-up. Am J Sports Med 2014. https://doi.org/10.1177/0363546514544682.
69. Boileau P, Saliken D, Gendre P, et al. Arthroscopic Latarjet: suture-button fixation is a safe and reliable alternative to screw fixation. Arthroscopy 2019. https://doi.org/10.1016/j.arthro.2018.11.012.
70. Lafosse L, Leuzinger J, Brzoska R, et al. Complications of arthroscopic Latarjet: a multicenter study of 1555 cases. J Shoulder Elbow Surg 2017. https://doi.org/10.1016/j.jse.2016.12.007.
71. Nourissat G, Neyton L, Metais P, et al. Functional outcomes after open versus arthroscopic Latarjet procedure: a prospective comparative study. Orthop Traumatol Surg Res 2016. https://doi.org/10.1016/j.otsr.2016.08.004.
72. Hurley ET, Lim Fat D, Farrington SK, et al. Open versus arthroscopic Latarjet procedure for anterior shoulder instability: a systematic review and meta-analysis. Am J Sports Med 2019. https://doi.org/10.1177/0363546518759540.
73. Provencher MT, Ghodadra N, LeClere L, et al. Anatomic osteochondral glenoid reconstruction for recurrent glenohumeral instability with glenoid deficiency using a distal tibia allograft. Arthroscopy 2009. https://doi.org/10.1016/j.arthro.2008.10.017.
74. Auffarth A, Schauer J, Matis N, et al. The J-bone graft for anatomical glenoid reconstruction in recurrent posttraumatic anterior shoulder dislocation. Am J Sports Med 2008. https://doi.org/10.1177/0363546507309672.
75. Scheibel M, Nikulka C, Dick A, et al. Autogenous bone grafting for chronic anteroinferior glenoid defects via a complete subscapularis tenotomy approach. Arch Orthop Trauma Surg 2008. https://doi.org/10.1007/s00402-007-0560-z.
76. Rahme H, Wikblad L, Nowak J, et al. Long-term clinical and radiologic results after Eden-Hybbinette operation for anterior instability of the shoulder. J Shoulder Elbow Surg 2003. https://doi.org/10.1067/mse.2002.128138.
77. Longo UG, Loppini M, Rizzello G, et al. Latarjet, Bristow, and Eden-Hybinette procedures for anterior shoulder dislocation: systematic review and quantitative synthesis of the literature. Arthroscopy 2014. https://doi.org/10.1016/j.arthro.2014.04.005.
78. Scheibel M, Kraus N, Diederichs G, et al. Arthroscopic reconstruction of chronic anteroinferior glenoid defect using an autologous tricortical iliac crest bone grafting technique. Arch Orthop Trauma Surg 2008. https://doi.org/10.1007/s00402-007-0509-2.
79. Taverna E, Garavaglia G, Perfetti C, et al. An arthroscopic bone block procedure is effective in restoring stability, allowing return to sports in cases of glenohumeral instability with glenoid bone deficiency. Knee Surg Sports Traumatol Arthrosc 2018. https://doi.org/10.1007/s00167-018-4921-7.
80. Plath JE, Henderson DJH, Coquay J, et al. Does the arthroscopic Latarjet procedure effectively correct "off-track" Hill-Sachs lesions? Am J Sports Med 2018. https://doi.org/10.1177/0363546517728717.
81. Buza JA, Iyengar JJ, Anakwenze OA, et al. Arthroscopic Hill-Sachs remplissage: a systematic review. J Bone Joint Surg Am 2014. https://doi.org/10.2106/JBJS.L.01760.
82. Lazarides A, Duchman K, Ledbetter L, et al. Arthroscopic remplissage for anterior shoulder instability: a systematic review of clinical and biomechanical studies. Arthroscopy 2019. https://doi.org/10.1016/j.arthro.2018.09.029.
83. Cho NS, Yoo JH, Juh HS, et al. Anterior shoulder instability with engaging Hill–Sachs defects: a comparison of arthroscopic Bankart repair with and without posterior capsulodesis. Knee Surg Sports Traumatol Arthrosc 2016. https://doi.org/10.1007/s00167-015-3686-5.
84. Robinson CM, Seah M, Akhtar MA. The epidemiology, risk of recurrence, and functional outcome

after an acute traumatic posterior dislocation of the shoulder. J Bone Joint Surg Am 2011. https://doi.org/10.2106/JBJS.J.00973.
85. DeLong JM, Jiang K, Bradley JP. Posterior instability of the shoulder: a systematic review and meta-analysis of clinical outcomes. Am J Sports Med 2015. https://doi.org/10.1177/0363546515577622.
86. McLaughlin H. Posterior dislocation of the shoulder. J Bone Joint Surg Am 1952;A(3):584–90.
87. Demirel M, Erşen A, Karademir G, et al. Transfer of the lesser tuberosity for reverse Hill-Sachs lesions after neglected posterior dislocations of the shoulder: a retrospective clinical study of 13 cases. Acta Orthop Traumatol Turc 2017. https://doi.org/10.1016/j.aott.2017.07.004.
88. Khira YM, Salama AM. Treatment of locked posterior shoulder dislocation with bone defect. Orthopedics 2017. https://doi.org/10.3928/01477447-20170308-07.
89. Shams A, El-Sayed M, Gamal O, et al. Modified technique for reconstructing reverse Hill–Sachs lesion in locked chronic posterior shoulder dislocation. Eur J Orthop Surg Traumatol 2016. https://doi.org/10.1007/s00590-016-1825-4.
90. Gerber C, Nyffeler RW. Classification of glenohumeral joint instability. Clin Orthop Relat Res 2002. https://doi.org/10.1097/00003086-200207000-00009.
91. Gupta AK, Chalmers PN, Klosterman E, et al. Arthroscopic distal tibial allograft augmentation for posterior shoulder instability with glenoid bone loss. Arthrosc Tech 2013. https://doi.org/10.1016/j.eats.2013.06.009.
92. Struck M, Wellmann M, Becher C, et al. Results of an open posterior bone block procedure for recurrent posterior shoulder instability after a short- and long-time follow-up. Knee Surg Sports Traumatol Arthrosc 2016. https://doi.org/10.1007/s00167-014-3495-2.
93. Tokish JM, Fitzpatrick K, Cook JB, et al. Arthroscopic distal clavicular autograft for treating shoulder instability with glenoid bone loss. Arthrosc Tech 2014. https://doi.org/10.1016/j.eats.2014.05.006.
94. Graichen H, Koydl P, Zichner L. Effectiveness of glenoid osteotomy in atraumatic posterior instability of the shoulder associated with excessive retroversion and flatness of the glenoid. Int Orthop 1999. https://doi.org/10.1007/s002640050316.
95. Inui H, Nobuhara K. Glenoid osteotomy for atraumatic posteroinferior shoulder instability associated with glenoid dysplasia. Bone Joint J 2018. https://doi.org/10.1302/0301-620X.100B3.BJJ-2017-1039.R1.
96. Hawkins RJ, Neer CS II, Pianta RM, et al. Locked posterior dislocation of the shoulder. J Bone Joint Surg Am 1987;69-A(1):9–18.
97. Basal O, Dincer R, Turk B. Locked posterior dislocation of the shoulder: a systematic review. EFORT Open Rev 2017. https://doi.org/10.1302/2058-5241.3.160089.
98. Burkhead WZ, Rockwood CA. Treatment of instability of the shoulder with an exercise program. J Bone Joint Surg Am 1992. https://doi.org/10.2106/00004623-199274060-00010.
99. Guerrero P, Busconi B, Deangelis N, et al. Congenital instability of the shoulder joint: assessment and treatment options. J Orthop Sports Phys Ther 2009. https://doi.org/10.2519/jospt.2009.2860.
100. Watson L, Balster S, Lenssen R, et al. The effects of a conservative rehabilitation program for multidirectional instability of the shoulder. J Shoulder Elbow Surg 2018. https://doi.org/10.1016/j.jse.2017.07.002.
101. Warby SA, Ford JJ, Hahne AJ, et al. Comparison of 2 exercise rehabilitation programs for multidirectional instability of the glenohumeral joint: a randomized controlled trial. Am J Sports Med 2018. https://doi.org/10.1177/0363546517734508.
102. Bateman M, Smith BE, Osborne SE, et al. Physiotherapy treatment for atraumatic recurrent shoulder instability: early results of a specific exercise protocol using pathology-specific outcome measures. Shoulder Elbow 2015. https://doi.org/10.1177/1758573215592266.
103. Warby SA, Pizzari T, Ford JJ, et al. The effect of exercise-based management for multidirectional instability of the glenohumeral joint: a systematic review. J Shoulder Elbow Surg 2014. https://doi.org/10.1016/j.jse.2013.08.006.
104. Gaskill TR, Taylor DC, Millett PJ. Management of multidirectional instability of the shoulder. J Am Acad Orthop Surg 2011. https://doi.org/10.5435/00124635-201112000-00006.
105. Warby SA, Pizzari T, Ford JJ, et al. Exercise-based management versus surgery for multidirectional instability of the glenohumeral joint: a systematic review. Br J Sports Med 2016. https://doi.org/10.1136/bjsports-2015-094970.
106. Longo UG, Rizzello G, Loppini M, et al. Multidirectional instability of the shoulder: a systematic review. Arthroscopy 2015. https://doi.org/10.1016/j.arthro.2015.06.006.
107. Toth AP, Warren RF, Petrigliano FA, et al. Thermal shrinkage for shoulder instability. HSS J 2011. https://doi.org/10.1007/s11420-010-9187-7.
108. Jansen N, Riet RPV, Meermans G, et al. Thermal capsulorrhaphy in internal shoulder impingement: a 7-year follow-up study. Acta Orthop Belg 2012; 78(3):304–8.
109. Waldt S, Burkart A, Imhoff AB, et al. Anterior shoulder instability: accuracy of MR arthrography in the classification of anteroinferior labroligamentous injuries. Radiology 2005. https://doi.org/10.1148/radiol.2372041429.

110. Bokor DJ, Conboy VB, Olson C. Anterior instability of the glenohumeral joint with humeral avulsion of the glenohumeral ligament. J Bone Joint Surg Br 1999. https://doi.org/10.1302/0301-620X.81B1.9111.
111. Owens BD, Nelson BJ, Duffey ML, et al. Pathoanatomy of first-time, traumatic, anterior glenohumeral subluxation events. J Bone Joint Surg Am 2010. https://doi.org/10.2106/JBJS.I.00851.
112. Hegedus EJ, Goode AP, Cook CE, et al. Which physical examination tests provide clinicians with the most value when examining the shoulder? Update of a systematic review with meta-analysis of individual tests. Br J Sports Med 2012. https://doi.org/10.1136/bjsports-2012-091066.
113. Farber AJ, Castillo R, Clough M, et al. Clinical assessment of three common tests for traumatic anterior shoulder instability. J Bone Joint Surg Am 2006. https://doi.org/10.2106/JBJS.E.00594.
114. van Kampen DA, van den Berg T, van der Woude HJ, et al. Diagnostic value of patient characteristics, history, and six clinical tests for traumatic anterior shoulder instability. J Shoulder Elbow Surg 2013. https://doi.org/10.1016/j.jse.2013.05.006.
115. Kim SH, Park JS, Jeong WK, et al. The Kim test: a novel test for posteroinferior labral lesion of the shoulder - a comparison to the Jerk test. Am J Sports Med 2005. https://doi.org/10.1177/0363546504272687.
116. Tzannes A, Murrell GA. Clinical examination of the unstable shoulder. Sports Med 2002;32(7):447–57.
117. Lafosse T, Fogerty S, Idoine J, et al. Hyper extension-internal rotation (HERI): a new test for anterior gleno-humeral instability. Orthop Traumatol Surg Res 2016. https://doi.org/10.1016/j.otsr.2015.10.006.
118. Whitehead NA, Mohammed KD, Fulcher ML. Does the Beighton score correlate with specific measures of shoulder joint laxity? Orthop J Sports Med 2018. https://doi.org/10.1177/2325967118770633.

Obesity is Associated with an Increased Prevalence of Glenohumeral Osteoarthritis and Arthroplasty: A Cohort Study

Kevin C. Wall, MD, MPH[a,*], Cary S. Politzer, MD[b], Jorge Chahla, MD, PhD[c], Grant E. Garrigues, MD[c]

KEYWORDS

• Arthritis • Shoulder • Obesity • Arthroplasty • Body mass index • Glenohumeral

KEY POINTS

- The relationship between obesity and glenohumeral osteoarthritis is relatively understudied and poorly understood.
- Individuals with a body mass index of greater than 25 are at significantly increased odds of developing glenohumeral osteoarthritis when compared with those with a normal body mass index.
- Individuals with a body mass index of less than 19 are significantly less likely to develop glenohumeral osteoarthritis than compared with individuals with a normal body mass index.
- A body mass index of greater than 30 confers an increased odds of undergoing arthroplasty among individuals with glenohumeral osteoarthritis.

INTRODUCTION

Osteoarthritis and obesity are widely recognized as 2 integrally associated pathologies, both with a rising incidence worldwide. The classic model of their relationship states that increasing body weight places a proportionally greater degree of mechanical stress on weight-bearing joints, leading to the development and progression of primary osteoarthritis.[1] An increased prevalence of osteoarthritis of the hip and knee in obese individuals is consistent with this theory,[2–5] and additional research has shown that, although the prevalence of osteoarthritis among all normal or underweight Americans is 16%, this number increases to 23% among overweight adults and to 31% for obese individuals.[6]

Globally, obesity has become an epidemic not only among high-income countries, but also in third-world countries. Between 1975 and 2016, the number of obese individuals tripled, such that now 1.9 billion adults are overweight and 650 million are obese.[7]

Economically, osteoarthritis is the leading cause of disability among American adults,[8] and annually results in $80.8 billion in direct medical costs and $47 billion in indirect costs, such as lost productivity.[9] Similarly, obesity's annual cost is $147 billion in medical spending alone, amounting to 42% more per capita medical spending than that which is spent on nonobese individuals.[10] Although these numbers are not as well-defined on global scale, it stands to reason that the medical and financial

[a] Department of Orthopaedic Surgery, University of Alabama at Birmingham, 1313 13th Street South, Birmingham, AL 35205, USA; [b] Department of Orthopaedic Surgery, University of California San Diego, 4150 Regents Park Row, La Jolla, CA 92037, USA; [c] Midwest Orthopaedics at Rush, Rush University Medical Center, 1611 West Harrison Street, Chicago, IL 60612, USA
* Corresponding author.
E-mail address: kcwall@uabmc.edu
Twitter: @grant_garrigues (G.E.G.)

Orthop Clin N Am 51 (2020) 259–264
https://doi.org/10.1016/j.ocl.2019.12.001

effect of the interplay between these diseases is profound and warrants further investigation.

Recent research into obesity has demonstrated that excess adipose tissue exerts an additional influence beyond the forces its mass applies to the body's susceptible joints. By a variety of mechanisms, obesity also induces a state of chronic, low-grade inflammation[11] with evidence of multiple systemic proinflammatory factors playing a role.[12] The adipokines (adipose tissue-secreted cytokines) are factors that have recently been reported to contribute to the pathophysiology of osteoarthritis affecting both cartilage loss in the knee[13–15] and pain.[16–18] In an attempt to further characterize the effect of obesity on the development of osteoarthritis, we analyzed a large joint classically described as non–weight-bearing, namely, the glenohumeral joint.

For these reasons, the purpose of this study was to determine the prevalence of glenohumeral osteoarthritis and arthroplasty when categorized by body mass index (BMI). Although the shoulder is a non–weight-bearing joint[19–22] and thus should not be as susceptible as the hip[2] and knee[4] to the increased mechanical forces secondary to obesity, we hypothesized that the obese state will still lead to an increased prevalence of shoulder osteoarthritis, and a greater number of shoulder arthroplasties when compared with nonobese individuals.

METHODS

Study Design

This retrospective review was conducted using the database of the United States private insurance payer, Humana, from 2007 to 2016 quarter 3 and was accessed with the PearlDiver Technologies user interface (Warsaw, IN). This database contains the entirety of the collected claims information from more than 25 million patients in the United States and is subjected to routine internal and external audits. Data available for analysis includes demographics, diagnoses, procedures performed, medications prescribed, and hospital admissions. This study was considered exempt from review by our institutional review board.

Database Query

The database was queried for BMI using *International Classification of Diseases, Ninth Revision, Clinical Modification* (ICD-9) diagnosis codes for a BMI of less than 19 kg/m^2 to a BMI of greater than 39 kg/m^2 in increments of 5 kg/m^2. The tenth edition (ICD-10) codes were also used for quarter 4 of 2015 to quarter 3 of 2016 (**Table 1**). Cases were grouped by BMI (<19, 20–24, 25–29, 30–34, 34–39, >39). To avoid any selection bias related to patients who are more likely to have a BMI diagnosis, all cohorts were matched by age and sex using PearlDiver command language. This resulted in 6 cohorts of 99,479 patients each, with identical age and sex makeup. Charlson Comorbidity Index (CCI), a measure of

Table 1
ICD codes

	Diagnosis vs Procedure	ICD-9 Code	ICD-10 Code
BMI <19	Diagnosis	V850	Z681
BMI 19–24	Diagnosis	V851	Z6820-Z6824
BMI 25–29	Diagnosis	V8521-V8525	Z6825-Z6829
BMI 30–34	Diagnosis	V8530-V8534	Z6830-Z6834
BMI 35–39	Diagnosis	V8535-V8539	Z6835-Z6839
BMI >39	Diagnosis	V8541-V8545	Z6841-Z6845
Shoulder osteoarthritis	Diagnosis	715.11	M19.011 (right), M19.012 (left), M19.019 (unspecified)
Total shoulder arthroplasty	Procedure	81.80	0RRJ07Z, 0RRJ0JZ, 0RRJ0KZ, 0RRK07Z, 0RRK0JZ, 0RRK0KZ
Reverse total shoulder arthroplasty	Procedure	81.81	0RRJ0J6, 0RRJ0J7, 0RRK0J6, 0RRK0J7
Hemiarthroplasty	Procedure	81.88	0RRJ0J6, 0RRJ0J7, 0RRK0J6, 0RRK0J7

10-year predicted mortality, was also calculated for each matched cohort.[23]

The prevalence of arthritis in each BMI cohort was attained using ICD-9 and ICD-10 diagnosis codes specifically for primary glenohumeral osteoarthritis. To determine how many patients with shoulder osteoarthritis underwent shoulder arthroplasty in each BMI cohort, ICD-9 and ICD-10 procedure codes for the various arthroplasty options were used (see **Table 1**). *Current Procedural Terminology* codes were not used because there is no code that identifies reverse total shoulder arthroplasty specifically, and we did want to systematically exclude these patients.

Statistical Analysis

When comparing BMI cohorts for osteoarthritis and arthroplasty incidence, odds ratios (ORs) and 95% confidence intervals (CIs) were calculated with an α of 0.05. Given that a BMI of 19 to 24 is considered normal, this cohort was used as the reference cohort to which all other cohorts were compared. CCI scores were grouped into values of 0, 1, 2 and at least 3 and Pearson's χ^2 was tested across all 6 BMI cohorts. Arthroplasty rates were calculated by dividing the number of shoulder arthroplasties performed in each BMI cohort by the number of patients in each respective cohort who have glenohumeral osteoarthritis, thus standardizing the rates across cohorts and minimizing any potential effect that changes in osteoarthritis rates may have on arthroplasty rates. Arthroplasty ORs were similarly calculated; only individuals who had glenohumeral osteoarthritis were included in the subanalysis sample so as to prevent any increased odds of osteoarthritis from also artificially increasing the odds of arthroplasty.

RESULTS

Demographics

Of the 2,748,702 patients with a BMI diagnosis code in the Humana database, 596,874 were able to be matched by age and sex into BMI cohorts so that each cohort had the same proportion of each age and sex group. Collectively, these age- and sex-matched BMI cohorts make up the primary cohort of this study. Of the primary cohort, 27,803 (4.66%) had a diagnosis of primary glenohumeral osteoarthritis. The BMI cohorts had statistically different CCI scores ($P<.001$), indicating each BMI cohort has a different average health status and 10-year estimated mortality (**Table 2**).

Primary Analysis

The underweight (BMI of <19) cohort and the cohorts above the normal range (25–29, 30–34, 35–39, and >39) were all compared with the normal BMI (19–24) cohort (see **Table 2**). Glenohumeral osteoarthritis was present in 3.76% of patients in the BMI 19 to 24 cohort versus 3.14% of patients in the BMI under-19 cohort (OR, 0.83; 95% CI, 0.79–0.87; $P<.001$), 4.4% of patients in the BMI 25 to 29 cohort (OR, 1.18;

Table 2
Glenohumeral osteoarthritis and arthroplasty prevalence and ORs by BMI cohort

	BMI (kg/m²)					
	<19	**19–24**	**25–29**	**30–34**	**35–39**	**>39**
Cohort count (n)	99,479	99,479	99,479	99,479	99,479	99,479
Mean CCI (SD)	3.31 (3.58)	2.40 (2.98)	2.46 (2.93)	2.73 (3.02)	3.03 (3.09)	3.44 (3.24)
GH OA (%)	3119 (3.14)	3740 (3.76)	4380 (4.40)	5082 (5.11)	5648 (5.68)	5834 (5.86)
OR (95% CI)	0.83[a] (0.79–0.87)	REF REF	1.18[a] (1.13–1.23)	1.38[a] (1.32–1.44)	1.54[a] (1.48–1.61)	1.59[a] (1.53–1.66)
GH Arthro (st %)	219 (7.02)	256 (6.84)	329 (7.51)	418 (8.23)	590 (10.45)	600 (10.28)
OR (95%CI)	1.03 (0.85–1.24)	REF REF	1.11 (0.93–1.31)	1.22[a] (1.04–1.43)	1.59[a] (1.36–1.85)	1.56[a] (1.34–1.82)

Abbreviations: GH arthro, number of patients who underwent glenohumeral arthroplasty (st % = the standardized arthroplasty rate - the percentage of patients in the cohort who underwent arthroplasty divided by the total number of patients in the cohort with GH OA); GH OA, number of patients in cohort with glenohumeral osteoarthritis (% of cohort with GH OA); REF, referent cohort for OR calculations; SD, standard deviation.

[a] Indicates significance at $\alpha = 0.05$.

CI, 1.13–1.23; $P<.001$), 5.11% of patients in the BMI 30 to 34 cohort (OR, 1.38; CI, 1.32–1.44; $P<.001$), 5.68% of patients in the BMI 35 to 39 cohort (OR, 1.54; CI, 1.48–1.61; $P<.001$), and 5.86% of patients in the BMI over-39 cohort (OR, 1.59; CI, 1.53–1.66; $P<.001$).

Of patients with glenohumeral osteoarthritis, the odds of undergoing shoulder arthroplasty in the BMI under-19 cohort (OR, 1.03; CI, 0.85–1.24) was not significantly different from the BMI 19 to 24 cohort. Similarly, the BMI 25 to 29 cohort was not found to be at increased odds of undergoing arthroplasty when compared with the reference cohort (OR, 1.11; CI, 0.93–1.31). However, the cohorts with a greater BMI did have higher standardized rates of arthroplasty. The 30 to 34 BMI cohort had a prevalence of 8.23% of shoulder arthroplasty, significantly higher than 6.84% of patients who underwent arthroplasty in the BMI 19 to 24 cohort (OR, 1.22; CI, 1.04–1.43; $P = .016$). Additionally, the 10.45% standardized rate in the BMI 35 to 39 cohort demonstrated a statistically significant OR of 1.59 (CI, 1.36–1.85; $P<.001$) when compared with the reference cohort, as did the standardized rate of the BMI over-39 cohort, 10.28% (OR, 1.56; CI, 1.34–1.82; $P<.001$).

DISCUSSION

We hypothesized that the prevalence of glenohumeral osteoarthritis and rate of shoulder arthroplasty would increase as BMI increased. To test this hypothesis, we mined 9 years of data from a large insurance database for patients with a recorded BMI. Six BMI cohorts of these individuals were generated in an age- and sex-matched fashion, and then each cohort was filtered for a diagnosis of glenohumeral osteoarthritis and subsequent arthroplasty. The overall prevalence of glenohumeral osteoarthritis was 4.66%. As hypothesized, there was a small but significant and progressive increase in osteoarthritis prevalence with increased BMI, relative to the normal BMI cohort. As a corollary, lower BMI (<19) served as a protective factor against glenohumeral osteoarthritis with a statistically significant OR of 0.83.

The fact that there exists an association between obesity and osteoarthritis in what has customarily been described as a non–weight-bearing joint[19–22] requires perhaps reconsidering the role of mechanical forces experienced by the shoulder in the obese individual, as well further study of other mechanisms that may predispose an obese individual to osteoarthritis. One such plausible explanation is that glenohumeral osteoarthritis is also a result of the chronic, systemic inflammatory state of obesity. As adipokines increase with the accumulation of additional adipose tissue, leptin, which has been discovered in glenohumeral synovial fluid,[19,24] may be mediating increased cartilage destruction.[14,17,25,26]

Leptin has proven destructive effects on cartilage and local differences in leptin concentration suggest that all joints are not equally affected. Leptin simultaneously slows chondrocyte proliferation while stimulating the same cells to increase synthesis of the proinflammatory molecules IL-1β, matrix metalloproteinase-9 and matrix metalloproteinase-13.[25] Although increased leptin levels have been observed in the infrapatellar fat pad of obese individuals,[24,27,28] and thus posited as a mechanism for osteoarthritis development in the adjacent knee joint, there is only weak evidence to show that the adipose tissue surrounding the shoulder may behave similarly.[29] As our data show, however, even in the absence of the fat pad that theoretically affects the knee joint, the shoulder nonetheless suffers higher osteoarthritis rates in individuals with more overall adipose tissue.

In addition, we found that the standardized rates of shoulder arthroplasty among patients with glenohumeral osteoarthritis was greater in patients with higher BMI levels. All BMI cohorts of greater than 30 kg/m^2 demonstrated significantly greater odds of having this procedure than our referent, the BMI 19 to 24 cohort. To attempt to contextualize this finding, we note the reason why the decision to progress to operative management is often made: failure of conservative therapy, often manifesting as refractory or increased pain.[3]

One plausible explanation for why patients with a higher BMI may experience worsened pain is the theoretically increased forces exerted across this joint in this population that may promote currently unrecognized degeneration. This effect is relatively understudied in the literature and future biomechanical studies are necessary to demonstrate such an effect. Another way by which the effect found in this study may be explained is the concurrent upregulation of central NMDA receptors and enhanced excitation of the same pathway in the presence of leptin.[18] It is possible that, with increased plasma leptin levels, as seen in the obese patient,[14] the central nervous system of the patient with a higher BMI is modulated in such a fashion, thus predisposing the patient to the resultant sensitivity to neuropathic pain.

As highlighted by Gandhi and colleagues,[19] shoulder osteoarthritis pain may present as constant, dull and aching pain or as what is presumed to be neuropathic pain, characterized as fleeting, but both physically and emotionally intense.[16] Gandhi and his colleagues additionally noted that synovial fluid leptin concentrations were predictive of scores on the short form of the McGill Pain Questionnaire (a patient-reported questionnaire for evaluating pain intensity, quality, and behavior), further reinforcing the leptin–pain hypothesis. Thus, the increased arthroplasty rates among the higher BMI cohorts may be a function of this modified pain pathway. This theory is supported by the numerous neuropathic pain medications already shown to be efficacious in osteoarthritis[30–38]; however, significantly more research is essential to establishing that this type of pain, and a possible, concurrent improved efficacy of medications that treat it, are present in the obese population.

This study was not without limitations. By accessing an existing database of insurance claims through PearlDiver, we were limited to only data based on ICD-9 and ICD-10 codes, hindering our ability to review charts for additional information or study any potentially confounding variables that were not collected for these claims. One such example of this limitation is the use of only postprocedure ICD codes to capture all arthroplasty events; indeed, some of these surgeries may have been performed but not captured by this specific coding for a myriad of reasons.

Similarly, it is possible that the indication for some of the reverse arthroplasties may have been rotator cuff disease concurrent with the requisite osteoarthritis. Issues such as these are theoretically mitigated by the auditing process that the PearlDiver database undergoes but it is difficult to fully assess the reliability of the data without access to the original medical records.

The difference in CCI scores across BMI cohorts also presents a source of potential confounding. However, the increase seen in these scores at the extremes of the BMI ranges is not entirely unexpected, because underweight and obese individuals generally tend to be more ill. Given that our cohorts were already matched for age and sex, we controlled for the main risk factors that predispose individuals to osteoarthritis, thus making it unlikely that any other comorbidity captured by the CCI scores would serve as a significant mediator of the BMI effect we found on osteoarthritis rates.

Despite these limitations, this study contributes to a better understanding of the influence that obesity has on the prevalence of glenohumeral osteoarthritis. Additionally, the previously unreported finding of an increased rate of glenohumeral arthroplasty performed on overweight and obese patients represents a novel source of a disproportionately high surgical burden among this segment of the population.

SUMMARY

Patients with a higher BMI are at increased odds of developing glenohumeral osteoarthritis, despite the conventional belief that such an association is limited to weight-bearing joints. There are also increased odds of undergoing arthroplasty in the higher BMI cohorts, disproportionate to the increase in osteoarthritis rates in these cohorts. These findings may prove to be useful in determining more targeted methods for treating osteoarthritis among the overweight and obese populations.

DISCLOSURE

The authors have nothing to disclose.

REFERENCES

1. Neogi T. The epidemiology and impact of pain in osteoarthritis. Osteoarthritis Cartilage 2013;21:1145–53.
2. Bourne R, Mukhi S, Zhu N, et al. Role of obesity on the risk for total hip or knee arthroplasty. Clin Orthop Relat Res 2007;465:185–8.
3. Chillemi C, Franceschini V. Shoulder osteoarthritis. Arthritis 2013;2013:370231.
4. Grotle M, Hagen KB, Natvig B, et al. Obesity and osteoarthritis in knee, hip and/or hand: an epidemiological study in the general population with 10 years follow-up. BMC Musculoskelet Disord 2008;9:132.
5. Litwic A, Edwards MH, Dennison EM, et al. Epidemiology and burden of osteoarthritis. Br Med Bull 2013;105:185–99.
6. Barbour KE, Helmick CG, Boring M, et al. Vital signs: prevalence of doctor-diagnosed arthritis and arthritis-attributable activity limitation — United States, 2013–2015. MMWR Morb Mortal Wkly Rep 2017;66:246–53.
7. Obesity and overweight. 2019. Available at: https://www.who.int/news-room/fact-sheets/detail/obesity-and-overweight. Accessed August 1, 2019.
8. Theis KA, Roblin D, Helmick CG, et al. Prevalence and causes of work disability among working-age U.S. adults, 2011-2013, NHIS. Disability and Health Journal; 2015.
9. CDC. Arthritis: cost statistics. Atlanta, GA: U.S. Department of Health & Human Services; 2017.
10. Finkelstein EA, Trogdon JG, Cohen JW, et al. Annual medical spending attributable to obesity:

payer-and service-specific estimates. Health Aff 2009;28:w822–31.
11. Saltiel AR, Olefsky JM. Inflammatory mechanisms linking obesity and metabolic disease. J Clin Invest 2017;127(1):1–4.
12. Mraz M, Haluzik M. The role of adipose tissue immune cells in obesity and low-grade inflammation. J Endocrinol 2014;222(3):R113–27.
13. Ding C, Parameswaran V, Cicuttini F, et al. Association between leptin, body composition, sex and knee cartilage morphology in older adults: the Tasmanian older adult cohort (TASOAC) study. Ann Rheum Dis 2008;67:1256–61.
14. Dumond H, Presle N, Terlain B, et al. Evidence for a key role of leptin in osteoarthritis. Arthritis Rheum 2003;48:3118–29.
15. Stannus O, Jones G, Cicuttini F, et al. Circulating levels of IL-6 and TNF-α are associated with knee radiographic osteoarthritis and knee cartilage loss in older adults. Osteoarthritis Cartilage 2010;18:1441–7.
16. Hawker GA, Stewart L, French MR, et al. Understanding the pain experience in hip and knee osteoarthritis - an OARSI/OMERACT initiative. Osteoarthritis Cartilage 2008;16:415–22.
17. Sowers MR, Karvonen-Gutierrez CA. The evolving role of obesity in knee osteoarthritis. Curr Opin Rheumatol 2010;22(5):533–7.
18. Tian Y, Wang S, Ma Y, et al. Leptin enhances NMDA-induced spinal excitation in rats: a functional link between adipocytokine and neuropathic pain. Pain 2011;152:1263–71.
19. Gandhi R, Perruccio AV, Rizek R, et al. Obesity-related adipokines predict patient-reported shoulder pain. Obes Facts 2013;6:536–41.
20. Hawellek T, Hubert J, Hischke S, et al. Articular cartilage calcification of the humeral head is highly prevalent and associated with osteoarthritis in the general population. J Orthop Res 2016;34: 1984–90.
21. Sankaye P, Ostlere S. Arthritis at the shoulder joint. Semin Musculoskelet Radiol 2015;19:307–18.
22. Wanner J, Subbaiah R, Skomorovska-Prokvolit Y, et al. Proteomic profiling and functional characterization of early and late shoulder osteoarthritis. Arthritis Res Ther 2013;15:R180.
23. Charlson M, Pompei P, Ales K, et al. A new method of classifying prognostic comorbidity in longitudinal studies: development and validation. J Chronic Dis 1987;40:373–83.
24. Gandhi R, Kapoor M, Mahomed NN, et al. A comparison of obesity related adipokine concentrations in knee and shoulder osteoarthritis patients. Obes Res Clin Pract 2015;9:420–3.
25. Simopoulou T, Malizos KN, Iliopoulos D, et al. Differential expression of leptin and leptin's receptor isoform (Ob-Rb) mRNA between advanced and minimally affected osteoarthritic cartilage; effect on cartilage metabolism. Osteoarthritis Cartilage 2007;15:872–83.
26. Wluka AE, Lombard CB, Cicuttini FM. Tackling obesity in knee osteoarthritis. Nat Rev Rheumatol 2013;9(4):225–35.
27. Gandhi R, Takahashi M, Virtanen C, et al. Microarray analysis of the infrapatellar fat pad in knee osteoarthritis: relationship with joint inflammation. J Rheumatol 2011;38:1966–72.
28. Presle N, Pottie P, Dumond H, et al. Differential distribution of adipokines between serum and synovial fluid in patients with osteoarthritis. Contribution of joint tissues to their articular production. Osteoarthritis Cartilage 2006;14:690–5.
29. Gandhi R, Takahashi M, Rizek R, et al. Obesity-related adipokines and shoulder osteoarthritis. J Rheumatol 2012;39(10):2046–8.
30. Abou-Raya S, Abou-Raya A, Helmii M. Duloxetine for the management of pain in older adults with knee osteoarthritis: randomised placebo-controlled trial. Age Ageing 2012;41:646–52.
31. Chappell AS, Desaiah D, Liu-Seifert H, et al. A double-blind, randomized, placebo-controlled study of the efficacy and safety of duloxetine for the treatment of chronic pain due to osteoarthritis of the knee. Pain Pract 2011;11:33–41.
32. Chappell AS, Ossanna MJ, Liu-Seifert H, et al. Duloxetine, a centrally acting analgesic, in the treatment of patients with osteoarthritis knee pain: a 13-week, randomized, placebo-controlled trial. Pain 2009;146:253–60.
33. Sullivan M, Bentley S, Fan MY, et al. A single-blind placebo run-in study of venlafaxine XR for activity-limiting osteoarthritis pain. Pain Med 2009;10: 806–12.
34. Sullivan MD, Bentley S, Fan M-Y, et al. A single-blind, placebo run-in study of duloxetine for activity-limiting osteoarthritis pain. J Pain 2009;10: 208–13.
35. Citrome L, Weiss-Citrome A. A systematic review of duloxetine for osteoarthritic pain: what is the number needed to treat, number needed to harm, and likelihood to be helped or harmed? Postgrad Med 2012;124:83–93.
36. Vonsy JL, Ghandehari J, Dickenson AH. Differential analgesic effects of morphine and gabapentin on behavioural measures of pain and disability in a model of osteoarthritis pain in rats. Eur J Pain 2009;13:786–93.
37. Beyreuther B, Callizot N, Stöhr T. Antinociceptive efficacy of lacosamide in the monosodium iodoacetate rat model for osteoarthritis pain. Arthritis Res Ther 2007;9:R14.
38. Rahman W, Dickenson AH. Antinociceptive effects of lacosamide on spinal neuronal and behavioural measures of pain in a rat model of osteoarthritis. Arthritis Res Ther 2014;16:509.

Elbow Hemiarthroplasty for the Treatment of Distal Humerus Fractures

Nicholas Chang, MBBS, MSc, FRCSC[1],
Graham J.W. King, MD, MSc, FRCSC*,[2]

KEYWORDS

• Distal humerus hemiarthroplasty • Fracture • Elbow

KEY POINTS

- Distal humerus hemiarthroplasty may be considered a surgical option for patients with nonreconstructable, intraarticular fractures of the distal humerus.
- Care should be taken to implant the prosthesis at the correct depth and rotation.
- The collateral ligaments should be preserved and/or the epicondyles repaired to maintain joint stability.

INTRODUCTION

The surgical management of displaced distal humerus fractures in adults generally consists of either open reduction internal fixation or arthroplasty. Although the first known distal humerus hemiarthroplasty was performed in 1925, the literature on arthroplasty options for distal humerus fractures has predominately focused on total elbow arthroplasty in the elderly population.[1] However, given the lifelong activity restrictions associated with total elbow replacements and concerns about implant longevity, there has been a recent resurgence of interest in distal humerus hemiarthroplasty. Other proposed advantages of distal humerus arthroplasty over total elbow arthroplasty include the absence of polyethylene and a potentially lower risk of component loosening.

Numerous implants have been used for distal humerus hemiarthroplasty. The first reported case was a custom implant composed of aluminum and bronze covered in a protective rubber coating.[1] Other earlier implant designs were produced from acrylic, nylon, or vitallium.[2–6] Street and Stevens[7] developed an anatomic stainless steel or titanium distal humeral implant without a stem. The system had 7 different size options. Ten distal humeral prostheses were implanted in their case series of 9 patients, which they reported on in 1954.

The introduction of more anatomically shaped commercially available distal humerus implants has significantly increased the use of these devices over the last 2 decades. Implants used include the humeral component of the capitellocondylar implant, the Sorbie-Questor implant (Wright Medical, Memphis, Tennessee, USA), the Kudo implant (Biomet, Warsaw, Indiana, USA), and the Latitude implant (Tornier is a subsidiary of Wright Medical). The capitellocondylar and Kudo implants were nonanatomical designs, whereas the Sorbie-Questor and Latitude humeral components were designed to closely replicate the anatomy of the capitellar and trochlear articulating surfaces. However, despite the increasing use of anatomic hemiarthroplasty

Roth | McFarlane Hand and Upper Limb Centre, St. Joseph's Health Care, Western University, 268 Grosvenor Street, Room D0-213, London, Ontario N6A4L6, Canada
[1] Primary author.
[2] Senior author.
* Corresponding author.
E-mail address: gking@uwo.ca

Orthop Clin N Am 51 (2020) 265–277
https://doi.org/10.1016/j.ocl.2019.11.009

designs worldwide, there are no commercially available implants that have been approved by the Food and Drug Administration to date. Of the aforementioned implants, only the Latitude EV implant is still commercially available (**Fig. 1**).

In vitro biomechanical studies have demonstrated that optimally sized distal humeral prostheses have the greatest ulnohumeral joint congruity, followed by an oversized implant.[8] Elbow kinematics were most affected by undersized implants, and native elbow kinematics were best simulated by an oversized implant.[9] Another biomechanical study reported a significant reduction in ulnohumeral contact compared with the native elbow joint, but no significant difference was detected for the radiocapitellar joint.[10] They did not observe a difference in contact area between implant sizes. These changes in contact are expected given the stiffer nature of the metallic implant relative to the native distal humeral cartilage and will likely have detrimental effects on ulna and radial head cartilage over time. It is unclear as to the extent that these alterations in contact will affect longer-term clinical outcomes.

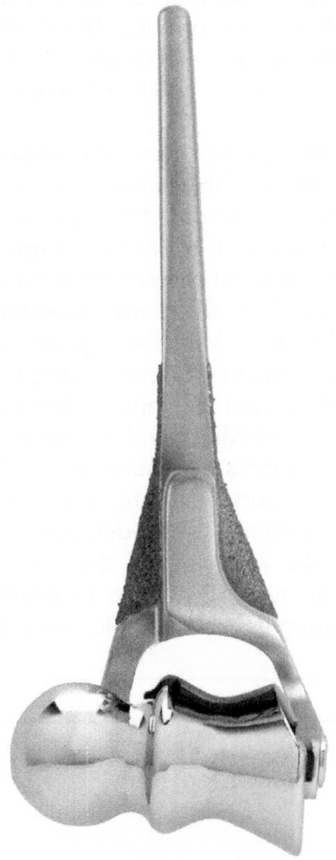

Fig. 1. Latitude EV distal humerus prosthesis from Wright Medical. (*Courtesy of* Wright Medical Group, N.V., Memphis, TN; with permission.)

INDICATIONS/CONTRAINDICATIONS

Indications to use distal humerus hemiarthroplasty in the setting of distal humerus fractures are not well defined. The general consensus is distal humerus hemiarthroplasty should be considered for patients with nonreconstructable intraarticular fractures, such as capitellar-trochlear and supracondylar fractures, who are too young or too active to consider a total elbow arthroplasty. Primary total elbow arthroplasty has traditionally been reserved for elderly, low-demand patients with distal humerus fractures, given the life-long 5- to 10-pound lifting restrictions. The age cutoff for choosing between distal humerus hemiarthroplasty and total elbow arthroplasty is not clear. Instead, the surgeon should account for the patient's overall health, functional status, and ability/inability to comply with the activity restrictions. Although acute trauma has been the most common indication for distal humerus hemiarthroplasty, other reported indications include failed open reduction internal fixation, nonunion, malunion, and capitellum/trochlea avascular necrosis.[11,12] Historically, distal humerus hemiarthroplasty was also used for posttraumatic arthritis, rheumatoid arthritis, and hemophilic arthropathy, but there are no long-term outcome studies to support these indications.[5,7,13]

Absolute contraindications include the presence of an active infection. Other contraindications include the lack of adequate bone stock of the condyles and nonreconstructable incompetence of the collateral ligaments. Patients with preexisting elbow arthritis are a relative contraindication for distal humerus hemiarthroplasty. The presence of a nonreconstructable radial head fracture requires a concomitant compatible radial head arthroplasty combined with a distal humerus hemiarthroplasty. Grade 1 open fractures may be considered for primary distal humeral hemiarthroplasty, but higher grades of open injuries should be debrided and are likely best managed with delayed arthroplasty after soft tissue healing.

SURGICAL TECHNIQUE/PROCEDURE

Preoperative Planning

A careful history and physical examination should be performed in all patients. Neurovascular status, especially the motor and sensory function of the ulnar nerve, should be documented. Orthogonal plain radiographs of the elbow are essential. Computed tomography (CT), including 3-dimensional (3D) reconstructions, may be beneficial to predict whether a fracture is amenable to open reduction internal fixation or better suited for arthroplasty. The timing of surgery should ideally be within 10 days of the fracture, as permitted by the status of the soft tissues.

Preparation and Patient Positioning

Patient positioning may be selected according to the surgeon's preference. Common positions include lateral decubitus or supine (with a bump under the ipsilateral scapula); the latter is the authors' preference. Regional anesthesia can be considered when performing surgery in the supine position, but general anesthesia is recommended when in the lateral decubitus position. If using a tourniquet, sterile tourniquets are preferred. Preoperative prophylactic antibiotics should be administered.

Surgical Approach

The surgical approach is left to the discretion of the surgeon. A posterior longitudinal skin incision is placed just medial to the tip of the olecranon. The ulnar nerve should be released and protected throughout the case. If the ulnar nerve is in contact with the implant, it should be transposed anteriorly. The authors routinely transpose the ulnar nerve when performing distal humeral hemiarthroplasty.

The most common surgical approach in the literature is the olecranon osteotomy.[11,14–17] Advantages of this approach are the excellent visualization of the distal humeral articular surface, and the preservation of the collateral ligaments and triceps. Disadvantages are risk of olecranon nonunion and prominent hardware. An olecranon osteotomy should be avoided if a total elbow arthroplasty may be inserted instead of a distal humerus hemiarthroplasty.

The triceps-splitting approach involves a midline split through the triceps with elevation of the triceps tendon insertion off the olecranon medially and laterally.[18] The Bryan-Morrey approach is a triceps-reflecting approach that elevates the triceps tendon from a medial to lateral direction.[19,20] An osteotomy of the medial and/or lateral epicondyle may also be considered to achieve exposure if these are not already fractured.[21,22] It is essential that the epicondyles are surgically fixed following implantation of the prosthesis to maintain functionality of the collateral ligaments. Another described approach is dislocation of the elbow following subperiosteal elevation of the lateral collateral ligament with subsequent repair.[12] However, the authors of this study reported that 2 of the 3 patients with this approach had postoperative valgus instability.[12]

Triceps-sparing approaches leave all or a portion of the triceps tendon attached to the olecranon at all times. Triceps preservation can be accomplished through a para-tricipital approach given the concomitant epicondyle fractures in most patients with distal humeral fractures.[23] This approach is the authors' preferred approach for distal humeral replacement in acute fractures. Phadnis and colleagues[24] used 2 variations for their triceps-split, the first at the junction between the lateral one-third and medial two-thirds of the triceps, and the second at the junction between the medial one-fourth and lateral three-fourths of the triceps. A lateral paraolecranon approach may also be considered.[25] The benefits of triceps-sparing approaches are the lack of postoperative restrictions for the triceps repair and the greater extension strength.[25]

Surgical Procedure

- Step 1: Exposure
  - Make a midline posterior elbow incision just medial to the olecranon
  - Raise full-thickness flaps on the deep fascia
  - Identify and protect and transpose the ulnar nerve
  - Use a paratricipital approach (Fig. 2)
  - Excise the capitellar and trochlear fracture fragments but save these for later use as bone graft

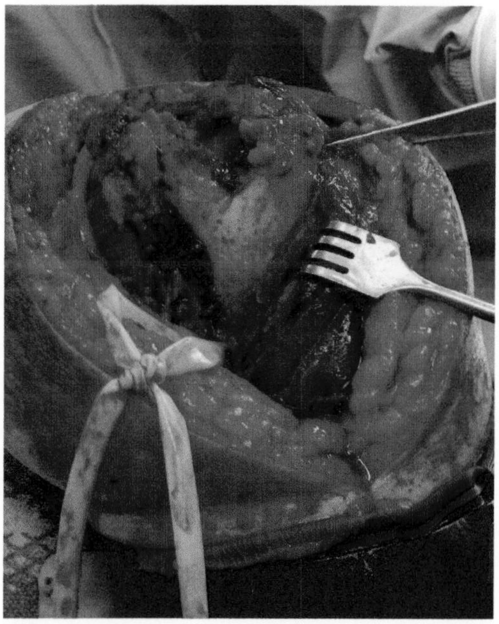

Fig. 2. Distal humerus exposure through a paratricipital approach (medial to triceps).

    - Preserve the medial and lateral condyles and epicondyles for later reconstruction
- Step 2: Implant sizing
    - The surgical technique of the Latitude EV implant system is used in this article because it is currently the only one commercially available
    - Place the sizing spool against the ulnar and radial head articular surfaces to determine the optimal implant size (**Fig. 3**)
    - When choosing between 2 implant sizes, select the larger one[8]
- Step 3: Humeral preparation
    - Enter the humeral canal with a burr
    - Use flexible reamers if the humeral canal is small to reduce the risk of fracture
    - Sequentially broach the humerus, matching the rotation of the broach to the flexion-extension axis of the elbow
        - Rotate the broach and humeral component 14° internally relative to the posterior humeral cortex[26]
        - Use the center of the capitellum and the anterior-distal aspect of the medial epicondyle when available to estimate the flexion-extension axis
    - Determine the correct depth of implant placement by:
        - Matching the component to an intact humeral condyle when present
        - Using the superior aspect of the olecranon fossa as the position of the anterior flange of the implant
        - Judging tension of the soft tissues with triceps-sparing approaches
    - Use implant-specific jigs to make the distal humeral cuts when necessary
- Step 4: Trial
    - Reduce the elbow and take it through a full range of motion (ROM) when the trial implant is in situ
    - Assess for blocks to motion and implant tracking; correct areas of impingement, such as the olecranon or coronoid process
    - Adjust the depth and rotation of the humeral component as required to achieve a full ROM with good articular congruity
- Step 5: Prosthesis implantation
    - Insert a cement restrictor
    - Prepare the humeral canal with pulse lavage
    - Inject polymethyl methacrylate cement retrograde using a cement gun and pressurize
    - Insert the prosthesis to the correct depth while maintaining appropriate rotation (**Fig. 4**)
    - Remove excess cement
    - Place a bone graft behind the anterior flange of the humeral component once the cement has cured

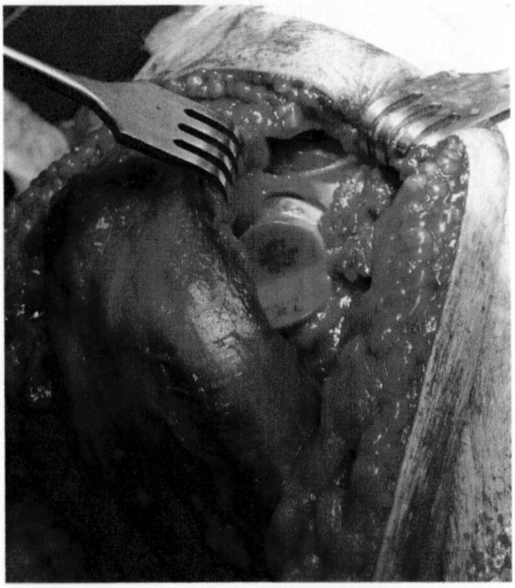

Fig. 3. Spool sizing shows a congruent fit at the radiocapitellar joint.

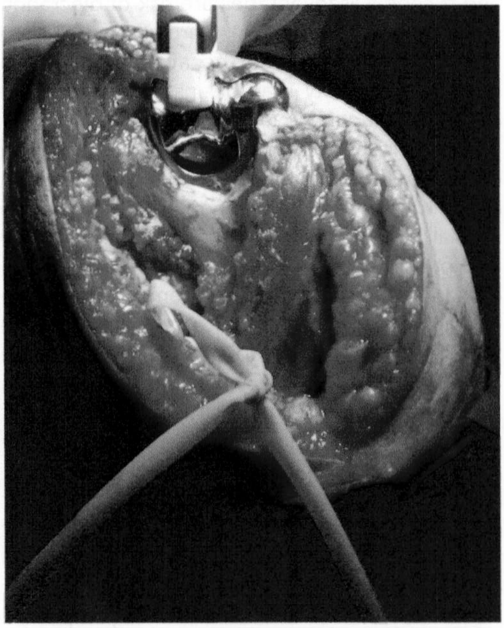

Fig. 4. Humeral component inserted to the correct depth.

- Step 6: Additional fixation
  - Fix concomitant condylar/epicondylar fractures with sutures, K-wires, or small plates; secure fixation is needed to maintain elbow stability
  - Repair the collateral ligaments if torn; a cannulation within the humeral component facilitates a secure repair
  - Fix the olecranon osteotomy, if used, with tension band wiring or a plate
- Step 7: Preclosure
  - Irrigate to remove debris in an effort to reduce risk of heterotopic ossification
  - Take the elbow through a final ROM to assess stability, articular tracking, and impingement
- Step 8: Closure
  - Repair the triceps mechanism/fascia as required (**Fig. 5**)
  - Transpose the ulnar nerve anteriorly
  - Close the elbow in layers after deflating the tourniquet, if used, while ensuring good hemostasis
  - Splint the elbow at 60° of flexion using an anterior splint to avoid posterior wound pressure

POSTOPERATIVE CARE

- Start hand motion immediately
- Perform a wound check at 10 to 14 days postoperatively
- Start active motion when the wound is healed. If the surgical approach required triceps repair, full flexion is delayed to avoid triceps disruption
- Begin passive motion at 6 weeks
- Commence strengthening as soon as healing of the epicondyles, collateral ligaments, and triceps is secure, typically at 8 to 12 weeks postoperatively
- Start static progressive extension splinting 4 weeks postoperatively if the recovery of extension is slow
- Educate patients about the need to protect their elbow arthroplasty to improve its longevity; specific restrictions are not provided as is typically done for a total elbow arthroplasty

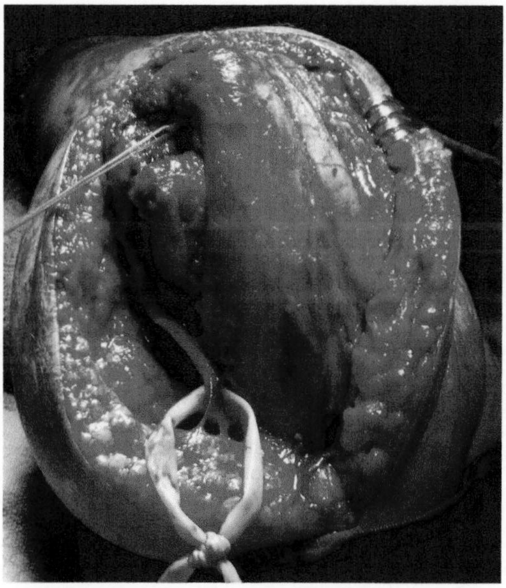

Fig. 5. Repair of the collateral ligaments through a cannulation in the humeral component.

COMPLICATIONS AND MANAGEMENT

Common complications reported in the literature are radiographic degenerative changes of the greater sigmoid notch or radial head, ulnar neuropathy, prominent hardware, stiffness/heterotopic ossification, and radiographic loosening (**Table 1**). Removal of prominent hardware is the most common reason for subsequent surgery. Elbow instability may also require further surgery to manage if this does not respond to splinting and directed physical therapy. Conversion to a total elbow arthroplasty may be required in patients with progressive arthritis, loosening, periprosthetic fracture, and persistent instability.

OUTCOMES

There are limited data on the long-term outcomes of distal humerus hemiarthroplasty for fracture. The highest-quality evidence thus far has been retrospective studies with small sample sizes. The heterogeneity of the studies makes it challenging to accurately compare and contrast them.

Historical case reports and case series used custom prostheses composed of various materials (**Table 2**). The patients generally reported good subjective outcomes, with 4 of the 22 patients developing complications that necessitated further surgery.

More recent studies that used commercially available implants displayed more promising results (**Table 3**). Only the Latitude EV implant is still available today (**Fig. 6**). Three studies used the Sorbie-Questor prosthesis.[11] This stemmed implant had an anatomic design but lacks an anterior flange. Parsons and colleagues[11] published their results on 8 patients, 4 for acute fractures and 4 for subacute management of

Table 1
Management of complications of distal humeral hemiarthroplasty

Timing	Complications	Possible Reasons	Management
Intraoperative	Instability	Malrotation of the implant	Correct implant rotation
		Incompetent collateral ligaments	Repair/re-tension collateral ligaments Ensure anatomic reduction of the condyles/epicondyles
	Tight in extension	Implant too distal	Ensure correct depth of the implant
		Tight anterior capsule	Limited anterior capsulectomy
	Incongruency of the ulnohumeral/radiocapitellar joints	Malrotation of the implant	Correct implant rotation
		Incorrect implant size	Ensure the spool is congruent with the greater sigmoid notch and the radial head Adjust implant size
Postoperative	Wound complications	Poor patient biology	Optimize patient factors for wound healing Immobilize elbow until wound heals
		Superficial wound infection	Oral or intravenous antibiotics Consider irrigation and debridement to rule out deep infection
		Elbow splinted in excess flexion	Splint with decreased flexion
	Stiffness	Insufficient/noncompliant therapy	Physiotherapy Static progressive splinting
		Capsular contracture/heterotopic ossification	Consider capsular release/HO excision if fails therapy and splinting
	Ulnar neuritis/neuropathy	Traction neurapraxia Perineural scarring	Clinical monitoring Consider EMG/NCS studies and imaging studies
		Compressive neurapraxia Subluxating ulnar nerve	Consider decompression ± transposition
	Nonunion of olecranon osteotomy	Patient factors Fixation factors	Optimize patient factors for union Revise fixation
	Painful elbow	Periprosthetic infection	Aspirate/inflammatory markers/staged revision arthroplasty
		Loosening Erosion of the radial head/greater sigmoid notch	Revise to total elbow arthroplasty
	Instability	Muscle atony Incompetent ligaments	Immobilization in more flexion Isometric biceps and triceps exercises to regain muscle tone Overhead rehabilitation protocol Revise fixation of condyles Revise ligament repair Revise to linked TEA

Abbreviations: EMG, electromyography; HO, heterotopic ossification; NCS, nerve conduction study; TEA, total elbow arthroplasty.

Table 2
Historical studies featuring custom implants

Author, y	Type of Study	Sample Size	Mean Age (Range)	Implant	Mean F/U (mo)	Indication	Flex-Ext. ROM	Complications
Robineau,[1] 1927	Case report	1	20	Custom aluminum-bronze implant, wrapped in rubber	N/A	Benign tumor	N/A	
Mellen & Phalen,[2] 1947	Case series	4	22.5 (19–28)	Custom acrylic implant	10.5	Nonunion	53°–142°	Instability, n = 1
Venable,[3] 1952	Case report	1	N/A	Custom vitallium implant	15	Fracture	0°–110°	
MacAusland,[4] 1954	Case series	4	38	Custom nylon implant		Failed ORIF	incomplete	Revision, n = 1
Barr & Eaton,[5] 1965	Case report	1	28	Custom vitallium implant	48	Posttraumatic OA	30°–125°	Radiographic osteolysis, broken screw
Street & Stevens,[7] 1974	Case series	10	39	Custom stainless steel or titanium implant	31	Posttraumatic OA, n = 1 RA, n = 3 Failed ORIF, n = 1 Heophilia, n = 1	40°–119°	Resection arthroplasty, n = 2 (loosening) HO, n = 2 Ulnar neuritis, n = 1 Stiffness, n = 1 Sup. infection, n = 1
Shifrin & Johnson,[6] 1990	Case report	1	19	Custom vitallium implant	240	Failed ORIF	40°-"full"	Radiographic wear

Abbreviations: Ext., extension; Flex, flexion; F/U, follow-up; N/A, not available; OA, osteoarthritis; RA, rheumatoid arthritis; Sup., superficial.

Table 3
Studies featuring commercial implants

Author, y	Type of Study	Sample Size	Mean Age (Range)	Implant	Mean F/U (mo)	Indication	Flex-Ext. ROM	Mean Outcome Scores	Complications
Swoboda & Scott,[13] 1999	Case series	7	33 (20–50)	Capitellocondylar (humeral component)	67	RA	46°–119°	N/A	Infection, n = 1 Stiffness, n = 1 Radiographic loosening, n = 1
Parsons et al,[11] 2005	Case series	8	61 (46–83)	Sorbie-Questor	N/A	Fracture (4) Fracture sequelae (4)	16°–126°	ASES: 81	Prominent hardware, n = 3 Ulnar neuritis, n = 1 Radiographic UH arthrosis, n = 1
Adolfsson & Hammer,[28] 2006	Case series	4	80 (79–89)	Kudo	10	Fracture	20°–126°	MEPS: 3 excellent, 1 good	Weakness, n = 2
Burkhart et al,[20] 2011	Case series	10	75 (62–88)	Latitude	12	Fracture (8) Failed ORIF (2)	18°–125°	MEPS: 91 DASH: 12	Ulnar neuritis, n = 1 Superficial infection, n = 1 HO, n = 1 Triceps weakness, n = 1 Revision to TEA, n = 1
Adolfsson & Nestorson,[29] 2012	Case series	8	79	Kudo	80	Fracture (7) Failed ORIF (1)	31°–126°	MEPS: 91	Radiographic UH arthrosis, n = 3 Periprosthetic number, n = 1 Stiffness, n = 1
Argintar et al,[14] 2012	Case series	10	73 (56–77)	Latitude	12	Fracture	22°–121°	MEPS: 77 DASH: 35	Intraoperative number, n = 1 Ulnar neuritis, n = 1 Prominent hardware, n = 1
Smith & Hughes,[27] 2013	Case series	17 (9 excluded)	63 (29–92)	Sorbie-Questor (12); Latitude (14)	80	Fracture (21) Failed ORIF (5)	116° arc	MEPS: 90 QuickDASH: 19	Radiographic UH wear, n = 13 (7 mild) Prominent hardware, n = 10 Revision to TEA, n = 4 (2 for infection, 2 for loosening) Ulnar neuritis, n = 4 Wound necrosis, n = 1 Stiffness, n = 1

Hohman et al,[32] 2014	Case series	7	64 (33–75)	Latitude	36	Fracture (5) Failed ORIF (2)	19°–120°	MEPS: 75 DASH: 13	Radiographic UH arthrosis, n = 7 (2 mild) Radiographic RH wear, n = 7 (5 mild) Prominent hardware, n = 3 Ulnar neuritis, n = 2 Intraoperative number ; n = 1 Radiographic loosening, n = 1
Heijink et al,[12] 2015	Case series	6	72 (56–84)	Latitude	54	Fracture (1) Nonunion (4) Capitellar AVN (1)	27°–123°	MEPS: 78 OES: 57 DASH: 8	Valgus instability, n = 3 Ulnar neuritis, n = 2 Radiographic UH arthrosis, n = 1 HO, n = 1
Lechasseur et al,[15] 2015	Case report	1	49	Latitude	19	Failed ORIF	30°–130°	MEPS: 100 DASH: 8	HO, n = 1 Prominent hard n = 1
Nestorson et al,[30] 2015	Case series	42	72 (56–84)	Latitude	34	Fracture	24°–127°	MEPS: 90 DASH: 20	Radiographic UH arthrosis, n = 5 (mild) Stiffness, n = 4 Ulnar neuritis, n = 2 Instability, n = 1 Revision for loosening, n = 1
Phadnis et al,[24] 2015	Case series	16	79 (60–90)	Latitude	35	Fracture	116° arc, 15° flex contracture	MEPS: 99 OES: 44 QuickDASH: 11	Radiographic lucency, n = 10 Radiographic UH wear, n = 10 (8 mild, 2 moderate) Radiographic RH wear, n = 3 (mild) Ulnar neuritis, n = 1
Smith et al,[17] 2016	Case series	6 (2 excluded)	44 (29–52)	Sorbie-Questor (3); Latitude (3)	81	Fracture (5) Failed ORIF (1)	23°–103°	MEPS: 88 QuickDASH: 12	Radiographic UH wear, n = 5 Prominent hardware, n = 4 Revision to TEA, n = 2 (loosening) Stiffness, n = 1

(*continued on next page*)

Author, y	Type of Study	Sample Size	Mean Age (Range)	Implant	Mean F/U (mo)	Indication	Flex-Ext. ROM	Mean Outcome Scores	Complications
Schultzel et al,[16] 2017	Case series	10	72 (56–81)	Latitude	73	Fracture	27°–129°	MEPS: 89 DASH: 34	Intraoperative number , n = 1 Prominent hardware, n = 1
Al-Hamdani et al,[18] 2019	Case series	24	65 (47–80)	Latitude	20	Fracture	110° arc	MEPS: 85 OES: 40	Stiffness, n = 3 Ulnar neuritis, n = 3 Radiographic UH wear (mild)/HO, n = 1
Nestorson et al,[31] 2019	Case series (registry data)	87	N/A	Kudo (9); Latitude (72)	90			N/A	HO, n = 4 Revision to TEA, n = 2 (1 loosening, 1 infection) Periprosthetic number, n = 3

Abbreviations: ASES, American shoulder and elbow surgeons; AVN, avascular necrosis; MEPS, mayo elbow performance score; OES, oxford elbow score; RH, radial head; UH, ulnohumeral.

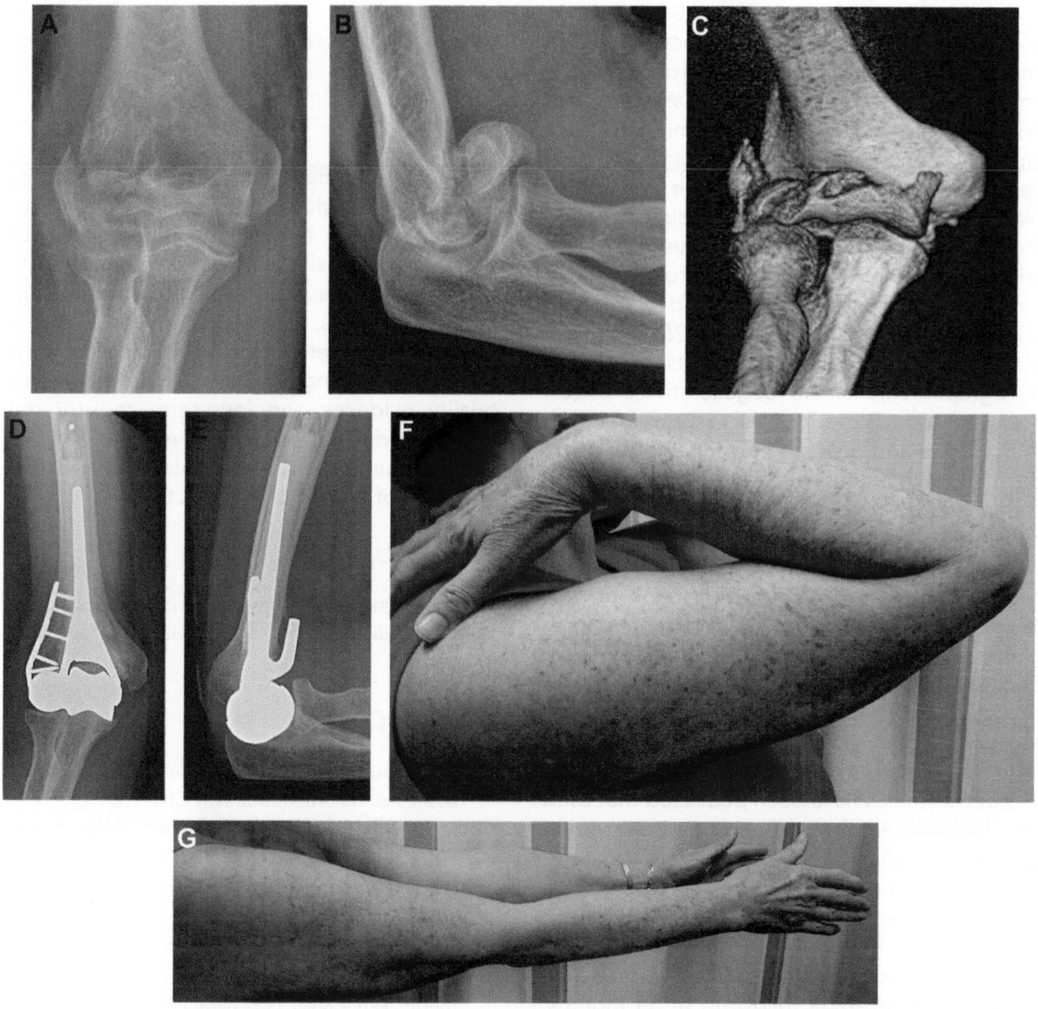

Fig. 6. An example case. (*A*) Preoperative anteroposterior (AP) radiograph, (*B*) lateral radiograph, and (*C*) 3D reconstruction computed tomography (CT) scan of a 63-year-old patient with a comminuted capitellum/trochlea fracture with an associated lateral epicondyle fracture. (*D*) Postoperative AP radiograph and (*E*) lateral radiograph of the patient 1 year following a distal humerus hemiarthroplasty and ORIF lateral epicondyle for a displaced capitellum/trochlea fracture. Clinical photographs demonstrating excellent elbow (*F*) flexion and (*G*) extension at 1 year postoperatively. ([*D, E*] *Courtesy of* Wright Medical Group, N.V., Memphis, TN.)

fracture sequelae. The average ROM was 16° to 126°, with a mean American Shoulder and Elbow Surgeons score of 81. One patient developed ulnohumeral arthrosis; 1 patient had self-limiting ulnar neuritis, and 3 patients required their olecranon tension band wires removed. Smith and colleagues[17,27] published 2 reports on their cohort of patients receiving distal humerus hemiarthroplasty for fractures or failed open reduction internal fixation (ORIF). Sorbie-Questor implants were used until mid-2005, when the authors switched to the Latitude implants. Their cohort averaged a flexion-extension arc between 16° and 131° and reported a mean Mayo score of 95 and QuickDash score of 10.5. Of note, the authors excluded 4 patients who required revision surgery to total elbow arthroplasty from their final analysis. Two elbows were revised for late periprosthetic fractures and 2 elbows were revised for aseptic loosening. All 4 revisions occurred in patients with the Sorbie-Questor implant. In addition, the patients with the Sorbie-Questor implants were more likely to develop moderate to severe radiographic degenerative changes to the ulnohumeral joint compared with those with the Latitude prosthesis; however, the duration of follow-up was longer for the Sorbie-Questor group. The pattern of wear also differed, with more medial-sided degeneration noted with the Sorbie-Questor patients.[17,27]

Adolfsson and colleagues[28,29] published short- and midterm results of patients receiving Kudo implants for trauma. The Kudo prosthesis is a nonanatomic total elbow system and was not originally designed for use as a hemiarthroplasty implant. The authors routinely performed a radial head excision in conjunction with the hemiarthroplasty. Despite the nonanatomic design, only 1 of the 8 patients required subsequent surgery following a complication (late periprosthetic fracture) after a mean follow-up period of 4 years. Their average motion was 31° to 126°, and their Mayo score was 91. Three patients developed radiographic ulnohumeral degenerative changes; however, no revisions for wear were required.[29]

Swoboda and Scott[13] reported the outcome of 7 distal humerus hemiarthroplasties for 7 young women with rheumatoid arthritis. They implanted the humeral component of the capitellocondylar implant, which featured a nonanatomic design. At a mean follow-up of 67 months, 1 patient had a resection arthroplasty for infection, and another patient had a triceps lengthening for stiffness. At final follow-up, no patients had radiographic evidence of erosion at the ulnohumeral joint and none required revision to a total elbow arthroplasty.

Twelve studies have been published that used the Latitude implant, including 1 analyzing Swedish registry data. Nestorson and colleagues[30] reported the largest series with a cohort of 42 patients. Using a triceps split leaving the medial half of the tendon still attached, the patients had an average motion from 24° to 127° at an average follow-up of 34 months. The mean Mayo score was 90, and the DASH (disabilities of the arm, shoulder, and hand) score was 20. Six patients developed complications necessitating further surgery. One patient was revised for component loosening; 4 had a capsular release for stiffness, and another patient required a lateral ligament reconstruction for instability. Five had mild radiographic ulnohumeral degenerative changes.[30]

Al-Hamdani and colleagues[18] reported their results on 24 patients receiving Latitude distal humerus hemiarthroplasties for fracture. The patients had an arc of motion of 110°, a Mayo score of 85, and Oxford elbow score of 40. Seven patients developed complications, including 3 with ulnar neuritis, 3 with stiffness requiring capsular release, and 1 patient with radiographic ulnar wear and heterotopic ossification.

The Swedish Registry Data from 1999 to 2014 includes 72 Latitude hemiarthroplasty.[31] Two patients required revision to total elbow arthroplasty, one for aseptic loosening and one for infection. Other complications included periprosthetic fracture (2), stiffness (4), and instability (1).

SUMMARY

Distal humerus hemiarthroplasty is a good option for the surgical management of nonreconstructable distal humeral fractures in selected patients. Care should be taken to preserve and/or repair the integrity of the collateral ligaments, condyles, and epicondyles. Short- to medium-term retrospective studies have reported promising results. However, higher-quality evidence and long-term registry data are needed to better understand the durability of distal humerus hemiarthroplasty for the management of distal humeral fractures.

DISCLOSURE

Dr G.J.W. King receives royalties and is a consultant for Wright Medical. Dr N. Chang has no conflicts of interest.

REFERENCES

1. Robineau R. Contribution à l'étude de prothèses osseuses. Bull Mem Soc Nat Chir 1927;53:886–96.
2. Mellen RH, Phalen GS. Arthroplasty of the elbow by replacement of the distal portion of the humerus with an acrylic prosthesis. J Bone Joint Surg Am 1947;29(2):348–53.
3. Venable CS. An elbow and an elbow prosthesis. Case of complete loss of the lower third of the humerus. Am J Surg 1952;83(3):271–5.
4. MacAusland WR. Replacement of the lower end of the humerus with a prosthesis; a report of four cases. West J Surg Obstet Gynecol 1954;62(11): 557–66.
5. Barr JS, Eaton RG. Elbow reconstruction with a new prosthesis to replace the distal end of the humerus. A case report. J Bone Joint Surg Am 1965;47(7): 1408–13.
6. Shifrin PG, Johnson DP. Elbow hemiarthroplasty with 20-year follow-up study. Clin Orthop Relat Res 1990;(254):128–33.
7. Street DM, Stevens PS. A humeral replacement prosthesis for the elbow. Results in ten elbows. J Bone Joint Surg Am 1974;56(6):1147–58.
8. Desai SJ, Lalone E, Athwal GS, et al. Hemiarthroplasty of the elbow: the effect of implant size on joint congruency. J Shoulder Elbow Surg 2016; 25(2):297–303.
9. Desai SJ, Athwal GS, Ferreira LM, et al. Hemiarthroplasty of the elbow: the effect of implant size on kinematics and stability. J Shoulder Elbow Surg 2014; 23(7):946–54.

10. Lapner M, Willing R, Johnson JA, et al. The effect of distal humeral hemiarthroplasty on articular contact of the elbow. Clin Biomech (Bristol, Avon) 2014; 29(5):537–44.
11. Parsons M, O'Brien RJ, Hughes JS. Elbow hemiarthroplasty for acute and salvage reconstruction of intra-articular distal humerus fractures. Tech Shoulder Elbow Surg 2005;6(2):87–97.
12. Heijink A, Wagener ML, de Vos MJ, et al. Distal humerus prosthetic hemiarthroplasty: midterm results. Strategies Trauma Limb Reconstr 2015;10(2): 101–8.
13. Swoboda B, Scott RD. Humeral hemiarthroplasty of the elbow joint in young patients with rheumatoid arthritis: a report on 7 arthroplasties. J Arthroplasty 1999;14(5):553–9.
14. Argintar E, Berry M, Narvy SJ, et al. Hemiarthroplasty for the treatment of distal humerus fractures: short-term clinical results. Orthopedics 2012;35(12): 1042–5.
15. Lechasseur B, Laflamme M, Leclerc A, et al. Incipient malunion of an isolated humeral trochlea fracture treated with an elbow hemiarthroplasty: case report. J Hand Surg Am 2015;40(2):271–5.
16. Schultzel M, Scheidt K, Klein CC, et al. Hemiarthroplasty for the treatment of distal humeral fractures: midterm clinical results. J Shoulder Elbow Surg 2017;26(3):389–93.
17. Smith GCS, Bayne G, Page R, et al. The clinical outcome and activity levels of patients under 55 years treated with distal humeral hemiarthroplasty for distal humeral fractures: minimum 2-year follow-up. Shoulder Elbow 2016;8(4):264–70.
18. Al-Hamdani A, Rasmussen JV, Sørensen AKB, et al. Good outcome after elbow hemiarthroplasty in active patients with an acute intra-articular distal humeral fracture. J Shoulder Elbow Surg 2019; 28(5):925–30.
19. Bryan RS, Morrey BF. Extensive posterior exposure of the elbow. A triceps-sparing approach. Clin Orthop Relat Res 1982;166:188–92.
20. Burkhart KJ, Nijs S, Mattyasovszky SG, et al. Distal humerus hemiarthroplasty of the elbow for comminuted distal humeral fractures in the elderly patient. J Trauma 2011;71(3):635–42.
21. Campbell WC. Incision for exposure of the elbow joint. Am J Surg 1932;15(1):65–7.
22. De Vos MJ, Wagener ML, Verdonschot N, et al. An extensive posterior approach of the elbow with osteotomy of the medial epicondyle. J Shoulder Elbow Surg 2014;23(3):313–7.
23. Alonso-Llames M. Bilaterotricipital approach to the elbow: its application in the osteosynthesis of supracondylar fractures of the humerus in children. Acta Orthop 1972;43(6):479–90.
24. Phadnis J, Banerjee S, Watts AC, et al. Elbow hemiarthroplasty using a "triceps-on" approach for the management of acute distal humeral fractures. J Shoulder Elbow Surg 2015;24(8):1178–86.
25. Studer A, Athwal GS, Macdermid JC, et al. The Lateral para-olecranon approach for total elbow arthroplasty. J Hand Surg Am 2013;38(11):2219–26.e3.
26. Sabo MT, Athwal GS, King GJW. Landmarks for rotational alignment of the humeral component during elbow arthroplasty. J Bone Joint Surg Am 2012;94(19):1794–800.
27. Smith GCS, Hughes JS. Unreconstructable acute distal humeral fractures and their sequelae treated with distal humeral hemiarthroplasty: a two-year to eleven-year follow-up. J Shoulder Elbow Surg 2013; 22(12):1710–23.
28. Adolfsson L, Hammer R. Elbow hemiarthroplasty for acute reconstruction of intraarticular distal humerus fractures: a preliminary report involving 4 patients. Acta Orthop 2006;77(5):785–7.
29. Adolfsson L, Nestorson J. The Kudo humeral component as primary hemiarthroplasty in distal humeral fractures. J Shoulder Elbow Surg 2012; 21(4):451–5.
30. Nestorson J, Ekholm C, Etzner M, et al. Hemiarthroplasty for irreparable distal humeral fractures: medium-term follow-up of 42 patients. Bone Joint J 2015;97-B(10):1377–84.
31. Nestorson J, Rahme H, Adolfsson L. Arthroplasty as primary treatment for distal humeral fractures produces reliable results with regards to revisions and adverse events: a registry-based study. J Shoulder Elbow Surg 2019;28(4): e104–10.
32. Hohman DW, Nodzo SR, Qvick LM, et al. Hemiarthroplasty of the distal humerus for acute and chronic complex intra-articular injuries. J Shoulder Elbow Surg 2014;23(2):265–72.

Foot and Ankle

Orthopedic Surgical Foot Management in Hansen Disease

Jose Carlos Cohen, MD[a,*],
Silvana Teixeira de Miranda, PT[b]

KEYWORDS

• Hansen disease • Leprosy • Drop foot • Neuropathy • Ulcers

KEY POINTS

- Leprosy is a chronic infectious disease caused by the *Mycobacterium leprae* with nerve injury being the central feature of its pathogenesis.
- Early diagnosis along with early detection and treatment of neuropathy remains the best method to prevent permanent primary impairments.
- Neuropathy of the tibial and common peroneal nerves is common, causing plantar forefoot ulcers, claw toes, and drop foot.
- Multidrug therapy and oral corticoids remain the mainstay in the treatment of neuropathy, but neurolysis of those major nerve trunks is considered in selected cases in order to improve nerve function.
- Tendon transfers are indicated in drop foot, using both the posterior tibial tendon and the peroneus longus, depending on the type of peroneal nerve injury (complete or partial).

INTRODUCTION

Leprosy is a chronic infectious disease caused by the *Mycobacterium leprae*. The terminology Hansen disease was adopted in 1976 by the Brazilian health ministry to minimize the secular prejudice related to the disease. The skin and nervous manifestations present a singular clinical picture that is easily recognized. Worldwide leprosy remains a common problem with 750,000 new cases being diagnosed each year. After India, Brazil is the country with the second greatest number of cases in the world.[1] Nerve injury is a central feature of the pathogenesis of leprosy because of the unique tendency of *M leprae* to invade Schwann cells and the peripheral nervous system, causing a "mononeuritis multiplex "of immunologic origin that results in autonomic, sensory, and motor neuropathy that can be permanent and develop into disabilities.

The role of the orthopedic surgeon in the care of those patients is important, both in the early stages of disease, and especially, in the final disease process with its known sequelae. The mainstay of treatment of Hansen disease is based on adequate multidrug therapy, because when detected and treated early, primary impairments may be reversible. However, a substantial proportion of patients have established nerve damage at the time of diagnosis, and therefore, orthopedic problems may be already present. In addition, the occurrence of recurrent neuritis and leprosy reactions can still damage the peripheral nerves in the postdischarge period.[2]

[a] Foot and Ankle Service, Federal University Hospital of Rio de Janeiro (UFRJ/HUCFF), Rua Rodolpho Paulo Rocco, 255, Cidade Universitária, Ilha do Fundão, Rio de Janeiro - RJ CEP 21941-913, Brazil; [b] Federal University Hospital of Rio de Janeiro (UFRJ/HUCFF), Rua Rodolpho Paulo Rocco, 255, Cidade Universitária, Ilha do Fundão, Rio de Janeiro - RJ CEP 21941-913, Brazil
* Corresponding author.
E-mail address: cohenorto@yahoo.com

Orthop Clin N Am 51 (2020) 279–291
https://doi.org/10.1016/j.ocl.2019.11.012
0030-5898/20/

The irreversible motor, sensory, and autonomic impairments caused by leprosy lead to increasing secondary impairments long after the disease process has been arrested. The progressive physical impairments caused by the disease process are compounded by the psychological and social consequences that adversely influence the participation in society of those affected.[3] Depending on the country and the regional control program, 16% to 56% of newly registered patients have clinically detectable impairments, often no longer amenable to drug treatment alone, at the time they are first seen. Early diagnosis of leprosy along with early detection and treatment of neuropathy remains the best method to prevent permanent primary impairments.[4]

Different forms of the disease have somewhat differing patterns of nerve involvement, but commonly involved nerves are the tibial, ulnar, peroneal, median, and superficial radial nerves. The variability of clinical presentations among patients with Hansen disease reflects differences in the extent of host resistance to infection with *M leprae*, and the disease can be classified accordingly, with tuberculoid type at 1 extreme, lepromatous type at the other, and a range of borderline forms in between. In the tuberculoid type, there is a strong cellular immune response to *M leprae*, which limits bacterial spread. As a result, few or no bacteria can be found within the affected tissues. Skin lesions are few and isolated damage of nerve trunks or more superficial dermal nerves are injured in the tuberculoid pole of the disease. In the lepromatous type, the immune response is antibody driven, and under these conditions, *M leprae* bacteria multiply freely and infiltrate the skin, with multiple nerves involved. The borderline form represents the spectrum between tuberculoid and lepromatous disease and is immunologically dynamic; if untreated, it often changes to the lepromatous end of the spectrum. These different patterns of host response can be explained partly by host genetic factors.The fact that *M leprae* multiplies best in cooler tissues might explain why more distal and superficial skin nerves are preferentially affected.

The World Health Organization (WHO) classification system is used to differentiate the clinical presentations of leprosy[5]; it has only 2 forms or classifications of leprosy. The 2009 WHO classifications are simply based on the number of bacilli per skin lesions as follows: paucibacillary (PB) leprosy: skin lesions with no bacilli (*M leprae*) seen in a skin smear; and multibacillary (MB) leprosy: skin lesions with bacilli (*M leprae*) seen in a skin smear.

However, the WHO further modifies these 2 classifications with clinical criteria because of the nonavailability or nondependability of the skin-smear services. The clinical system of classification for treatment includes the use of number of skin lesions and nerves involved as the basis for grouping patients with leprosy into MB and PB leprosy. Investigators state that up to about 4 to 5 skin lesions and/or 1 or no nerve involved constitutes PB leprosy, whereas about 5 or more lesions and/or more than 1 nerve involved constitute MB leprosy.

CLINICAL MANIFESTATIONS IN THE FOOT AND ANKLE CAUSED BY HANSEN DISEASE

The bacilli are mainly located in Schwann cells, but also are encountered in hystiocytes, and in perineural and endothelial cells. The infection occurs in both peripheral neurologic trunks and small neural fibers with involvement of sensitive and autonomic nerves in skin lesions.[6] The neuritis represents a primary inflammation of the nerve, causing spontaneous or induced pain in the peripheral nerve trunk with palpation, generally accompanied with local edema and nerve dysfunction with muscular weakness and cutaneous sensory disturbance. Fibrosis and nerve thickening might occur with disease progression, predisposing to recurrent episodes of acute neuritis and pain because of nerve compression within their tunnels.[7]

Silent neuritis, on the other hand, is nerve dysfunction without pain.[8,9] Asymptomatic neuropathy of common peroneal nerve is not rare and diagnosis is frequently done when the patient already presents with partial or complete muscle paralysis with drop foot. Tibial nerve involvement is the most common and more disabling neuropathy in Hansen disease with its compression in the tarsal tunnel, which produces loss of protective sensation on the sole of the foot. Besides, tibial nerve innervates the intrinsic muscles of the foot, which is responsible for the balance between the extrinsic extensors and flexors of the toes, because they act to keep the toes well aligned and in contact with the ground. With involvement of the intrinsic muscles (intrinsic minus deformity), there will be clawing of the toes, initially only observed when the patient stays on his or her tiptoes, but in more advances stages, it will become rigid deformities, increasing the pressure beneath both the metatarsal heads and the tip of the toes, predisposing the development of plantar forefoot ulcers. When both nerves are damaged, weight-bearing falls on the anesthetic forefoot

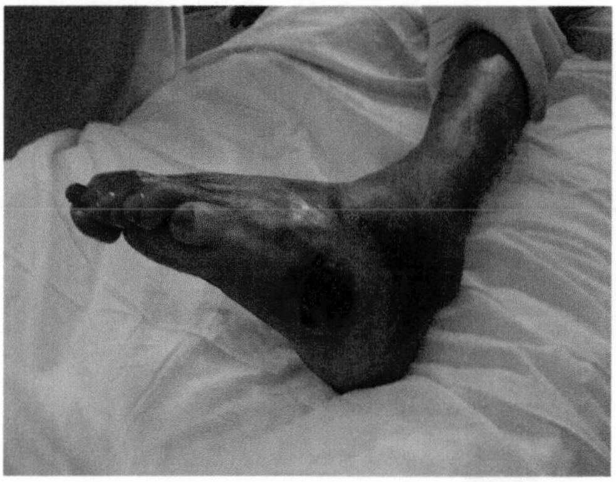

Fig. 1. The classic appearance of equinus, varus, and supination of the foot caused by concomitant involvement of the common peroneal and tibial nerves. Note the ulceration on the lateral border of the foot because of excessive pressure and clawing of the toes.

rather than on the heel and causes trophic ulceration (Fig. 1).

Drop foot is found in 2% to 5% of newly diagnosed patients with leprosy.[10] When there is complete involvement of the common peroneal nerve (deep and superficial portions), the clinical picture is similar to the traumatic injury with paralysis of the anterior and lateral compartments of the leg, causing the classic equinovarus deformity. However, in Hansen disease, there is the possibility of isolated involvement of the deep peroneal nerve branch, sparing the superficial peroneal branch. The classic clinical manifestation of supinated equinovarus deformity associated with injury of the common peroneal nerve owing to overpull of plantarflexors and inverters associated with loss of dorsiflexors and everters, is replaced by a selective paralysis of the anterior compartment of the leg with preservation of function of both peroneal tendons in the lateral compartment. In addition, the peroneus longus (PL) can overpower the weak anterior tibial tendon (its antagonist on the first metatarsal) and produces marked plantar flexion in the first metatarsal that can cause secondary varus in the hindfoot.

ORTHOPEDIC PROCEDURES IN HANSEN DISEASE

Treatment of Neuropathic Ulcers

Primary neuropathic ulcer prevention is by patient health education and self-awareness; hygiene of the insensate foot with attention to cracks and fissures; awareness of potential injury mainly during work; and appropriate footwear.When present, the treatment of plantar ulceration includes debridement of devitalized tissue, non-weight-bearing by means of a total-contact cast or bed rest, and the vigorous treatment of secondary infection, which is most commonly caused by *Staphylococcus aureus*. The ulcers should be examined for infection and probed to detect any bony involvement. If there is slough or necrotic material, it should be thoroughly debrided. Bony involvement may require multiple debridements and sometimes excision. Leprous ulcers heal well if weight-bearing is prevented because they have good vascular supply unlike those in diabetic neuropathy. Once healing takes place, walking must be limited and only increased slowly. Extradepth or custom-made shoes with molded inserts are required to prevent recurrence. Areas of bony prominence that may lead to ulceration should be removed surgically. Alternatively, in cases of noninfected ulcers, the use of percutaneous osteotomies could be used to alleviate the pressure without the need of removing the prominent bone under the plantar surface of the foot (Figs. 2 and 3) Amputation may be indicated if there is gross destruction of bones and joints.[11]

Neurolysis of the Tibial and Peroneal Common Nerves

The neurologic approach is based on the premise that releasing the constricting structures

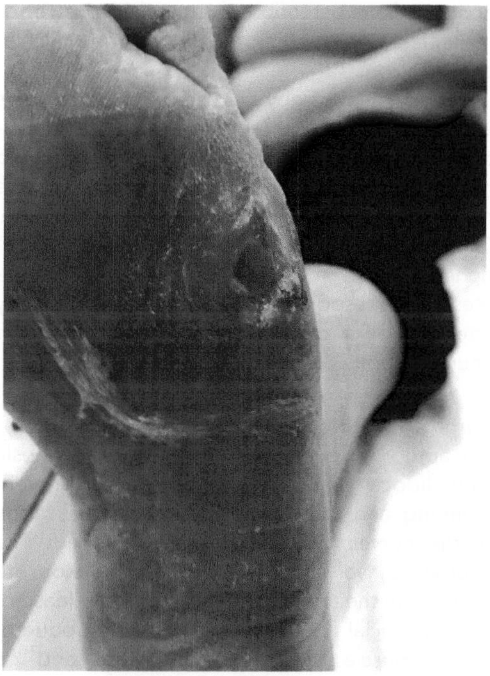

Fig. 2. Noninfected superficial ulcer caused by plantar prominence under the fifth metatarsal head.

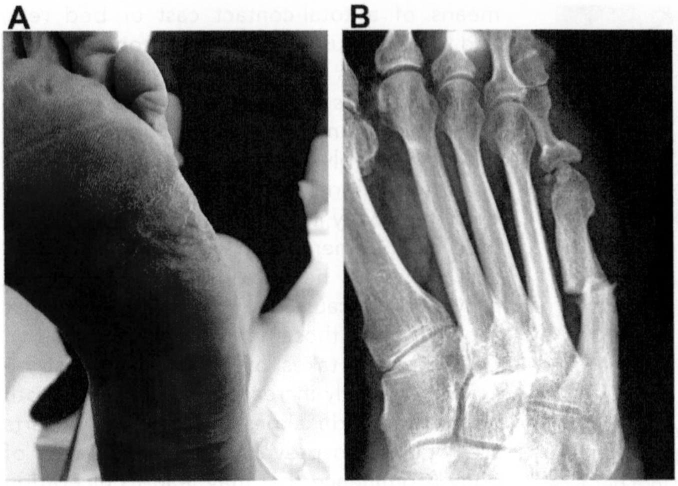

Fig. 3. (*A, B*) Ulcer healed with percutaneous osteotomy of the fifth distal metatarsal.

around the damaged nerves caused by the inflammation and immune response along with late development of perineural fibrosis might improve their sensitive motor and autonomic functions. Although there is still controversy related to the real benefits of surgical decompression in comparison with isolated treatment with oral corticoids, the author believes the neurolysis is effective because it improves the vascularization of the nerve (vasa nervorum), especially the tibial nerve, which is anatomically confined together with vascular plexus in a tight noncompliant osteofibrous tunnel in the retromalleolar area, leading to neural and vascular compression.[12–14]

In patients whereby the use of corticosteroids is contraindicated, there is an absolute indication for the surgical release of the affected nerve, because the decompression of the nerve may prevent definitive and irreversible damage. Other indications for the surgical release of peripheral nerves in Hansen disease are nerve abscess, nonresponsive peripheral neuropathy after 4 weeks of clinical treatment, recurrent neuritis, and neuropathic chronic pain.

Surgical technique

The author advocates the use of local anesthesia with lidocaine and epinephrine to prevent bleeding and thus provide better visualization of the nerves; no tourniquet is required. The neurolysis involves the release of the flexor retinaculum in the tarsal tunnel along with release of the superficial and deep fascia of the abductor hallux muscle for the tibial nerve and its branches (Figs. 4 and 5). The common peroneal nerve is released at the neck of the fibula, where both the fibrous band of the deep crural fascia and the fibrous arcade of the peroneal longus muscle belly are cut (Figs. 6 and 7).

SURGICAL CORRECTION FOR DROP FOOT IN HANSEN DISEASE

Preoperative Planning

It is of paramount importance that the disease process is controlled and the patient adequately treated with multidrug therapy for Hansen disease according to specific protocols determined by the WHO.[5] Also, it must be established that there has been at least 1 year without inflammatory reactions (reverse reaction or erythema nodosum) because the surgical procedure itself might cause those reactions, compromising the surgical results. The neurologic damage must be irreversible, which is considered after 1 year without

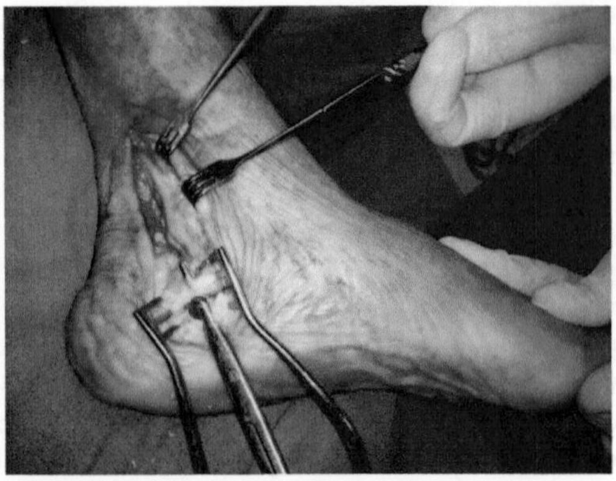

Fig. 4. The flexor retinaculum was released, and the neurovascular bundle is easily visualized; the tip of the scissors is under the superficial fascia of the abductor hallucis.

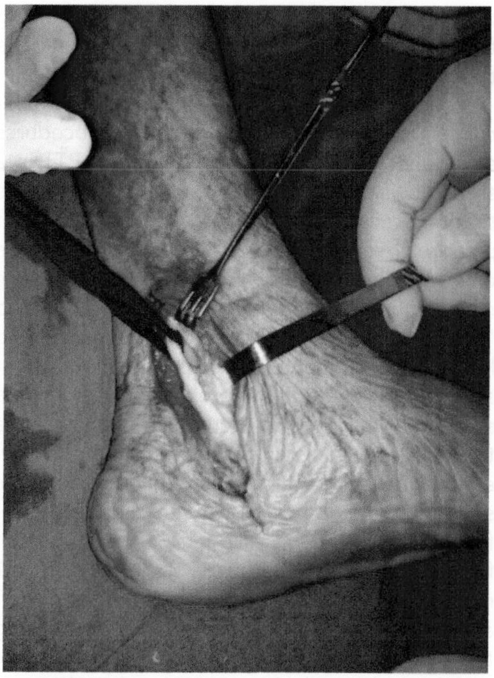

Fig. 5. Complete release with sectioning of both the superficial and the deep components of the abductor hallucis fascia.

improvement of the motor function or established earlier with eletroneuromuscular studies.

Equinus contracture of the Achilles tendon should be tested. Patients with passive

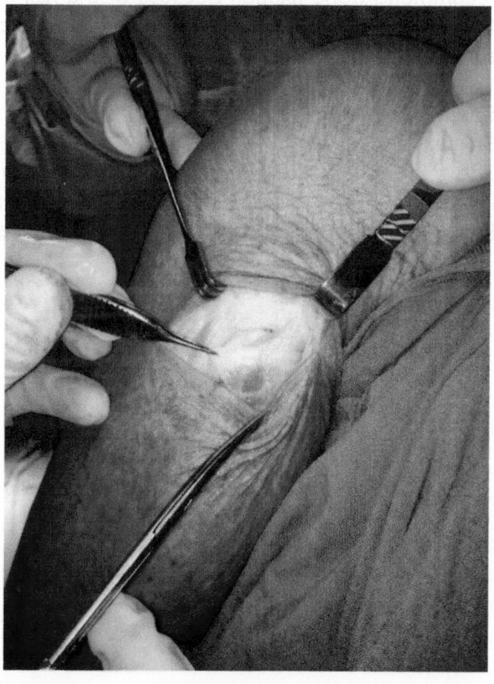

Fig. 6. Deep crural fascia being released.

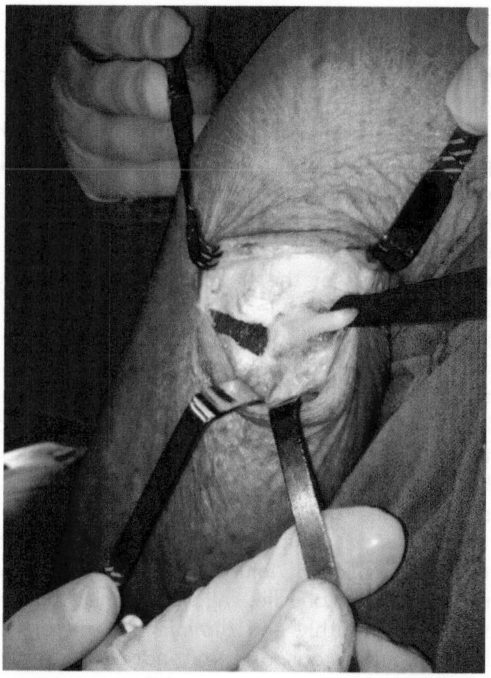

Fig. 7. Final release of the common peroneus nerve after sectioning the fibrous arcade of the PL muscle belly.

dorsiflexion of less than 20° should have percutaneous lengthening of the Achilles at the same time as the transfer. Indeed, it may be advisable to perform percutaneous lengthening in all patients, because the much more powerful Achilles tendon will overcome the transferred tendon in the long run. The ideal patient has normal motor strength in the tendon to be transferred, but motor strength of at least +4 is also acceptable and will provide enough power for ambulation out of a brace. As in all tendon transfers, any fixed joint deformities must be corrected to gain a successful result, requiring arthrodesis, osteotomy, or soft tissue release. The presence of clawing of the toes should be noted and treated if necessary.

The author always tries to instruct his patients on how to contract the tendon to be transferred in an isolated manner in the preoperative period to maximize results. Factors such as motivation, self-care, and whether the patient is able to strictly follow the postoperative recommendation are important to consider.

TRANSFER OF THE POSTERIOR TIBIAL TENDON TO THE DORSUM OF THE FOOT

The objectives of tendon transfer for the treatment of drop foot are to improve functional deficit by restoring or reinforcing lost functions, to neutralize deforming forces, and to gain stability, eliminating the need for bracing during gait.[15,16]

The correction of drop foot in leprosy with posterior tibial tendon (PTT) transfer is well established in the literature, although there is still some debate concerning the need to use the interosseus route. The author advocates the use of the technique described by Srinivasan and colleagues,[17] consisting of anterior transposition of the PTT subcutaneously, dividing the tendon in 2 slips, and suturing the medial slip to the extensor hallucis longus (EHL) and the lateral slip to the extensor digitorum longus. The author believes it is unnecessary to use the interosseus route, because the circumtibial (CT) transfer is easier and safer to perform, and there is no risk of injury or tethering of the neurovascular bundle, allowing the tendon to glide smoothly and diminishing the possibility of adhesions of the tendon or muscle belly in the interosseous (IO) membrane. Despite the routine use of the subcutaneous route, bow-stringing of the tendon under the skin as it crosses the ankle has not been a problem to his patients so far.

On the other hand, advocates for the IO transfer state some advantages, such as the direct pull of the tendon, producing less inversion deformity and the possibility of having a greater length of tendon for insertion and thus preventing the tenodesis effect related to an overly high tension of the suture transfer. Hall[18] reported that the subcutaneous route gave greater dorsiflexion (25°–30° compared with only 17°) than the IO route, but in the opposite direction, Soares[10] in a long-term study comparing the PTT transfer using the CT with the IO route for drop foot in patients with leprosy reported an unacceptably high rate of recurrent inversion in the CT group even in those cases with the peroneal tendons intact, leading to ulceration of the lateral border of the foot, and recommends that the CT route should be reserved for patients with a calcified and unyielding IO membrane. He also reported better active dorsiflexion in the IO group, although less active plantar flexion than the CT route. The peroneal strength was recommended by Das and colleagues[19] as an indicator in selecting route of tibialis posterior transfer for footdrop correction in leprosy, using the CT when the peroneals were intact, whereas selecting the IO in cases of paralysis of the lateral compartment, thus minimizing the risk of inversion deformity after the transfer.

Tendon-to-tendon suture addresses the difficulties related to tendon-to-bone procedures and donor tendon length. Dividing the PTT in 2 slips allows the surgeon to adjust and modulate tendon tension, appropriately verifying foot posture before suturing is completed. The more distal attachment to the EHL and extensor digitorum comunis (EDC) allows a better leverage and "reactivation" of extension of the hallux and lesser toes. The bone fixation provides a stronger attachment site and theoretically prevents the stretching that might occur over time when a tendon-to-tendon transfer is performed. However, despite the possibility of a minor degree of stretching, the author feels that it might be beneficial because it will allow for better plantar flexion power with adequate push off, while still maintaining the dorsiflexion action of the PTT, allowing adequate clearance of the foot during the swing phase. In addition, the occurrence of Charcot arthropathy as a consequence of a creation of a bone tunnel in patients with leprosy should be observed.[20,21] In fact, some investigators state that the presence of leprosy is a contraindication for bone fixation, and that all those cases should be managed with tendon-to-tendon procedures. The author's recommendation is that in PB cases, the transfer could be to bone, and in MB cases, the author does not recommend bone fixation because of the risk of Charcot arthropathy, anchoring the tendon to soft tissues in the dorsum of the foot.

Surgical Technique (as Described by Srinivasan)

The PTT is harvested through a small medial incision in its insertion site on the navicular (**Fig. 8**). A second posteromedial incision is

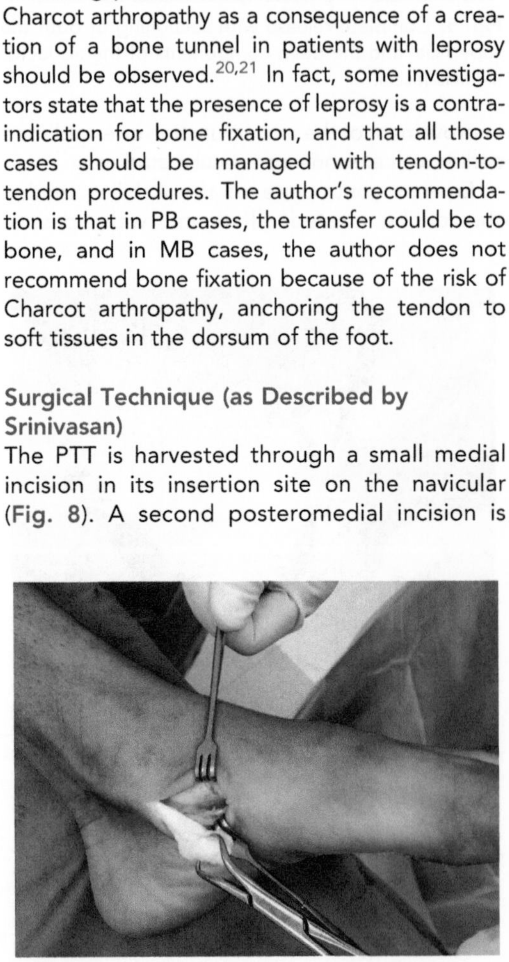

Fig. 8. Harvesting of the PTT.

made proximally in the leg to expose the muscle belly of the PTT. Note that it is necessary to retract the muscle belly of the flexor digitorum longus (FDL) medially to expose the deeper PTT muscle belly. One must be careful with the neurovascular bundle because it might be visible during the blunt dissection. The PTT tendon is delivered proximally and is divided into 2 slips with a number 11 scalpel. (It is important to keep both halves with the same thickness dividing the tendon from proximal to distal; Fig. 9.) A transverse dorsal incision is performed, taking care not to injure the intermediate branch of the superficial peroneal nerve, and the EHL and the EDC tendons are identified. A special tunnelization clamp is passed subcutaneously from this incision, grasping both halves of the PTT (Fig. 10). The medial slip is attached with a pulvertaft-type suture to the EHL while maintaining maximum tension on both tendons (PTT pulled distally and EHL proximally) with a nonabsorbable stitch. The lateral slip is attached in the same manner to the EDC (Figs. 11 and 12). The tenodesis is performed at least 5 to 7 cm distal to the ankle mortice, to improve the mechanical advantage of the transferred tendon. At the final step of the procedure, the foot should rest ideally in 5° to 10° of dorsiflexion (Fig. 13). The incisions are closed, and a well-padded below-the-knee cast is applied, keeping the ankle in slight dorsiflexion. Figs. 14 and 15 demonstrate a postoperative result with 1 year follow-up.

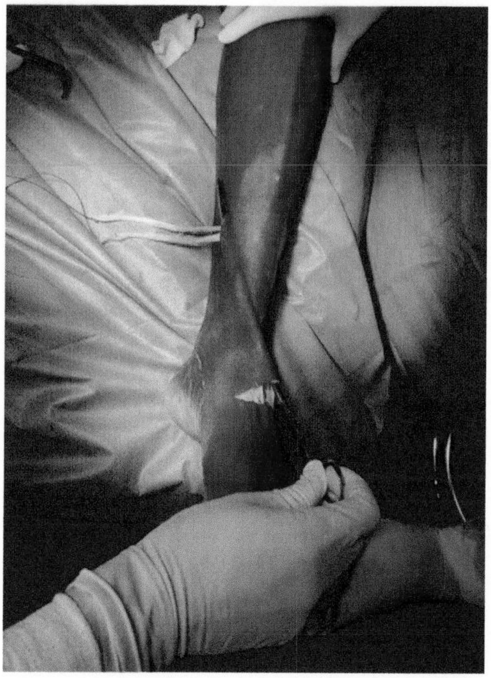

Fig. 10. Subcutaneous transposition of the PTT to the dorsum of the foot.

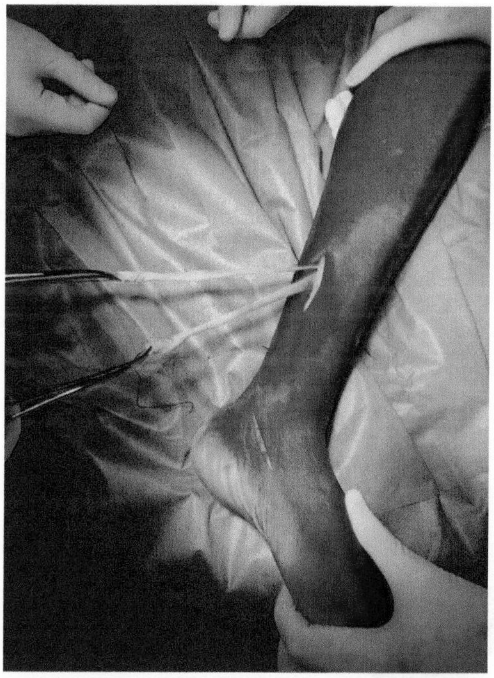

Fig. 9. Splitting the PTT into 2 -halves.

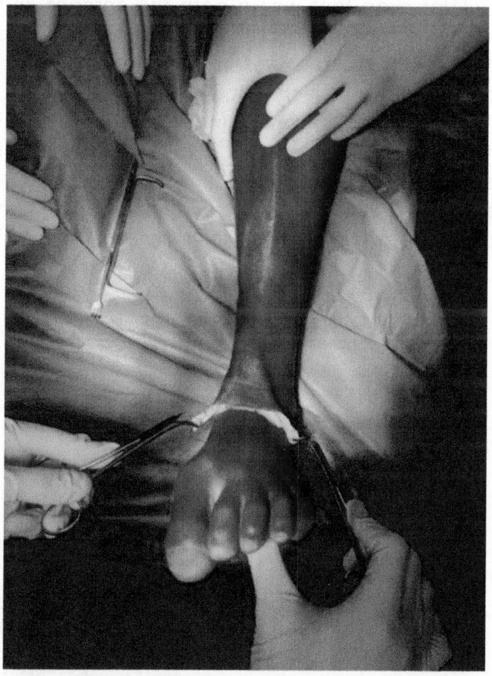

Fig. 11. Maximum tension at both slips of the PTT to be transferred.

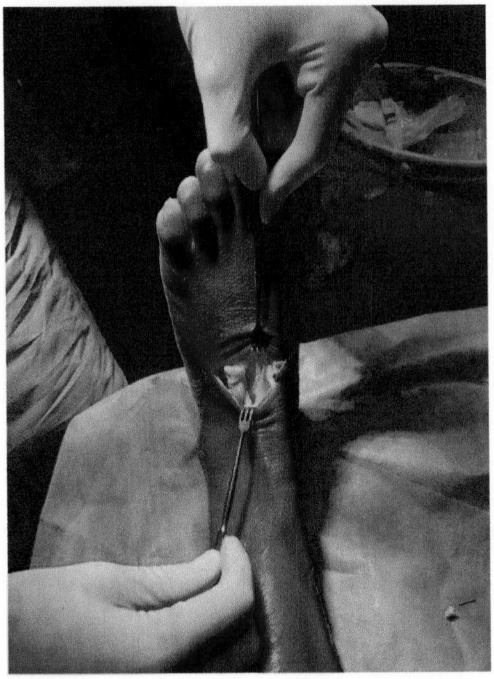

Fig. 12. Medial slip sutured to the EHL and the lateral slip to the EDC.

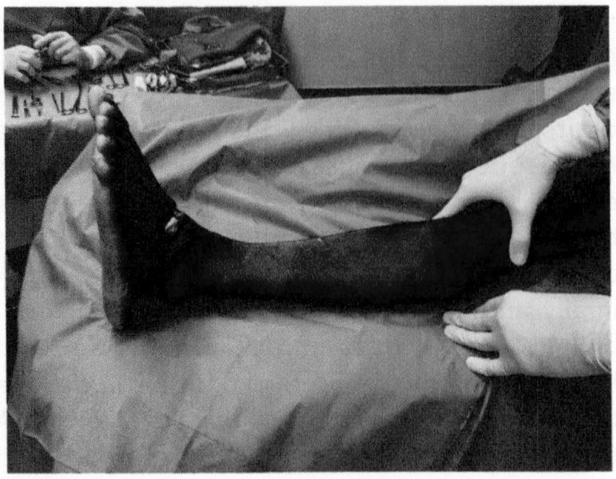

Fig. 13. Final position of the foot with 5° to 10° of dorsiflexion.

THE USE OF THE PERONEUS LONGUS TENDON AS A MAJOR DORSIFLEXOR OF THE FOOT

The occurrence of flatfoot after havesting the PTT for drop foot where both the anterior and lateral compartments of leg are paralyzed is rare in the literature; this may be explained because of the fact that, in the palsied foot, loss of peroneus brevis function (as a result of nerve injury) and loss of PTT (as a result of tendon transfer) result in a new dynamic balance,[15] preventing the arch breakdown. In contrast, in the presence of normal function of the superficial peroneal nerve, the primary evertor of the foot, the peroneus brevis muscle, is unopposed after the PTT transfer, leading to an imbalance between the inversion and eversion muscles, which could cause the development of flatfoot, because the deforming force exerted by the peroneus brevis is a well-recognized feature in the adult-acquired flatfoot, leading to hindfoot valgus and midfoot collapse[22] (Fig. 16). Thus, when the lateral compartment of the leg is intact (in cases of isolated paralysis of the deep peroneal nerve), the authors advocate the use of the PL tendon transfer to the dorsum of the foot.

The use of the peroneal longus tendon as the single dorsiflexor of the foot in leprosy was first reported by Srinivasan and colleagues,[17] where Srinivasan felt that "with the peronei tendons intact, removal of the tibial posterior from the medial side of the ankle might cause instability of the foot." Leaving the PTT intact on the medial side has the advantage to counteract the peroneus brevis on the lateral side, thus balancing the hindfoot

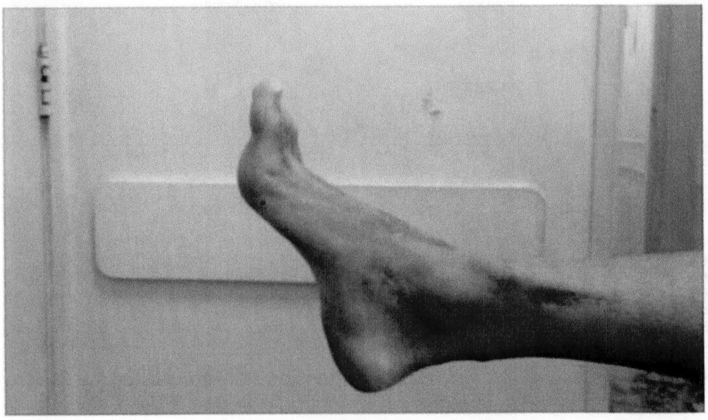

Fig. 14. Clinical example of active plantar flexion.

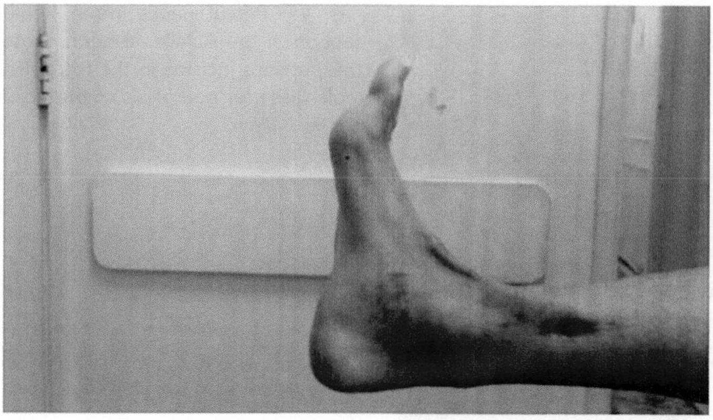

Fig. 15. Active dorsiflexion (same case as Fig. 14).

properly. They also quoted that if the patient later developed paralysis of the peroneals, the tibialis posterior could still be used as a motor. In their original technique, Srinivasan split the tendon into 2 halves and performed a tendon-to-tendon transfer into the EHL, extensor digitorum longus, and peroneus tertius. In the author's surgical procedure, he uses the entire tendon, uses a subcutaneous route, and anchors it to the intermediate cuneiforme with a drill hole (PB cases) or to the intercuneifom ligaments (MB cases). Two benefits are derived from this tendon transfer. A deforming force (plantar flexion of the first metatarsal producing forefoot-driven hindfoot varus) is eliminated, because there is an unopposed pull of the PL against the weak tibialis anterior tendon, and a correcting force (dorsiflexion in the ankle) is established. Morton[23] pointed out that the PL had been a lateral dorsiflexor in early evolutionary stages, justifying its use as a dorsiflexor muscle.

The Bridle procedure was described by Riordan and later modified by Rodriguez.[24] It also uses the PL tendon, combining the transfer of the PL with the PTT in order to balance the foot in dorsiflexion. However, in this surgery, the PL is not used as the primary active dorsiflexor, because it is divided proximally, rerouted anteriorly to the lateral malleolus, and anastomosed with the anterior and posterior tibialis tendons in the anterior leg.

Surgical Technique

With the patient lying supine on the operating table, a pneumatic tourniquet is applied to the thigh. The entire lower limb is prepared and draped in a regular fashion. If the limb is overly externally rotated, an ipsilateral bump is placed under the buttock to internally rotate the leg. Patients are given preoperative intravenous antibiotics. This procedure may be performed with the patient under spinal, epidural, or general anesthesia. Testing for equinus contracture is

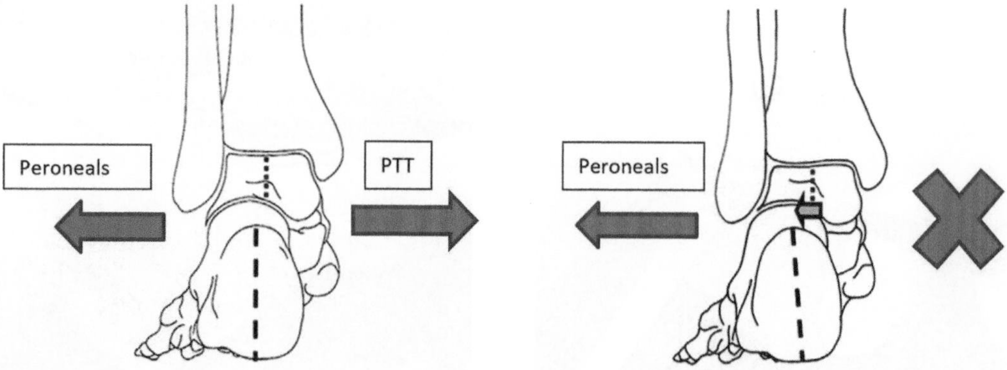

Fig. 16. Hindfoot alignment is influenced directly by the harmonious balance between peroneals and the PTT. In the presence of active peroneals, the surgically removed PTT will no longer counteract, possibly causing hindfoot valgus.

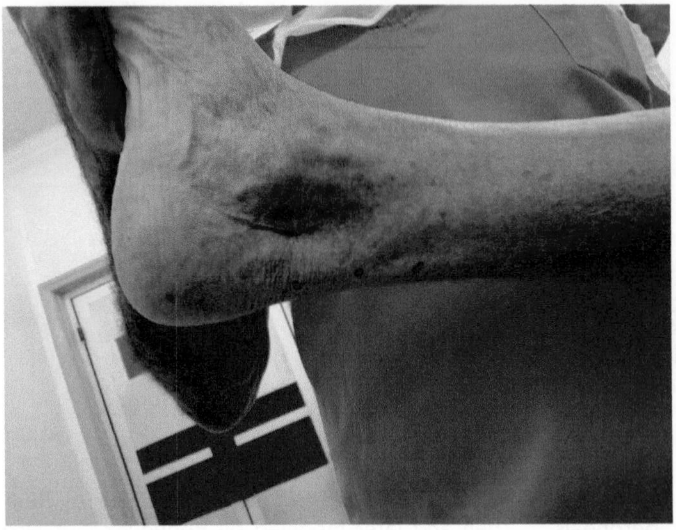

Fig. 17. Percutaneous triple hemisection of the Achilles tendon. Note the previous incision in the retromalleolar area for neurolysis of the tibial nerve.

performed. If present, a percutaneous lengthening of the Achilles is performed (Fig. 17). The peroneal tendons are accessed through a short incision at the level of the base of the fifth metatarsal aimed approximately 3 cm toward the lateral maleolus, parallel to the plantar surface of the foot. The dissection is carried down to the level of the paratenon. The sural nerve usually runs more cranially; if identified, it is retracted. The peroneal tendon sheath is then opened, and the PL can typically be seen beneath the peroneus brevis. The PL is pulled using an elevator and secured by a suture. It is important to tenodese the distal stump of the PL with the peroneus brevis tendon using a side-by-side suture (Ethibond no. 2) (Fig. 18) before cutting the tendon, thus preventing the occurrence of elevation of the first metatarsal (dorsal bunion) because of the unopposed pull of the tibialis anterior tendon. Although this tendon is theoretically weak in drop foot, the author always tenodeses the distal stump of the PL to the PB tendon. Now the PL tendon can be sectioned as distally as possible in the cuboid tunnel, and the proximal stump is tagged with a whipstitch suture.

A second incision is then made proximally on the lateral compartment in the distal third of the leg, about 8 cm proximal to the tip of the fibula at the level of the PL' musculotendinous junction. The superficial peroneal nerve should be protected. The tendon sheath of the PL is incised, and the PL tendon is identified and pulled proximally in the wound (Fig. 19). The tendon is kept moist with a moist sponge or allowed to remain in its sheath during dissection

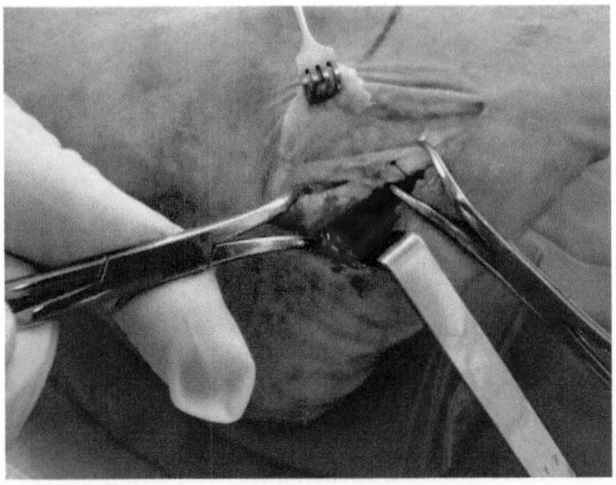

Fig. 18. Tenodesis of the distal stump of the PL to the peroneus brevis before cutting the tendon.

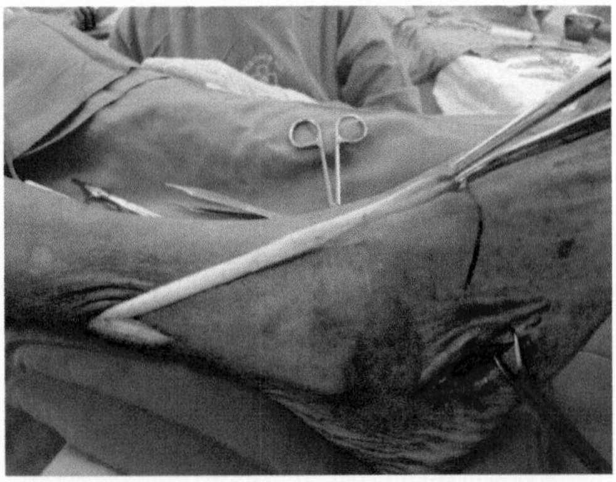

Fig. 19. Delivery of the PL tendon through the lateral incision in the lower leg after cutting it in the distal wound.

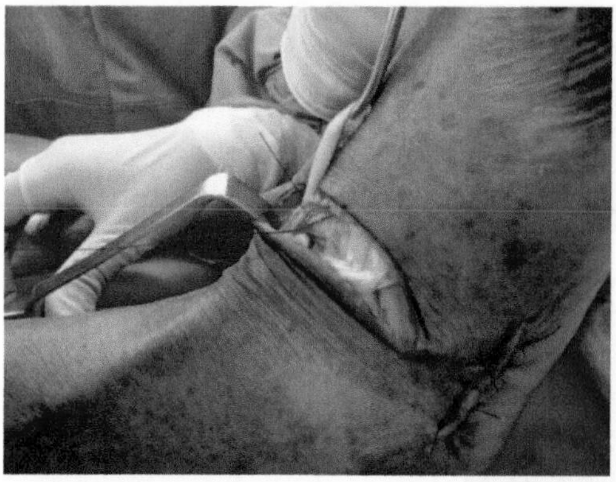

Fig. 20. After rerouting the PL tendon through the subcutaneous route.

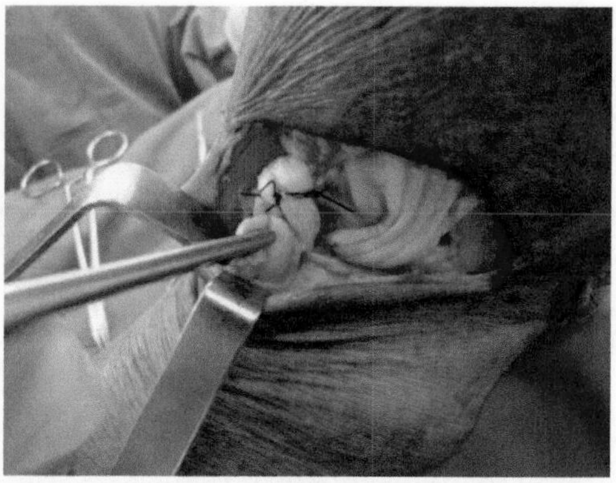

Fig. 21. Suture of the PL tendon to the intertarsal ligaments with nonabsorbable stitches.

of the dorsal tarsus. A third 3-cm transverse incision is finally made on the dorsum of the foot over the intermediate cuneiform. Care is taken with the superficial peroneal nerve and extensor tendons. The deep neurovascular bundle, usually encountered in this approach, should be protected because it is directly deep to the muscle of the extensor hallucis brevis. The intermediate cuneiform should be identified, leaving the periosteum and capsular tissue intact. A tunnelization clamp is passed subcutaneously from this incision to the proximal lateral wound, and the tagged peroneal longus tendon is delivered distally (Fig. 20). Using a fluoroscopic image is helpful to confirm the exact position for creation of the bone tunnel in the intermediate cuneiform. The bone tunnel is made from dorsal to plantar using drill bits and curettes as necessary to accommodate for the tendon. A straight Keith needle is used to pass the tag suture through the bone tunnel, exiting the sole of the foot. The foot is then held in maximal dorsiflexion (if possible in 30° of dorsiflexion), and the tag suture in the plantar aspect of the foot should be pulled distally, thereby pulling the tendon end into the tunnel. The proximal stump of the PL is then fixed to the bone tunnel using staples, biotenodesis screws, or anchors. If possible, the author augments the anchor point with several nonabsorbable sutures from the periosteum surrounding the tunnel to the tendon directly at the entrance of the tunnel. In MB cases, the author avoids using the bone insertion because of the potential for Charcot arthopathy. In this situation, the author inserts the PL transfer in the lateral margin of the intertarsal ligaments (Fig. 21). The entire wound is irrigated and closed in a regular fashion. At the final step of the procedure, the foot should rest in neutral to 5° of dorsiflexion (Fig. 22), and a well-padded short leg cast is applied to hold the foot in the desired dorsiflexion position. Figs.

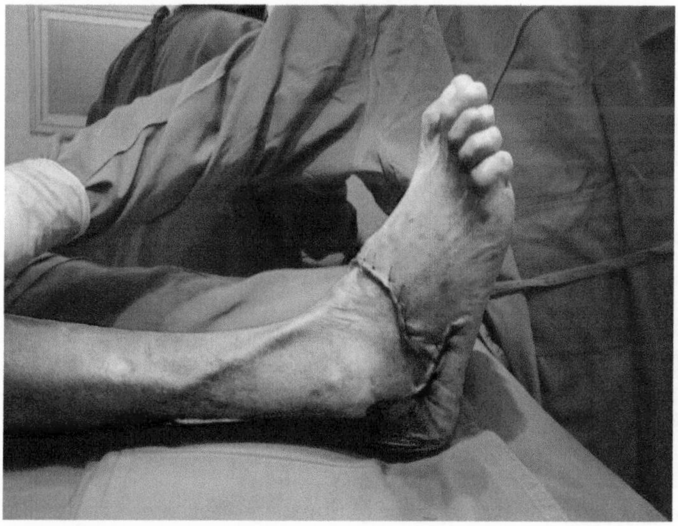

Fig. 22. Wounds closed; the transferred PL can be seen under the skin.

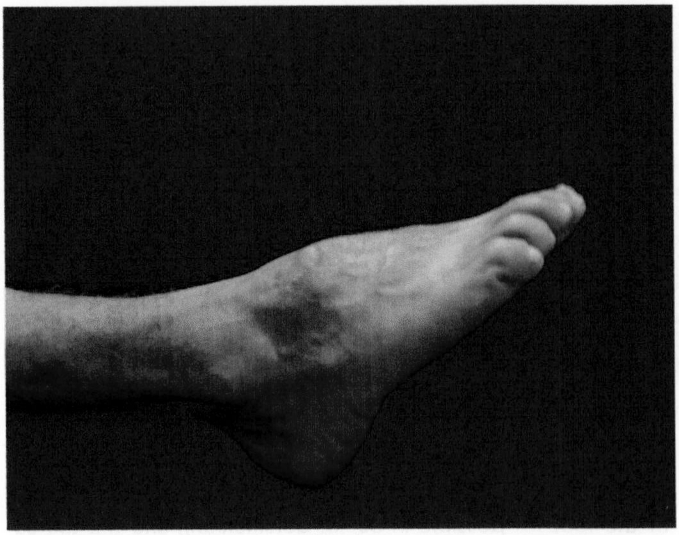

Fig. 23. Postoperative example of active plantar flexion.

23 and 24 show clinical examples of active plantarflexion and dorsiflexion.

POSTOPERATIVE MANAGEMENT FOR BOTH PTT AND PL TRANSFER

The cast is maintained for 2 weeks. The cast is then removed, and stitches are taken out. The patient is then placed in a weight-bearing cast, and he or she is allowed to partial weight-bear with use of crutches. Six weeks after the procedure, the cast is removed, and the patient is instructed to ambulate in an ankle-foot orthosis brace or walker boot. At 8 weeks, the rehabilitation program to improve strengthening, proprioception, gait, and range of motion is started, but the protected ambulation is continued for 4 months. Also, the patient should use a CAM boot for sleeping until 4 months after surgery. Physical therapy is beneficial to train the PL in its new phase, and the patient is encouraged to walk as much as possible. If the muscle fails to adapt to its new function, electrical stimulation should be added to the physical therapy program.

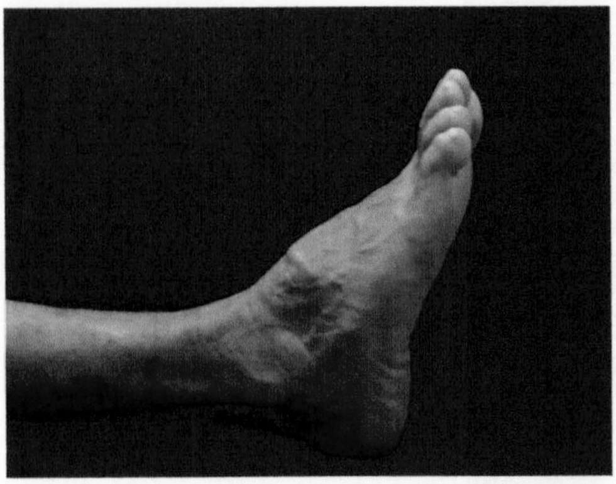

Fig. 24. Postoperative example of active dorsiflexion.

SUMMARY

Despite significant improvements in leprosy (Hansen disease) treatment and outlook for patients since the introduction of multidrug therapy 3 decades ago, the global incidence remains high, and patients often have long-term complications associated with the disease. The presence of bacilli in the skin produces the dermatologic manifestations of the disease, and nerve infection produces axonal dysfunction and demyelination, leading to sensory loss and its consequences of disability and deformity.[25] In this sense, the degenerative changes associated with infection of the peripheral sensory nerves are considered a crucial event in the natural history of Hansen disease. The deformities and disabilities caused by Hansen disease, as well as religious and social meanings associated with the disease or the physical changes that might result from it, have resulted in and continue to generate stigmatizing attitudes toward and negative beliefs about people affected by the disease. The orthopedic surgeon has an important role in the multidisciplinary approach because he or she can improve limb function and prevent the development of secondary disabilities caused by Hansen disease. Aggressive treatment of neuropathic ulcers with debridement followed by the use of custom shoes and adequate insoles, off-loading shoes, and total-contact weight-bearing cast are effective in most cases of noninfected ulcers. Neurolysis of the tibial nerve is frequently performed to improve nerve function, providing better protective sensation and potentially decreasing plantar ulcer formation. Surgical techniques described for the treatment of drop foot caused by paralysis of the common peroneal nerve caused by Hansen disease can also be used in the more common scenario of traumatic nerve injury seen in developed countries, because biomechanically, the functional impairment is the same in both clinical situations, despite the different pathophysiological mechanisms. Unlike traumatic common peroneal nerve injury, whereby both components of the nerve are injured, in Hansen disease, a selective paralysis of the deep component of the common peroneal nerve is possible, making the PL transfer to the dorsum of the foot a viable option in these exceptional cases.

DISCLOSURE

The author has nothing to disclose.

REFERENCES

1. Araujo MA. Leprosy in Brazil. Rev Soc Bras Med Trop 2003;36(3):373–82.
2. Harboe M, Aseffa A, Leekassa R. Challenges presented by nerve damage in leprosy. Lepr Rev 2005;76(1):5–13.
3. Van Brakel WH. Peripheral neuropathy in leprosy and its consequences. Lepr Rev 2000;71(suppl):S146–53.
4. Smith WC. Review of current research in prevention of nerve damage in leprosy. Lepr Rev 2000; 71(suppl):s138–44 [discussion: s145].
5. WHO EXPERT COMMITTEE ON LEPROSY. Seventh Report. Geneva: World Health Organization; 1998. Tech. Rep. Ser. 874.
6. Scollard DM, Adams LB, Gillis TP, et al. The continuing challenges of leprosy. Clin Microbiol Rev 2006;19(2):338–81.
7. Talhari S, Neves RG, de Oliveira MLW, et al. Manifestações cutâneas e diagnóstico diferencial. In: Talhari S, et al, editors. Hanseníase. 2006. p. 21–50. Manaus (Brazil), 4th edition,Dermatologia Tropical.
8. Job CK. Nerve damage in leprosy. Int J Lepr Other Mycobact Dis 1989;57(2):532–9.
9. van Brakel WH, Khawas IB. Silent neuropathy in leprosy: an epidemiological description. Lepr Rev 1994;65(4):350–60.
10. Soares D. Tibialis posterior transfer for the correction of foot drop in leprosy. Long-term outcome. J Bone Joint Surg Br 1996;78(1):61–2.
11. Moonot P, Ashwood N, Lockwood D. Orthopaedic complications of leprosy. J Bone Joint Surg Br 2005;87(10):1328–32.
12. Pandya NJ. Surgical decompression of nerves in leprosy. An attempt at prevention of deformities. A clinical, electrophysiologic, histopathologic and surgical study. Int J Lepr Other Mycobact Dis 1978;46(1):47–55.
13. Chaise F, Roger B. Neurolysis of the common peroneal nerve in leprosy. A report on 22 patients. J Bone Joint Surg Br 1985;67(3):426–9.
14. Bernardin R, Thomas B. Surgery for neuritis in leprosy: indications for and results of different types of procedures. Lepr Rev 1997;68(2): 147–54.
15. Vigasio A, Marcoccio I, Patelli A, et al. New tendon transfer for correction of drop-foot in common peroneal nerve palsy. Clin Orthop Relat Res 2008; 466:1454–66.
16. Yeap JS, Birch R, Singh D. Long-term results of tibialis posterior tendon transfer for drop-foot. Int Orthop 2001;25:114–8.
17. Srinivasan H, Mukherjee SM, Subramaniam RA. Two-tailed transfer of tibialis posterior for correction of drop-foot in leprosy. J Bone Joint Surg Br 1968;50(3).
18. Hall G. A review of drop-foot corrective surgery. Lepr Rev 1977;48:185–92.
19. Das P, Kumar J, Karthikeyan G, et al. Peroneal strength as an indicator in selecting route of tibialis posterior transfer for foot drop correction in leprosy. Lepr Rev 2013;84(3):186–93.
20. Anderson JG. Foot drop in leprosy. Lepr Rev 1964; 35:41–6.
21. Warren AG. The correction of foot drop in leprosy. J Bone Joint Surg Br 1968;50-B:629–34.
22. Mizel MS, Temple HT, Scranton PE, et al. Role of the peroneal tendons in the production of the deformed foot with posterior tibial tendon deficiency. Foot Ankle Int 1999;20(5):285–9.
23. Morton DJ. The human foot: its evoluition, physiology, and functional disorders. Morningside Heights (NY): Columbia University Press; 1935.
24. Rodriguez RP. The bridle procedure in the treatment of paralysis of the foot. Foot Ankle 1992; 13(2):63–9.
25. White C, Franco-Paredes C. Leprosy in the 21st century. Clin Microbiol Rev 2015;28(1):80–94.

Brazilian Total Ankle Replacement Experience

Caio Nery, MD, PhD[a], André Vitor Kerber C. Lemos, MD[b], Cesar Eduardo Castro Ferreira Martins, MD[c], Daniel Baumfeld, MD, PhD[d,*]

KEYWORDS

• Replacement • Ankle • Arthrosis • Arthritis • Post-traumatic arthritis

KEY POINTS

- Mobile-bearing total ankle arthroplasty and fixed-bearing implants are available in Brazil.
- Ankle arthroplasty is still a technically demanding procedure despite improvements in surgical techniques and implant design.
- Although there is no national registry in Brazil, and few data sets are available to consult and report, the number of TAR procedures is growing every year in the country.
- Survivorship of ankle implants in Brazil is similar to those found in the literature for other countries.

INTRODUCTION

There are several alternatives available for the operative treatment of ankle arthritis.[1,2] Although some may consider ankle arthrodesis the gold standard, the stimulus for total ankle replacement (TAR) in the last 40 years is derived from the partial dissatisfaction with ankle arthrodesis and the success obtained with total hip and knee arthroplasties.[3–5]

When gait analysis of patients with ankle arthrodesis is performed, we learn that the ankle motion is compensated for by increased motion of the small joints of the ipsilateral foot and altered motion of the contralateral ankle.[6,7] Consequently, degenerative changes may be seen at the subtalar and midtarsal joints as a consequence of these changes. Ideally, total ankle arthroplasty will spare joints adjacent to the ankle from developing arthritis, and the gait will be less compromised.[8]

Even though many aspects are still being defined (indications, long-term outcomes of the newer designs, etc.), TAR should no longer be considered inferior to ankle fusion or as an experimental procedure.[9] However, surgeons should remember that TAR is not for every patient and the appropriate indication, based on the evidence available, is fundamental to obtain durable and predictable outcomes.

BRIEF HISTORY IN BRAZIL

The first series of TARs in Brazil were performed in the National Institute of Orthopedics and Traumatology (INTO, Rio de Janeiro) with the Agility (DePuy Synthes, US). Between October 2002 and January 2006, 13 patients, 10 women, and 3 men were enrolled in this first experience. Eight patents present posttraumatic arthritis, two with rheumatoid arthritis, and three with arthritis secondary to other causes. Two patients were revised to ankle arthrodesis before 2 years after the surgery, whereas other 2 are still functioning for more than 13 years after the surgery. Eight implants were revised to ankle arthrodesis after 2 years, with 6.5 years of survivorship. One patient, with rheumatoid arthritis, presents a post-surgical complication with arterial occlusion and a below-knee amputation.

[a] Foot and Ankle Clinic, UNIFESP – Federal University of São Paulo, São Paulo, São Paulo, Brazil; [b] UNIFESP – Federal University of São Paulo, São Paulo, São Paulo, Brazil; [c] Curitiba, Paraná, Brazil; [d] Department of the Locomotor Apparatus, Federal University of Minas Gerais, Belo Horizonte, Brazil
* Corresponding author. Rua engenheiro albert scharle, 30, 701, Belo Horizonte, Minas Gerais 30380370, Brazil.
E-mail address: danielbaumfeld@gmail.com

Orthop Clin N Am 51 (2020) 293–302
https://doi.org/10.1016/j.ocl.2019.11.013

In 2005, a pilot study on TARs—The HINTEGRA Experience—was started in Brazil. The first 10 surgeries were performed by the Federal University of São Paulo and the State University Of São Paulo. Data regarding this experience were published in 2010.[10]

After this pilot study, the country remained without any implant available in the market for more than 8 years. Obstructions and difficulties in implant approval by the Brazilian National Agency of Sanitary Vigilance (ANVISA) and the high cost to import new technology were the main factors related to this gap. Only in 2013 ankle replacements were performed again with the approval of 2 different implants, Taric TAR (implantcast, Germany) and Zenith TAR (Corin Group, UK).

Currently, there are mobile-bearing (TARIC, Zenith) and fixed-bearing (Inbone II, Infinity—Wright Medical) implants available in the country. The most commonly used TARs in Brazil are all unconstrained, 3-component mobile-bearing designs. These include the Taric and Zenith prosthesis.

Table 1 presents all the implants registered in the National Agency of Sanitary Vigilance (ANVISA) and the actual availability.

BRAZILIAN MARKET AND PROFESSIONAL TOTAL ANKLE REPLACEMENT SURVEY: WHO DOES WHAT IN BRAZIL?

TAR market in Brazil report observes different predilections, obstructions, and difficulties. Two hundred sixty-three TAR procedures were performed in Brazil since 2005, but the country experienced a long period without any implant available and no surgery was performed. As a consequence, Brazil experienced a significant delay in the development of the ankle replacement in relation to the Latin America and worldwide. **Table 2** represents the number of procedures per year and the type of replacement implanted.

Total ankle arthroplasty remains a technically demanding surgery highly influenced by the surgeon's experience. Some reports in the literature states that 50 ankle replacements are needed to consider a surgeon proficient, whereas other reports demonstrate that a surgical learning curve does indeed exist when performing total ankle arthroplasty.[11,12] Most of the operative variables as well as clinical and radiological outcomes stabilize after a surgeon has performed an average of 28 cases. The number of ankle replacements is growing in Brazil, but until now, there are few surgeons who have performed more than 30 replacements, and the whole country performs an average of fewer than 40 ankle replacements per year.

CAUSES AND INDICATIONS AND PATIENT SELECTION AROUND THE COUNTRY

Patient selection is an important issue to achieve good outcomes. Each surgeons must decide who the ideal candidate for an ankle replacement is, identify potential risks and determine whether there are contraindications for the procedure. The best candidate is older than 50 years with posttraumatic arthritis or inflammatory arthropathies with a stable, neutrally aligned ankle in the coronal plane; however, this patient is not easy to find.[12–15]

An important factor that needs to be taken into account is the presence of degenerative changes in other joints, such as the subtalar, midtarsal, and proximal joints and the contralateral ankle. These patients seem to benefit more from TAR than from arthrodesis because ankle arthrodesis shifts abnormal loads onto the neighboring joints and thus accelerates degenerative changes.[6,14,16] In fact, it has been shown that at an average of 8 years after ankle fusion, approximately 50% of the patients have clinically significant hindfoot arthritis and after an average

Table 1
Total ankle replacement with National Agency of Sanitary Vigilance approval

Total Ankle Replacement System	Registry	Availability	Year
Agility TAR (DEPUY—J&J, US)	10132590603	No	2002
Waldemar Link TAR (Waldemar Link, Ger)	10247530033	No	2004
Zenith TAR (Corin, UK)	80012450017	Yes	2009
Salto-Tallaris TAR (US)	80240590032	No	2010
TARIC TAR (Implant Cast, Ger)	80454380015	Yes	2010
INBONE II (Wright Medical Group N.V., US)	80043770011	Yes	2015
INFINITY (Wright Medical Group N.V., US)	80043770011	Yes	2017

Table 2
Number of replacements per year in Brazil until 2019

Implant/Year	2002	2003	2004	2005	2006	2007~2012	2013	2014	2015	2016	2017	2018	2019
Agility	1	4	1	0	7	0	0	0	0	0	0	0	0
HINTEGRA	—	—	—	10	—	0	0	0	0	0	0	0	0
TARIC	—	—	—	0	—	0	8	13	21	32	36	37	10
Zenith	—	—	—	0	—	0	8	6	7	5	—	—	—
INBONE	—	—	—	0	—	0	0	0	0	0	12	23	9
INFINITY	—	—	—	0	—	0	0	0	0	0	0	6	20
Total	1	4	1	10	7	0	16	19	28	37	48	66	39

of 22 years, virtually all patients develop hindfoot arthritis.[17,18]

In patients with posttraumatic arthritis where the ankle soft tissue envelope may have been damaged by trauma or successive treatment attempts, the planning of incisions and scar debridement is especially important.

Relative contraindications to TAR include osteoporosis, smoking, diabetes mellitus, immunosuppression, neurologic disease, vascular disease, age, severe malalignment, instability, and avascular necrosis (AVN) of the talus. Absolute contraindications are active infection, Charcot neuroarthropathy, and peripheral vascular disease.[13]

In Brazil, indications for TAR are not so different from around the world, and the available data demonstrate 65% of posttraumatic arthritis, 26% of inflammatory arthritis, 2% post-infectious arthritis, and 7% of primary arthritis. In Brazil there are three segments for payment of healthcare: private (out-of-pocket) payment, private health care insurance, and public insurance. Only with the first 2 is there a possibility to have a TAR, and the procedure is expensive and quite rare. Brazil's public insurance does not currently cover TAR, because it is found to be cost-prohibitive. The largest part of the population who experience post-traumatic ankle arthritis are on public insurance and consequently do not have access to this type of treatment. This helps explain the lower number of posttraumatic arthritis indication for TAR in Brazil as compared to the literature.

PREOPERATIVE PLANNING

Surgical planning begins with a detailed patient history and physical examination including the following: muscle function, ankle range of motion, tendon excursion, standing limb alignment, gait, strength, peripheral vascular examination, and skin quality. Hindfoot alignment evaluation (valgus, varus, or neutral) is critical and is assessed from behind, with the patient standing. Stability can be determined with the patient seated, using the talar tilt test and the anterior drawer test. Mobility of the ankle and subtalar joint is also measured manually using a goniometer underload and/or seated. Additional information such as body mass index, physical activity levels, previous and/or current treatment, severity of pain, limitations in everyday private and/or occupational activities, intake of analgesics, and concomitant diagnoses (diabetes mellitus, osteoporosis, polyneuropathy, etc.) should be recorded.[19,20]

Radiographic assessment with full-length limb alignment covering coronal plane malalignment and extraarticular malalignment is an important tool to define coexistent deformities. It is advisable to have dorsoplantar and lateral views of the foot, anteroposterior (mortise) and lateral views of the ankle, and Saltzman view to assess the rearfoot alignment. A long axial view of the hind foot can be used instead of the Saltzman view. Supramalleolar alignment should to be determined using the medial distal tibial angle. In patients with proximal joints deformities (knee, femur, or hip) a whole leg radiograph is also taken. Optionally, computed tomography or MRI may be performed. It can provide important additional information as subchondral cyst formation, intraarticular pathology, AVN, and periarticular coexistent pathology.[21–23]

IMPLANTS RESULTS AND COMPLICATIONS

HINTEGRA Total Ankle Replacement

The HINTEGRA (Newdeal SA, Lyon, France) total ankle prosthesis, a 3-component mobile-bearing implant (flat tibial component, ultra-high-molecular-weight polyethylene [UHMWPE] inlay, and a convex conic talar component), designed by a group of European doctors, has been in clinical use since 2000. It relies on minimal bone resection to allow placement of the prosthesis in the very distal, better-quality cancellous subchondral bone. The talar and tibial components have ventral shields to allow screw placement, although the current trend is not to use screws for fixation because they could lead to loosening of the prosthesis during the initial phase of osteointegration. Side borders on the talar component should prevent dislocation of the polyethylene. The anterior tibial flange aims to reduce postoperative heterotopic ossification and soft tissue adherence. The designers of the prosthesis reported a relatively high complication rate of 14% (39 complications in 278 implantations and 13 failures) in his earlier case series (prostheses implanted before 2000), whereas the failure rate dropped after 2003. Overall survivorship in 340 primary total ankle replacements at 6 years was 98.2%, being 97.9% for the talar component and 98.8% for the tibial component.[5,18,20]

The Brazilian experience with this model started in 2005 with only in 10 surgeries performed. The results were published in 2010.[10] The patients (6 women and 4 men), aged between 29 and 66 years, underwent a surgical procedure according to Hinterman technique, from January to June 2005. There were 30% of post-traumatic arthritis, 10% of postinfection arthritis, and 60% inflammatory arthritis. The surgery led to a significant improvement in ankle mobility. Radiological studies showed no signs of loosening or failure in the prosthetic components in any of the patients studied (Fig. 1). Although the rate of complications was high, it was equivalent to that of other investigators and directly represents the long, steep learning curve associated with this kind of procedure. The investigators reported around 80% of minor and major complications. Intraoperative complications included 1 fracture of the medial malleolus and 1 of the lateral malleolus. Minor complications were one superficial infection and two wound dehiscence cases. Major complications were 1 vasculitis of the inferior limb which required a below-knee amputation and 1 dehiscence that was treated with a microsurgery free flap. At

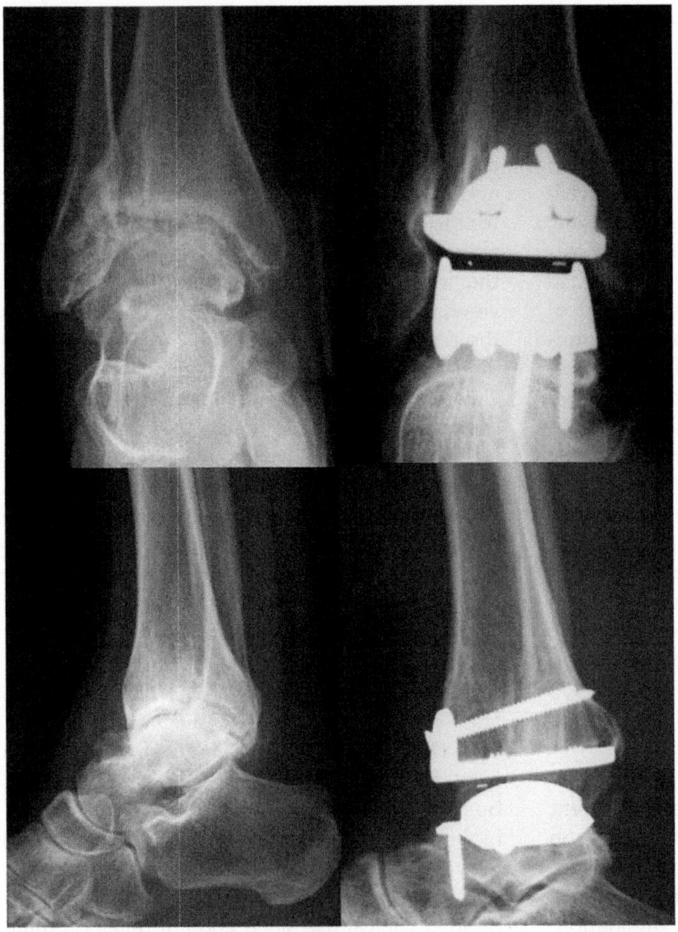

Fig. 1. HINTEGRA TAR. Preoperative plain ankle radiographs. Right-hand images: 4-year postoperative control radiographs showing good implants position with no signs of loosening. (*Courtesy of* Newdeal SA, Lyon, France.)

the end of 4 years, there was a significant reduction in pain and an improvement in functional pattern, with AOFAS and Hinterman scores indicating 20% excellent, 70% good, and 10% poor results.

TARIC Total Ankle Replacement

The TARIC ankle system is designed as a cementless mobile-bearing system. Two fins are configured for the primary fixation of the tibial and talar components. These fins are configured so that they clamp the host bone. The additional applied cpTi- and HA-coating allows a solid secondary fixation of the metal components to the bone. The system includes 5 sizes of tibial implants and 4 sizes of talar components. The highly congruent polyethylene inlays are made of UHMWPE.[5]

This model of ankle replacement is currently the most chosen by the surgeons in Brazil until now. This can be explained because it was one of the first ones available since 2013 and dominated the market from 2013 to 2017 when others models with more published results in the literature became available in the country (Fig. 2). In 7 years 157 surgeries were performed, in different parts of the country, but only 1 surgeon performed 43 cases (27.3% of the total). Table 2 demonstrates the number of procedures performed per year. Currently there are no published results in the literature regarding this procedure in Brazil. Unpublished data from a study report that survivor rate in the first year was 95.3%, 87% in the second year, 85.7% in the third year, 85.7% in the fourth year, and 77.7% in the fifth year.

Zenith Total Ankle Replacement

The Zenith (Corin Group) ankle system is designed as a cementless mobile-bearing system that minimizes constraint to maintain ROM, promoting tibial freedom for rotational and translational movements. The tibial component is fixed to the bone with a stem placed inside the tibia through an anterior window. Zenith incorporates titanium porous coating combined with a calcium phosphate (CaP) coating with a microcrystalline structure that provides substrate surface roughness with a large area for osteointegration.[5,18]

The system includes 4 sizes of tibial implants and 4 sizes of talar components. The highly congruent polyethylene inlays are made of UHMWPE in 6 different heights.

Mean 3 year follow up of 26 patients treated with the Zenith TAR system was collected by the investigators. These patients were treated between 2013 and 2016 by 4 different surgeons.

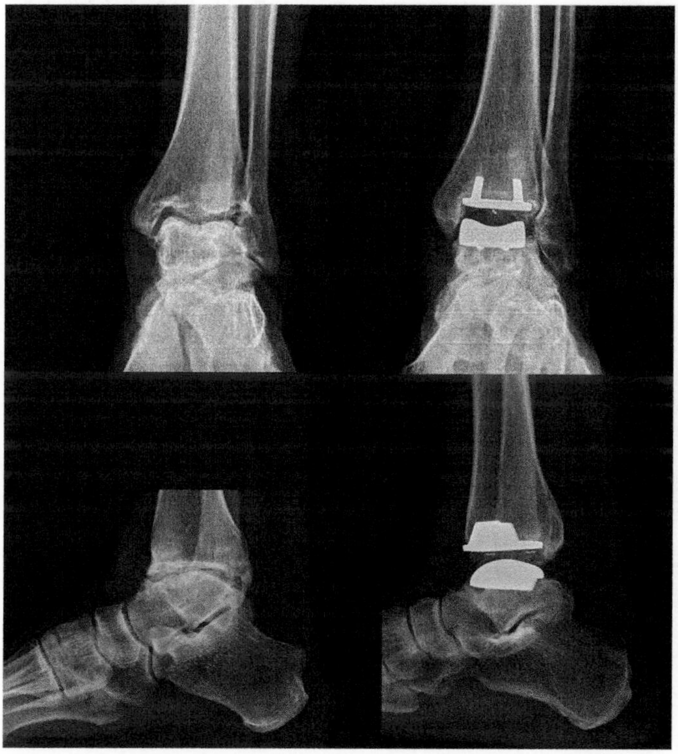

Fig. 2. TARIC TAR. Preoperative plain left ankle radiographs. Three-year postoperative control radiographs showing good implants position with no signs of loosening. (*Courtesy of* implantcast GmbH, Buxtehude, Germany.)

Patients had a significant improvement in VAS and AOFAS score (40 points) after 3-year follow-up. There was a significant improvement in ankle mobility (13°) with improved mobility in 92% of patients (Fig. 3).

The occurrence of surgical wound complications was present in 3 patients (11%), but only 2 patients required procedures (graft or skin flap) to close the surgical wound.

Malleolus fractures occurred in 5 patients (19%), all identified during the primary procedure and promptly treated with internal fixation, and were considered only as surgical occurrence and not as complications.

During the postoperative follow-up, 8 (30%) patients complained of ankle pain and presented periprosthetic cysts or subsidence around the talus or tibia components, leading to revision with Inbone II in 2 cases and a revision to arthrodesis in 1 case.

A positive correlation between the measurement of lateral talus positioning variation lateral talus surface (LTS) and the variation of the tibial distal sagittal articular angle was found in pre- and postoperative radiographs, confirming findings published in the literature previously. Surgeon should customize the sagittal distal tibial cut to the individual patient based on the preoperative LTS in order to achieve neutral TAR alignment.[24]

In this sample the investigators found a consistent increase from 39% to 62% in the anterior position of talar center of rotation that could contribute to high early failure rate of this implant.

INBONE Total Ankle Replacement

The INBONE II total ankle system (Wright Medical Group N.V., US) uses unique intramedullary alignment instrumentation, combined with modular titanium tibial and talar stems. The stem consists of small, interconnecting pieces and can be built up piece-by-piece. This creates the theoretic advantage of better fixation in osteoporotic tibial bone and the possibility of subtalar fusion via the implant for revision cases. The fundamental design concept is that of increased vertical fixation in the tibia and and broad cortical coverage in the talus. The modularity of the implants, stems, differing polyethylene thicknesses, flat cut approach to the talus, and the optional use of longer calcaneal stems offer the possibility of revising another total ankle prosthesis to INBONE II. This is a fixed bearing model of TAR. It received Food and Drug Administration approval in 2005.[5,18]

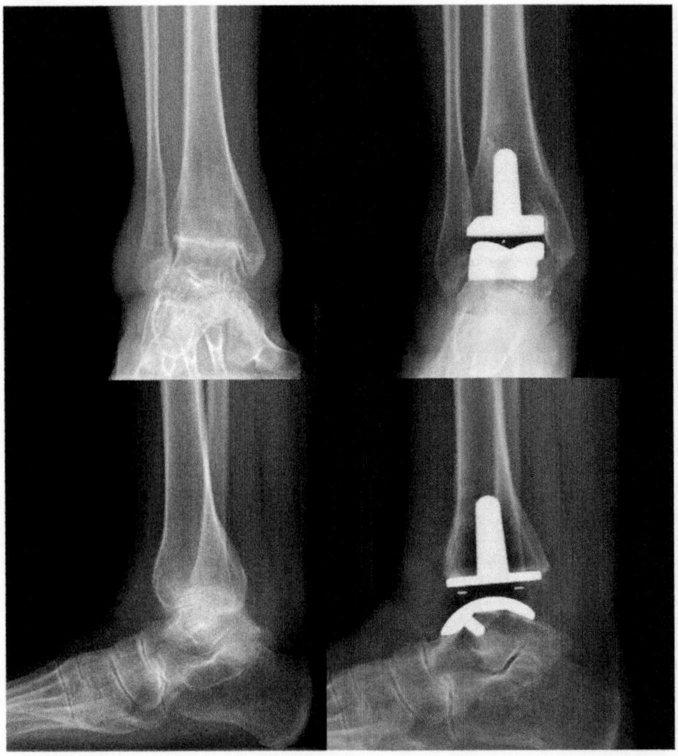

Fig. 3. Zenith TAR. Left-hand images: preoperative plain ankle radiographs. Right-hand images: 2-year postoperative control radiographs showing good implant position and osteointegration with no signs of loosening. (*Courtesy of* Corin Group, Cirencester, United Kingdom.)

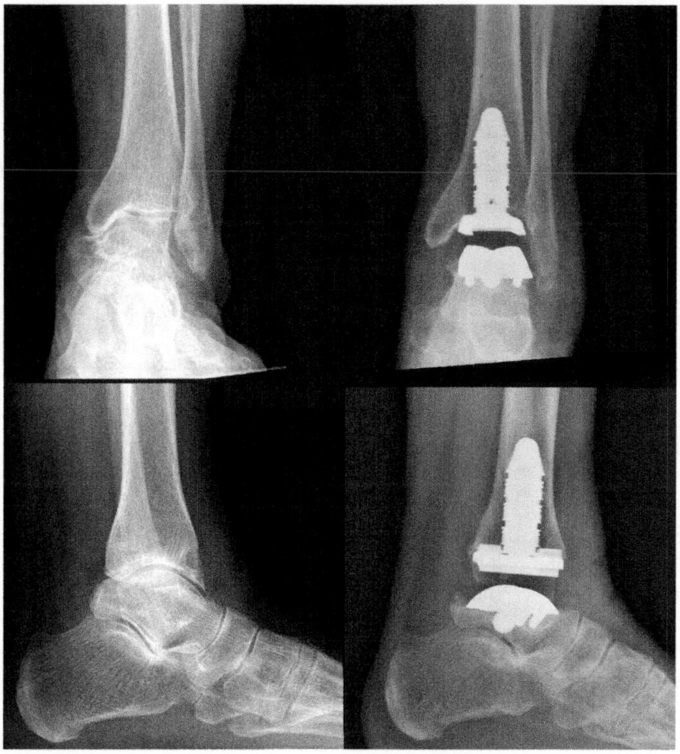

Fig. 4. INBONE II TAR used as a primary case. Left-hand images: preoperative plain ankle radiographs. Right-hand images: 1.5-year postoperative control radiographs showing good implant position and integration with no signs of loosening or subsidence. (*Courtesy of* Wright Medical Group N.V., Memphis, TN.)

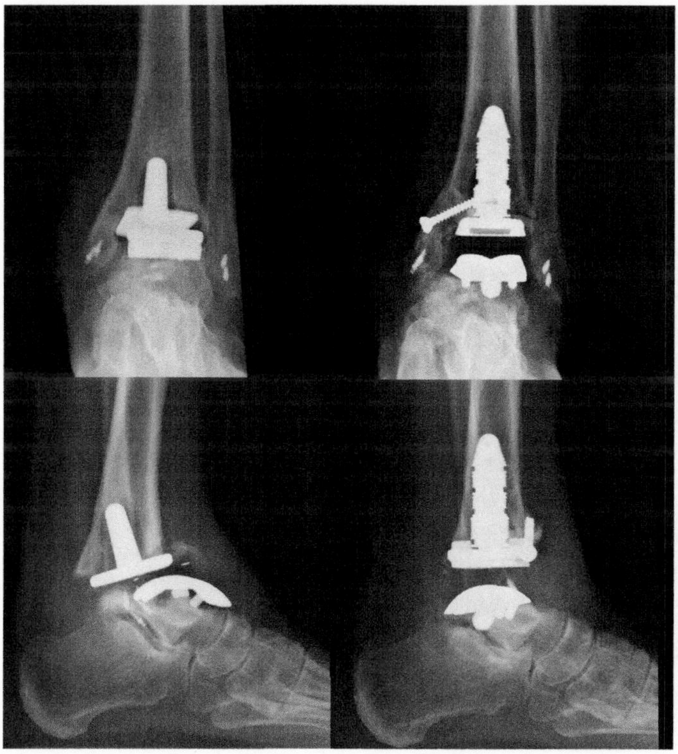

Fig. 5. INBONE II TAR used for a revision case. Male patient: 2 years postop of a Zenith TAR. Left-hand images: plain radiographs showing tibial and talar components subsidence and loosening with a gross anterior talar subluxation. Right-hand images: 1-year postoperative control radiographs showing acceptable implant positioning with no signs of loosening. (*Courtesy of* Wright Medical Group N.V., Memphis, TN.)

Table 3
Survival rate per year of each implant available in the country

Survival Rate	1 y	2 y	3 y	4 y	5 y
Agility	92.00%	76.00%	69.00%	69.00%	61.00%
Hintegra	90.00%	90.00%	90.00%	90.00%	—
Taric	95.35%	83.87%	85.71%	80.95%	77.78%
Zenith	96.15%	96.15%	85.71%	85.71%	75.00%
Inbone	92.31%	85.71%	—	—	—
Infinity	100.00%	—	—	—	—
TOTAL	94.00%	86.19%	82.84%	81.62%	71.47%

This implant has been available in Brazil since 2017 for use in both primary procedures and revision for other TAR systems. In our country, this implant was performed as primary indication in more cases than in revision (70% vs 30%) (Figs. 4 and 5). Tables 2 and 3 represent the number of procedures per year of this ankle system, totaling 44 surgeries. An unpublished data of this total ankle prosthesis-demonstrates a survivor rate of 92.3% in first year and 85.7% in the second year.

INFINITY Total Ankle Replacement

The INFINITY total ankle system consists of a highly polished metal talar dome, a titanium alloy tibial tray, and a fixed-bearing UHMWPE insert.

The INFINITY prosthesis was purposefully designed without tibial flanges or barrels and without talar dome sidewalls that would obscure fluoroscopic imaging. This implant also provides a talar design that is interchangeable with the INBONE II allowing surgeon preference to dictate talar preparation option.

The literature demonstrates promising early clinical and radiographic outcomes and comparable results in 2 to 4 years for both fixed- and mobile-bearing third-generation total ankle arthroplasty designs, even when used in cases with deformity and increased case complexity.[25]

The INFINITY total ankle replacement became available in Brazil in 2017, but the first

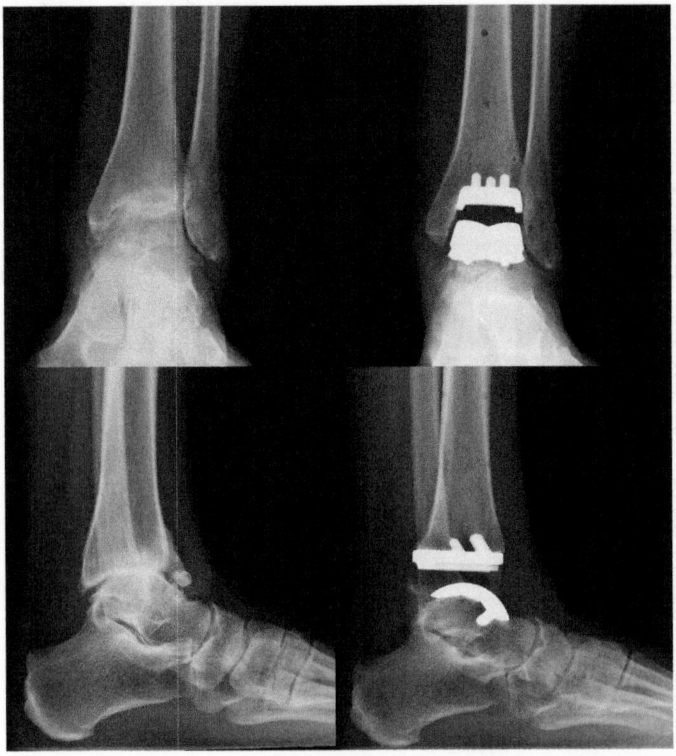

Fig. 6. INFINITY TAR. Left-hand images: preoperative plain radiographs. Right-hand images: 8-month postoperative radiographs showing good implant position and integration and no signs of loosening. (*Courtesy of* Wright Medical Group N.V., Memphis, TN.)

procedure was not performed until November of 2018 (Figure 6). To date, 26 INFINITY procedures have been performed with no complications reported and with an early survival rate at of 100% at <1 year.

LIMITATION AND OVERALL RESULTS OF TOTAL ANKLE REPLACEMENT IN BRAZIL

Many aspects of total ankle replacement are still being defined in Brazil: the option of TAR is subject to more limitations due to implant availability in each state, patient healthcare coverage and learning curve of each TAR system. Distribution of the various implant systems through the country is unequal and is determined by sales volumes rather than individual necessity of the surgeon or patients.

Limitations of these results include lack of independent review of the patient records; the number of concominant procedures and functional score could not be retrieved for all procedures performed in the country. Table 3 presents the actual survival rate per implant in the past 5 years.

Brazil is a huge country with good medical education, and there is a strong growth potential for total ankle replacement. There is an ongoing need for clinical data, and the Brazilian medical societies are advocating for this data.

SUMMARY

TAR is a surgical treatment alternative to arthrodesis of the ankle joint in a select group of patients. Progress in the design of implants has been made over the past few years. The implantation technique has improved as well. Increased experience has led to a higher survival rate and lower complication rate as compared with first-generation prostheses. Over time, the constrained, cemented, first-generation ankle replacements have been eliminated. Although some two-component, anatomic, designs are still used, it seems that three-component mobile-bearing ankle prostheses are winning the race of evolution. Not only have the implants changed over the years, but so have surgeons and their patients. The ankle replacement procedures are still subject to continuous modifications.[5,14,18]

Our country experiences a late participation in total ankle arthroplasty, which could have positive and negative aspects. The positive argument is that Brazil has skipped the early TAR generation that presents more complications and low survival rate in the literature. The negative aspects are related to gap of experience, inability of Brazilian surgeons to participate in the development of technique and implant designs over the years.

In Brazil there are limited and different ankle arthroplasty systems available for use. The procedure itself continues to be technically demanding and requires surgical sophistication and expertise. A national registry to justify the procedure indication reports the outcomes and survivorship has not been developed. For this reason, there are no long-term prospective studies regarding all the implants available and only a few surgeons have their own data available for consult. This procedure is growing around the county, as well as the surgeon experience, but we should remember that TAR is not for every patient and that the appropriate indication, based on the evidence available, is fundamental to obtaining durable and predictable outcomes. Ankle fusion is still a valid alternative for patients who are not amenable to TAR. A thorough knowledge of ankle anatomy, pathologic anatomy, and biomechanics together with a careful preoperative planning are mandatory to successful technical performance of TAR surgery.

DISCLOSURE

D. Baumfeld—Arthrex consultant/speaker; MSD (Merck sharp dome) speaker, Geistlish Speaker. C. Nery—Arthrex consultant/speaker; Wright medical consultant/speaker, Geistlish Speaker.

REFERENCES

1. Barg A, Pagenstert GI, Hügle T, et al. Ankle osteoarthritis: etiology, diagnostics, and classification. Foot Ankle Clin 2013;18(3):411–26.
2. Santos ALG, Demange MK, Prado MP, et al. Cartilage lesions and ankle osteoarthrosis: review of the literature and treatment algorithm. Rev Bras Ortop 2014;49(6):565–72.
3. Krause FG, Schmid T. Ankle arthrodesis versus total ankle replacement: how do I decide? Foot Ankle Clin 2012;17(4):529–43.
4. Esparragoza L, Vidal C, Vaquero J. Comparative study of the quality of life between arthrodesis and total arthroplasty substitution of the ankle. J Foot Ankle Surg 2011;50(4):383–7.
5. Gougoulias NE, Khanna A, Maffulli N. History and evolution in total ankle arthroplasty. Br Med Bull 2008;89(1):111–51.
6. Wang H, Brown SR. The effects of total ankle replacement on ankle joint mechanics during walking. J Sport Health Sci 2016;1–6. https://doi.org/10.1016/j.jshs.2016.01.012.

7. Arno F, Roman F. The influence of footwear on functional outcome after total ankle replacement, ankle arthrodesis, and tibiotalocalcaneal arthrodesis. Clin Biomech (Bristol, Avon) 2016;32:34–9.
8. Schuh R, Hofstaetter J, Krismer M, et al. Total ankle arthroplasty versus ankle arthrodesis. Comparison of sports, recreational activities and functional outcome. Int Orthop 2011;36(6):1207–14.
9. Ellis SJ, Moril-Peñalver L, Deland JT. The Scandinavian total ankle replacement (STAR) system. Semin Arthro 2010;21(4):275–81. Available at: https://books.google.com.br/books?id=DYErAQAAQBAJ&pg=PA1156&lpg=PA1156&dq=ellis+star+total+ankle+replacement&source=bl&ots=-OmgmiyPuc&sig=ACfU3U2_3Z5ryEDe44k7YTy86QnBUUGOKQ&hl=en&sa=X&ved=2ahUKEwj9tdqMge_mAhUtE7kGHcS3Ar4Q6AEwAXoECAgQAQ#v=onepage&q=ellis%20star%20total%20ankle%20replacement&f=false.
10. Nery C, Fernandes TD, Réssio C, et al. Total ankle arthroplasty: Brazilian experience with the hintegra prosthesis. Rev Bras Ortop 2015;45(1):92–100.
11. Usuelli FG, Maccario C, Pantalone A, et al. Identifying the learning curve for total ankle replacement using a mobile bearing prosthesis. Foot Ankle Surg 2016;1–8. https://doi.org/10.1016/j.fas.2016.02.007.
12. Skyttä ET, Koivu H, Eskelinen A, et al. Total ankle replacement: a population-based study of 515 cases from the finnish arthroplasty register. Acta Orthop 2010;81(1):114–8.
13. Bonasia DE, Dettoni F, Femino JE, et al. Total ankle replacement: why, when and how? Iowa Orthop J 2010;30:119–30.
14. Latham WC, Lau JT. Total ankle arthroplasty: an overview of the Canadian experience. Foot Ankle Clin 2016;21(2):267–81.
15. Saltzman CL, Mann RA, Ahrens JE, et al. Prospective controlled trial of STAR total ankle replacement versus ankle fusion: initial results. Foot Ankle Int 2009;30(7):579–96.
16. Barg A, Wimmer MD, Wiewiorski M, et al. Total ankle replacement. Dtsch Arztebl Int 2015;1–21. https://doi.org/10.3238/arztebl.2015.0177.
17. Besse JL, Colombier JA, Asencio J, et al. Total ankle arthroplasty in France. Orthop Traumatol Surg Res 2010;96(3):291–303.
18. Gougoulias N, Maffulli N. History of total ankle replacement. Clin Podiatr Med Surg 2013;30(1):1–20.
19. Prusinowska A, Krogulec Z, Turski P, et al. Total ankle replacement – surgical treatment and rehabilitation. Reumatologia 2015;1:34–9.
20. Barg A, Knupp M, Henninger HB, et al. Total Ankle replacement using HINTEGRA, an unconstrained, three-component system: surgical technique and pitfalls. Foot Ankle Clin 2012;17(4):607–35.
21. Brunner S, Barg A, Knupp M, et al. The Scandinavian total ankle replacement: long-term, eleven to fifteen-year, survivorship analysis of the prosthesis in seventy-two consecutive patients. J Bone Joint Surg Am 2013;95(8):711–8.
22. Barg A, Pagenstert GI, Leumann AG, et al. Treatment of the arthritic valgus ankle. Foot Ankle Clin 2012;17(4):647–63.
23. Dodd A, Daniels TR. Total ankle replacement in the presence of talar varus or valgus deformities. Foot Ankle Clin 2017;1–24. https://doi.org/10.1016/j.fcl.2017.01.002.
24. Veljkovic A, Norton A, Salat P, et al. Sagittal distal tibial articular angle and the relationship to talar subluxation in total ankle arthroplasty. Foot Ankle Int 2016;37(9):929–37.
25. Penner M, Davis WH, Wing K, et al. The infinity total ankle system: early clinical results with 2- to 4-year follow-up. Foot Ankle Spec 2019;12(2):159–66.

Printed and bound by CPI Group (UK) Ltd, Croydon, CR0 4YY
03/10/2024
01040306-0019